Surgical Nursing

M. Merriman

CW01603404

M. Merriman

Surgical Nursing

Joan Bickerton, BA, SRN, SCM, RNT

Director of Nurse Education,
Winchester and Basingstoke School of Nursing;
ENB Examiner

Heinemann Nursing
London

First published 1985 by
William Heinemann Medical Books Ltd
23 Bedford Square, London WC1B 3HH

ISBN: 0-433-02832-7

© 1985 Joan Bickerton

Typeset by
Macmillan India Ltd., Bangalore.
and printed by Butler & Tanner Ltd
Frome, Somerset
in Great Britain

Contents

Preface

Books have different purposes and are meant to be used in a variety of ways. Apart perhaps from novels, it is rare to gain the most from a book, particularly a textbook, by reading solidly from page one right through to the end. In fact research with university students has shown how ineffective this method is and yet how widely used.

This book is primarily meant to be used for study purposes by student nurses, although I am sure that qualified nurses will also find it useful to refer to. I would suggest that the student adapts the following strategy to her learning style. To start with, the student should write down what she already knows about the subject, after which she will be able to decide what questions she needs answered. An overall picture of the contents should then be gained by looking at the various headings, illustrations and tables, and then the chapter should be read through rapidly. (A book on rapid reading will help with this.)

The table at the beginning of the chapter may then be studied. This is not a synopsis of what is in the chapter, but rather a way of highlighting information to trigger off the memory process in revision. I would suggest that reference be made to the book *Use Your Head* (Buzan, 1982) for guidance in making flow charts.

Once the student has followed the above approach to the book, she is in a position to work through the passage, making her own diagrams and flow charts to help her when she revises.

No tutor or book ever gives the complete picture on a subject and therefore it is essential that the student follows up at least some of the references or reads other books on the subject. Journals are the most up-to-date sources of information, and this information may be added to the margins of the book or to the study notes. Some of the books referred to give more detailed information on the subject, or are examples of research in that field.

The nursing care plans are very brief examples of care related to a condition covered in the chapter. The student can develop her own care plans for conditions not covered, by referring back to the text.

Learning is not a passive process; reading a book is not sufficient to learn about nursing. The information has to be used in an active way. Comparing and contrasting the information in the book with that in practice in her own hospital should help the student nurse to ask the surgeon or senior nursing staff relevant questions and if the book achieves this, I shall be satisfied.

The nurse has been referred to throughout the book as 'she', and it should be noted that this has been done for reasons of clarity and convenience only.

REFERENCE AND FURTHER READING

Buzan T. (1982). *Use Your Head.* London: BBC.

James D. E. (1967). *A Students' Guide to Efficient Study.* London: Pergamon Press.

Introduction

Nursing has always been considered as a generic occupation, the basic concepts of which could be applied to the care of patients whatever the reason for their admission to hospital. This approach may have been adequate when the nurse was only required to carry out the doctor's instructions, and nursing care was very basic. However, as surgery has advanced, so the need for a highly trained nurse with specialist skills has become apparent.

In the early days of surgery the problems of haemorrhage, pain and sepsis were paramount and surgical procedures had to be kept as simple and quick as possible. Because accurate diagnosis of the condition was rarely possible, surgery was not attempted in many cases or was carried out inappropriately.

In 1536 Ambroise Pare demonstrated that by ligating the severed blood vessels during surgical procedures it was possible to control bleeding (Cox, 1983). Since then surgeons have discovered even quicker and more effective ways of sealing the blood vessels, such as diathermy.

It was not until 1846 that anaesthetics were introduced, so controlling the pain and reducing shock. Nitrous oxide (laughing gas), ether, and chloroform were applied to open masks and produced their own hazards. Anaesthetics have now improved to such an extent that patients who would once have been considered too great an operative risk can now be operated on safely, but skilled nursing care is required. Opium and morphia became available for the control of postoperative pain but caused vomiting and led to addiction if administered for long periods. We now have a wide variety of analgesics, ranging from the mild to the potent, and can therefore choose the most appropriate one.

In the latter half of the nineteenth century, infection was recognised for what it was. Robert Koch (1843–1910) established the science of bacteriology, and Louis Pasteur (1822–95) showed that the 'laudable pus', without which no wound was expected to heal, could be prevented. By maintaining strict surgical cleanliness and using carbolic acid to spray the operating field, he was able to reduce the incidence of infection dramatically. Since then aseptic and non-touch techniques have been applied to dressing procedures, and strict cleaning routines and the filtering of air in the theatre have been introduced, as well as nurses responsible for the control of infection. The range of anti-bacterial agents for local application or internal administration is enormous, so ensuring that even if infection does occur it is no longer a major problem. This has also allowed the performance of more complex surgery.

Diagnostic procedures were a little later in developing, x-rays being introduced in 1896 by Röntgen. Since then, x-ray procedures have become progressively more refined, with tomograms to pinpoint a lesion and contrast media to outline systems which otherwise would not be seen. The ventricles of the brain, the arterial system and the lymphatic system can all be demonstrated on x-rays with the aid of these media. Even more sophisticated diagnostic procedures, such as radioactive isotopes, scans and fibreoptic endoscopy, are now in common use. The use of the computer in diagnostic techniques enables them to be more accurate and less dangerous and unpleasant.

Once it was possible to control the three main hazards of surgery, and more sophisticated and accurate diagnostic procedures were available, surgeons were able to concentrate on more complex surgical techniques. Some surgical procedures, such as tracheostomy and colostomy, have been carried out for many years, in fact there are records of a tracheostomy being performed in 124 BC. The development of the heart–lung machine has enabled great advances to be made in cardiac surgery and this has been assisted by using anaesthesia under hypothermia which increases the time available to the surgeon when operating. The use of synthetic materials has enabled new procedures to be attempted in arterial surgery, as well as in the replacement of joints, or the tiny bones in the ear. Organ transplants have become more common as tissue typing and the control of rejection have progressed. The use of microscopic surgery, laser beams and cryosurgery has increased the complexity of some procedures and simplified others.

It can be seen that surgical procedures cover a wide range of activities and do not always require an incision through the skin with a scalpel. They may involve the removal of a foreign body, a benign or malignant growth, or even localised infection. Frequently an organ itself, or another part of the body, has to be removed. However, at times the removal of the offending part is insufficient and the surgeon has to use a graft or refashion the part. Drainage techniques are frequently part of an operation, but may also be the sole purpose for surgical intervention.

Surgery is obviously only one method of treatment and although it may be the only method for some conditions, for others it is only used after medical treatment has been found to be insufficient. It is frequently used in conjunction with radiotherapy for malignant growths.

Approaches to patient care have also changed. For example, the patient no longer has to be kept semi-recumbent for 24 hours and in bed for 2 weeks because it is now recognised that this causes more complications rather than preventing them. In fact, some operations require vigorous physiotherapy. Recovery rooms and intensive care units are responsible for the very ill patients and therefore the nurse on the general surgical ward may never nurse a patient requiring this care. Five-day wards, progressive patient care and mixed male and female wards all influence the way nursing care is delivered. Many tasks which were traditionally considered to be nursing responsibilities have been taken over by other people, so freeing the nurse for the organisation of patient care. Sterile equipment is supplied in packs from the CSSD; meals may also be supplied from a central kitchen already plated up.

Because doctors are involved in more complex surgery, they can no longer spend time carrying out some of the routine tasks that have traditionally been seen as their province, and so the role of the nurse has had to be extended. This is particularly so in highly technical areas such as the intensive care unit where immediate attention may be life saving and the doctor may not be constantly available. Many of these life and death decisions have ethical considerations and therefore the nurse has to become much more aware of the issues involved.

Each surgical ward has its own identity, nevertheless they all have much in common. Although the general surgical ward does exist, there is an increasing tendency amongst surgeons to specialise. This means that many wards will have a limited range of conditions frequently related to one or two systems. Because many minor operations are carried out on a day basis or by admitting the patient to a five-day ward, other surgical wards may deal predominantly with major operations. Early discharge means that the patients are dependent on the nursing staff. A large proportion of patients will have been seen in out-patients and will therefore have been prepared for their admission and for the fact that they will be having surgery. Others will have been affected by a sudden condition necessitating an emergency admission and possibly also an emergency operation. Most hospitals try to control the number of emergency admissions to a ward by having particular days when they are 'on take'.

All this has meant that the role of the nurse in the surgical ward has changed and has become much more technical, so it is important that she should take great care not to forget the total needs of the patient. In order to do this in the limited time available to her, it is essential that she has the responsibility for the total care of particular patients and that this is not divided up among many nurses. She needs to have a good knowledge of the resources available to her and the best way of caring for the patient. Continuing education and up-to-date information on research findings are essential.

THE NURSING PROCESS

The nursing process is one way of carrying out nursing care in any type of ward or unit. Its aim is to improve the standard of nursing care by:

1. ensuring that the total needs of the patient are properly assessed so that both short-term and long-term problems are identified and dealt with;
2. planning care in a systematic way, implementing it and evaluating its effectiveness;
3. involving the patient in decisions about his own needs and care and therefore improving the communication between the patient and the nurse;
4. making one nurse responsible for the management of the total care of a patient throughout his stay in hospital;
5. improving the standard of communication between the nurse and others involved in the care of the patient so that information given is more accurate.

The elements of the nursing process

Assessment

This requires a nursing history to highlight the patient's needs and problems. Some of this information may be gained when the doctor is examining the patient, so avoiding repetitive questions. Not all the information has to be gathered at once and some of it will be gleaned from observation rather than questioning. Relatives and others involved in the previous care of the patient may give useful information. The nurse will be systematically assessing the ability of the patient to manage the activities of daily living.

Table 1.1 The nursing process

		Activities of daily living				People involved		Outcome
Details on admission from patient	ASSESSMENT	Sleep Temperature control Respiratory function	NURSING CARE PLAN	Short-term objectives	IMPLEMENTATION	Nurses Patient Relatives	EVALUATION	Completed successfully
Medical information		Elimination Sexuality Social Hygiene				Friends Doctor Physiotherapist Social worker		Successful but needs to continue
Information from relatives		Occupation Religion Nutrition				Dietition Speech therapist Occupational therapist		Unsuccessful—needs a new approach
Observation		Culture Attitudes Leisure pursuits Mobility		Long-term objectives		Other carers Statutory bodies Voluntary bodies		Causing unforeseen problems—deal with problems and try new approach
Information from other carers		**Other needs** Recent care including drugs Pain						

Planning

The nurse will plan the nursing care, setting short-term and long-term objectives to deal with the needs of the patient and the problems that have been identified in the assessment. These will cover the physical, psychological and social aspects of the care.

Implementation

The plan is carried out using the resources available in the best way. This includes using the latest information on how to deal successfully with a particular problem.

Evaluation

At this point the nurse assesses the effectiveness of the care with the help of the patient. Following evaluation it may be necessary to change the nursing care plan and to start the process over again. This will probably mean that with some patients several stages of the nursing process are occurring at the same time with different problems.

SUGGESTED WORK

1. Take a nursing history you have compiled and discuss it with your clinical teacher or a more senior colleague. Is there any information you have omitted or that would not be understood in 6 months time?

2. With the patient's help, plan his care for the next span of duty. Discuss with your colleagues how they would have planned his care.

SUGGESTED READING

Cox C. (1983). *Sociology*. London: Butterworth.
Kratz C. R., ed. (1979). *The Nursing Process*. London: Baillière Tindall.
McFarlane, Professor Baroness of Llanduff (1982). *A Guide to the Practice of Nursing Using the Nursing Process*. London: C. V. Mosby.
Marriner A. (1983). *The Nursing Process*. St Louis, Miss.: C. V. Mosby.
Roper N., Logan W. W., Tierney A. J. (1981). *Learning to Use the Process of Nursing*. Edinburgh: Churchill Livingstone.

ACKNOWLEDGEMENTS

It would have been impossible to write a book of this size without a great deal of support from my colleagues, both in teaching and on the clinical side. In particular, I am grateful for their help in checking that the surgical and nursing approaches I have described are the most up-to-date. Undoubtedly, however, the greatest influence on the style and presentation of the book came from the questions posed over the years by the students at the Winchester and Basingstoke School of Nursing.

I am greatly indebted to Deidre Keeble, Fran Boxall and Jenny Millward for the chapters on ENT, theatre nursing and the nursing care of the patient having eye surgery, and to Mr Toy for the photographs in the chapter on theatre nursing.

Joan Bickerton

Section I

1

The Psychological, Spiritual and Social Needs of the Surgical Patient

It must always be remembered that to the patient being admitted to hospital for surgery, the physical aspects of his condition may be only part of his problem. He is a complete person and this must not be forgotten. He will also have psychological, spiritual and social needs which will have to be taken into account when planning his care. A patient lacking the will to live may die as a result of an operation which a mentally fit person would quickly recover from. His spiritual needs will become highlighted when he has to face an operation and an anaesthetic. Above all, the patient is part of a family and social situation which influence the way he reacts.

THE NEED FOR RESPECT

Although physical age gives some indication of the maturity of the individual, there are wide variations at any age. Someone in their fifties may appear old, whereas a person in their eighties may have an alert lively mind. The intelligence of patients entering hospital will also vary from the mentally handicapped to the university professor, the majority falling between these two extremes. The nurse should be sensitive to these differences and treat the patient as an individual. Explanations given by the nurse to the patient need to take these differences into account.

Good communications are vital. The patient should be given adequate information that he can understand. He has a right to know what treatment is being offered to him and to be involved in decisions regarding examinations and surgery, whatever his age or his level of intelligence.

This respect for him as a person will show in the way that the nurse avoids causing him embarrassment. Privacy when being washed or using a bedpan is essential. There are some examinations which cause considerable discomfort to the patient, who may be concerned at the way he behaves in front of the nurse.

In hospital there is the tendency to remove the autonomy of patients by removing their clothes and expecting them to conform to hospital routine. If the patient stays for any length of time, he becomes hospitalised and finds it difficult to revert back to making his own decisions. A patient who is fit enough to be up, can be dressed, which will help him to feel much better. Challenging the established routine is the patient's way of showing his independence. He should not be thought of as difficult, but his opinion sought and adequate reasons given for what is being done. The nurse should respect differences in personality. Not every patient enjoys the company of a group of people, they may prefer to be on their own.

THE NEED FOR SECURITY

Most of us feel happier in an environment which is familiar, and the patient is no exception to this. He needs to know where to find the various facilities, who he can call upon when in doubt, and what is expected of him. The nurse admitting him and responsible for his daily care will need to develop a good relationship with him so that he will share those things that are worrying him. As the nurse in charge does her round, there will be further opportunities to ask questions. These opportunities must be created for the patient to talk as he may be reluctant to take the initiative in case the nurse is too busy.

Many operations affect the body image a person has of himself, and if this is so, the patient must be adequately prepared beforehand and given support afterwards. A woman having a mastectomy may feel that she is no longer attractive to her husband. It is therefore important not only to prepare the woman herself for the effects of the operation, but also her husband. He will need to know how he can best support her. If the patient is to have an ileostomy or colostomy, he may find this physically repugnant and require a lot of support both before and after the operation. An amputation of a limb may interfere with future plans, so causing frustration and bitterness. In each of these conditions the patient may grieve for what is lost and feel revulsion at his condition. He must be given the opportunity to work through these feelings. He may also be helped by meeting someone who has undergone a similar experience.

Before any examination, the nurse must explain exactly what should be expected, and how the patient may help to make it easier for himself. In the same way he should be prepared for any equipment that may be present postoperatively. Pain that is recognised as a normal part of the procedure is easier to bear than the anxiety that something may be wrong.

THE NEED TO BE LISTENED TO

It is surprising how difficult people find it, to listen properly to others. Watch a conversation between several people and you will find each one is just waiting for the opportunity to jump in and have his say. Too frequently it is assumed that we know what the other person is going to say. If the patient has the impression that he has not got the nurse's or doctor's full attention, he will cease to give information, and a vital part of his care may be overlooked. The patient's way of seeing and interpreting the situation may be rather different from that of the doctor or nurse. Inaccurate, prejudiced information gained from unreliable sources may cause him to behave in what appears to the staff to be an inappropriate way. Frustration may occur if no one seems to take heed of what he is saying, so causing him to appear stubborn, difficult or even aggressive to the staff.

Body language is just as important as what is actually being said, revealing embarrassment or anxiety. The patient may start to say something but then change the subject. If so, it is important to come back to what he was saying at a later point. Some patients will withhold information which would help the doctor in his diagnosis because they are frightened of being labelled as neurotic, or they may want to avoid a particular investigation or treatment.

THE NEED FOR MENTAL STIMULATION

Experiments have been carried out depriving a small group of university students of all stimulation. The students developed hallucinations and found the experience intolerable. The right amount of stimulation from the environment is particularly important in the elderly. Many elderly people have a diminished sensory input due to some degree of deafness and visual impairment. Add to this admission to the unfamiliar surroundings of hospital and any other minor disorder, and it may be sufficient to make them confused. A slight disturbance of electrolyte balance may cause few problems in the younger person, but to the elderly it may be sufficient to disturb a precarious mental balance. Night-time, with less visual input and the influence of night sedation, may also upset this balance.

The younger patient may have the problem of boredom, particularly the patient who has to remain in bed and stay in hospital for a long period of time. The work of occupational therapists needs to be augmented by the relatives and voluntary workers. The relatives can use their knowledge of the patient's interests to provide suitable material for him to work on.

SPIRITUAL NEEDS

Faced with situations he has never met previously, the patient may call upon resources he has never fully used before. He may start to question beliefs he has never really thought about. If he follows a particular faith, then it is important that he has the opportunity to discuss these issues with the relevant minister, or another person of the same faith. Although there may be a chaplain, non-conformist minister or Roman Catholic priest attached to the hospital, the patient may prefer to have the minister from his own church. Many patients like to celebrate Holy Communion and it should be possible to arrange this, either with a small group or individually. A devout person may wish to have the opportunity to pray without being disturbed, and this wish should be respected. If a patient is too weak to read the Bible for himself, he will appreciate it if a relative or nurse offers this service to him.

SOCIAL NEEDS

The patient is part of the community in which he lives and, in particular, part of a family. He may come from a close-knit village where everyone knows everyone else or from a lonely bedsitter in the heart of town; from a highly respectable professional family or a hippy commune. His relationships with his family will influence how much they can be involved in his care. If he has a close supportive family, they will help him to come to terms with very traumatic experiences. However, a relationship already in danger of disintegrating may be tried to the limit by his condition. The nurse should be able to find out enough of his background to assist her in his care. On discharge from hospital, the individual living on his own may need more services and follow-up than one who has relatives to support him. These services will need to be arranged well before the patient's discharge.

SUGGESTED WORK

1. Discuss with a patient who is ready for discharge what aspects of hospital care he or she found most difficult or worrying. Could modifications of nursing have helped to prevent this?
2. Take a patient who has different needs from the majority in the ward, such as a person from abroad or someone who is incapacitated in some way, and check how well his or her needs have been met.

SUGGESTED READING

Henderson V. (1969). *Basic Principles of Nursing Care*, revised edition. Geneva: International Council of Nurses.

Henley A. (1979). *Asian Patients in Hospital and at Home*. Oxford: Kings Fund, Oxford University Press.

Hewitt F. S. (1981). The nurse and the patient; communication skills. Getting it across. *Nursing Times*; 77(35), Suppl.: 29–32.

Leonard C. (1981). Understanding sexuality: talking through a taboo. *Nursing Mirror*; **153**(5): 19–20.

Nesbitt Blondis M., Jackson B. E. (1982). *Non-Verbal Communication with Patients*. Chichester: John Wiley.

Schain W. S. (1980). Patients' rights in decision making; the case for personalities versus paternalism in health care. *Cancer*; **46**(4), Suppl.: 1035–41.

Wienburg J. S. (1982). *Sexuality. Human Needs and Nursing Practice*. London: Baillière Tindall.

2

Pathological Investigations

Before surgery is attempted, the patient has to undergo various investigations. These have two main purposes. First, to define what exactly is wrong with the patient, where it is and its extent. Second, to ensure that the patient is fit enough for surgery. These investigations may be of a general type, such as those involving the blood, or may relate to a particular tract or organ. Some of them are uncomfortable for the patient or require specific preparation or after-care.

When collecting specimens from patients it is important that the request form is adequately filled in with the name of the hospital and ward, patient's full name and hospital number and date of birth, because in any pathological laboratory there are thousands of specimens passing through each day. Although the nurse is not usually responsible for filling in these forms, it is up to her to make sure that each specimen leaving the ward has the appropriate form filled in legibly in black ink, as they are frequently photocopied.

BLOOD SPECIMENS

The correct bottle or container should be selected for each test and this must be adequately and accurately labelled. Many specimens need to be intimately mixed with the preservative in the collecting bottle but not shaken.

Great care should be taken in the handling of blood taken from patients having repeated blood transfusions, drug addicts and those suffering from acquired immune deficiency syndrome (AIDS), hepatitis or on renal dialysis. Within each district there are strict instructions on how to handle material which is considered to be a hepatitis or AIDS risk. The specimens should be given a distinctive label and placed in a protective polythene bag. The accompanying request form should not be put in the bag. After handling any contaminated material, the hands must be washed.

In the surgical ward many blood tests will be taken prior to operation to ensure that the patient is in the best possible condition for it. If he is to have a major operation or an investigation which involves the risk of haemorrhage, blood will be taken for blood grouping and cross-matching. The blood grouping is done to ascertain which ABO and Rhesus group the patient belongs to. Before blood can be transfused it must also be cross-matched against the patient's blood to ensure that it is compatible.

In cases of septicaemia or subacute bacterial endocarditis, a blood culture may be necessary. The specimen is taken when the patient's temperature is raised, under strictly aseptic conditions, the blood being added to a bottle containing broth in which it is incubated.

Blood tests

Table 2.1 gives details of some of the main blood tests.

Glucose tolerance test

For those patients in which the diagnosis of diabetes is not clear. No food is given from midnight the night before the test. A fasting blood sugar is taken in the morning and 75 g glucose given in a glassful of water. Blood is then taken after 1 hour and again after 2 hours. The first specimen of blood may be omitted if it is thought from the symptoms that the second specimen will provide sufficient information. If both the blood tests are 10 + mmol/l, this is diagnostic of diabetes. If after 1 hour the result is 10 + mmol/l but after 2 hours it is between 7 and 10 mmol/l, this indicates an impaired glucose tolerance which could develop into diabetes at a later date if care is not taken with the diet.

EXAMINATION OF THE URINE

On admission and prior to operation, ward specimens of urine will be collected to test for albumin, sugar, acetone, blood and bile with the appropriate reagent tablets or strips, the instructions for which are on the containers. It is important that these reagents are kept dry and are not handled. Equipment must be clean and dry and the instructions carefully followed. Fluid balance charts will also be kept for many patients and these must be accurate.

The midstream specimen of urine for the presence of bacteria

The midstream flow of urine is collected in a sterile container following cleansing of the glans penis or vulva. The specimen is kept in a refrigerator until it is taken to the laboratory to prevent the bacteria multiplying and giving a false reading. The doctor will state on the request form if the patient is receiving antibiotics.

Table 2.1 Blood tests

Test	Normal value	Lowered	Raised
Absolute values			
Red blood cells (RBCs)	$5.00 \times 10^{12}/l$	Iron deficiency anaemia	Polycythaemia
White blood cells	$10 \times 10^{9}/l$	Agranulocytosis	Infection Inflammation Leukaemia
MCHC (mean cell haemoglobin concentration) = amount of haemoglobin in cells	30.0 g/dl	Iron deficiency anaemia	
MCD (mean cell diameter) = diameter of the RBC	6.7–7.7 μm	Iron deficiency anaemia	Pernicious anaemia
MCV (mean cell volume) = average volume of one RBC	90 fl	Iron deficiency anaemia	Pernicious anaemia
MCH (mean cell haemoglobin) = amount of haemoglobin in each RBC	30 pg	Iron deficiency anaemia	Pernicious anaemia
Size and colour of RBCs			
Normocytic	Normal size		
Microcytic	Small	Iron deficiency anaemia	
Macrocytic	Large	Pernicious anaemia	
Normochromic	Normal colour		
Hypochromic	Less colour	Iron deficiency anaemia	
Colour index	1	Iron deficiency anaemia	

Table 2.1 (*Continued*)

Test	Normal value	Lowered	Raised
Tests to exclude haemorrhagic conditions			
Thrombocytes	$150–350 \times 10^9/l$	Haemorrhagic disorders	
Bleeding time (time taken for prick to stop bleeding)	3–5 min		Haemorrhagic disorders
Clotting time (time taken for blood to clot in tube)	4–7 min		Haemorrhagic disorders
Prothrombin ratio (patients on anticoagulants)	If increased to more than twice the control, bleeding will take place		
ESR (erythrocyte sedimentation rate)	3–5 mm in 1 hour		Infection Inflammation
Electrolytes (salts present in the blood which on their own carry electrical charge)			
Sodium	133–146 mmol/l	These values may be altered in diarrhoea and vomiting, following aspiration from a nasogastric tube and the administration of intravenous fluids	
Chloride	96–106 mmol/l		
Potassium	3.5–5.5 mmol/l		
Bicarbonate	23–31 mmol/l		
Blood urea (level of nitrogenous waste)	2.5–7.5 mmol/l		Kidney damage
Liver function tests			
Van den Bergh test Serum bilirubin	20 μm/l		Jaundice
Fasting blood sugar	3.6–5.6 mmol/l	Hypoglycaemia	Diabetes*
Glucose tolerance test (see text)			

* The Expert Committee on Diabetes Mellitus of the World Health Organisation recommends that a random blood sugar of 10+ mmol/l or a fasting blood sugar of 7+ mmol/l is diagnostic of diabetes in the presence of typical symptoms.

Specimens may also be taken from a catheter, nephrostomy drain or via a suprapubic catheter. In infants a bladder puncture may be done when the bladder is full, with a needle and syringe. If a specimen is being taken from an indwelling catheter, the catheter is clamped off for half an hour prior to taking the specimen with a syringe and needle through the appropriate part of the tubing. If there is any difficulty in transporting the specimen to the laboratory, a culture spoon or slide containing culture media may be dipped into the urine.

Twenty-four-hour specimen of urine

Urine may be examined for blood, casts, protein, cells, chemicals etc. If a quantitive test is to be done, then a 24-hour specimen of urine must be taken. In suspected phaeochromocytoma a 24-hour specimen is necessary to measure for an increase in the catecholamines.

To collect a 24-hour specimen of urine, the bladder is emptied and this specimen is discarded. The time is noted, and all urine is collected into the special container for the next 24 hours. At the end of this time the patient voids urine and this specimen is added to the collection.

Renal biopsy

To do this test the co-operation of the patient is necessary and therefore it is not carried out on confused patients or children. If there is any difficulty in obtaining a specimen of the kidneys by closed renal biopsy, an operation will be done under a general anaesthetic to obtain an open biopsy. Before the procedure, tests will be carried out to rule out urinary infection and bleeding disorders and to test renal function. X-rays are taken to show the position of the kidneys, and blood is cross-matched. After the doctor has explained the nature of the procedure a consent form is signed. A raised blood pressure is reported to the doctor. The specimen is taken with the patient in the prone position, a Vim–Silverman biopsy needle being used. Following the procedure the patient remains in bed for 24 hours. He is observed for any indication of bleeding including haematuria, infection and loin pain. Fluids are encouraged and a fluid chart maintained. A check midstream specimen of urine is collected.

Renal function tests

These are done in order to test the efficiency of the kidney in excreting various substances. Water, urea or creatinine is used. The most popular is creatinine as it is more sensitive and easier to do. In the creatinine clearance test a 24-hour collection of urine is made. During this time 10 ml of blood are collected. If the patient is a child, or his height or weight varies considerably from normal, these figures should be supplied so that a correction factor can be applied. In the normal patient, 70–130 ml of blood are cleared of creatinine in 1 minute. This value may be considerably reduced in renal failure.

DIAGNOSTIC TESTS OF THE GASTROINTESTINAL TRACT

Gastric test meals

These are done to investigate the level of hydrochloric acid and other substances in the gastric juice, which may be altered in the presence of peptic ulceration, carcinoma of the stomach, pernicious anaemia or following a vagotomy.

After fasting the night before, a nasogastric tube is passed and the complete contents of the stomach aspirated (resting juice). The patient is then given 100 ml of 7% alcohol. Every 15 minutes, 5–10-ml samples of gastric juice are aspirated for six specimens. Finally the remaining contents of the stomach are aspirated (residual juice). All specimens are labelled with the actual time of collection. If the reaction of the first specimen is not acid, histamine 0.5 mg will be ordered by the doctor. This is noted on the request form.

Pentagastrin test meal

The patient is starved from midnight. On the morning of the test a nasogastric tube is passed. Four specimens of gastric juice are collected at 15-minute intervals for the basal acid output. The patient is then given a subcutaneous injection of pentagastrin. Four further specimens are collected at 15-minute intervals.

Gastrotest or tubeless test meal (diagnex blue)

The patient is given the dye in the form of tablets after a control urine has been collected. A 2-hour collection of urine is then made. The amount of dye excreted in the urine indicates the level of acid.

Insulin test meal

This is done to test the efficiency of a vagotomy. The day prior to the test the patient is given a light diet. He is then starved from midnight. The following morning a nasogastric tube is passed and the stomach completely aspirated. A specimen of blood is taken and 15 units of soluble insulin injected intravenously. The stomach is then aspirated every 15 minutes for 2 hours. Blood samples are also taken at half-hourly intervals. The amount of acid secreted should be reduced after a vagotomy.

Test for occult blood in faeces

This laboratory test is used to look for blood that is not visible to the eye. It is not necessary if the blood is seen as bright red streaks on the surface of the faeces or if there is melaena (the passage of black, tarry stools). Any bleeding in the gastrointestinal tract will result in some blood being excreted in the faeces. This will occur in patients with suspected peptic ulcers, carcinoma in the tract and ulceration. Because any blood will give a positive result, the patient should not have any food which is rich in blood for 3 days prior to the test.

Liver biopsy

A liver biopsy may be required in the investigation of liver disorders where physical and laboratory tests have failed, or to estimate the degree of liver damage. Before the procedure is carried out it is most important that a haemoglobin test, platelet count and prothrombin index have been done. If the last-mentioned is low, or the patient is confused, the procedure is not carried out. Two units of blood should be grouped and cross-matched. Abdominal x-rays may also be done. The biopsy is taken with a Menghini or Vim–Silverman needle (Fig. 2.1). The patient may be given a sedative such as diazepam 30 minutes before the procedure.

The procedure is carried out with the patient on his back and his right arm extended (Fig. 2.2). After the procedure he will remain in bed for 24 hours, observations being made for any evidence of bleeding. The most common complications are haemorrhage, biliary peritonitis and a small pneumothorax.

THE RESPIRATORY TRACT

Sputum

In the surgical patient this is most likely to be examined for organisms or malignant cells. An early morning specimen before any food is taken is the best. Physiotherapy and hot drinks may help the patient to expectorate.

Chest aspiration

Normally the amount of fluid between the two layers of the pleura is just enough to allow them to glide over one another in respiration, but not enough to separate them. If it is increased due to inflammation, malignancy or diseases which alter

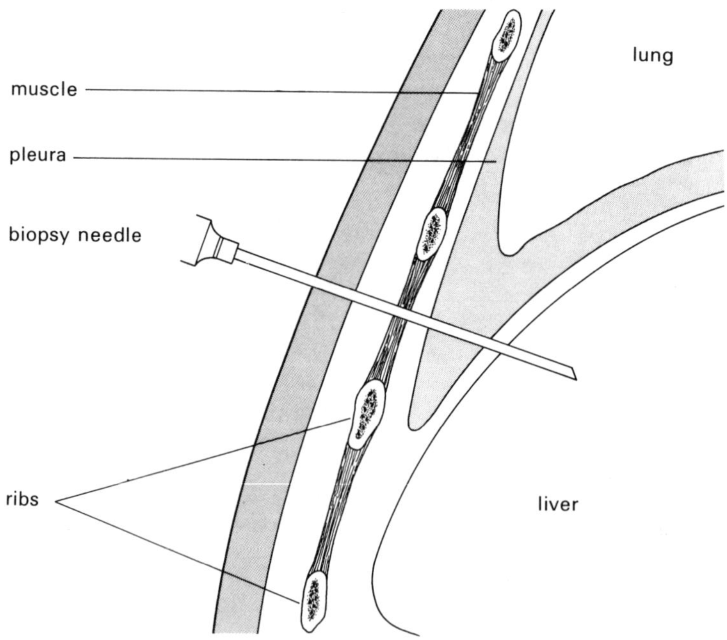

Fig. 2.1 *Liver biopsy.*

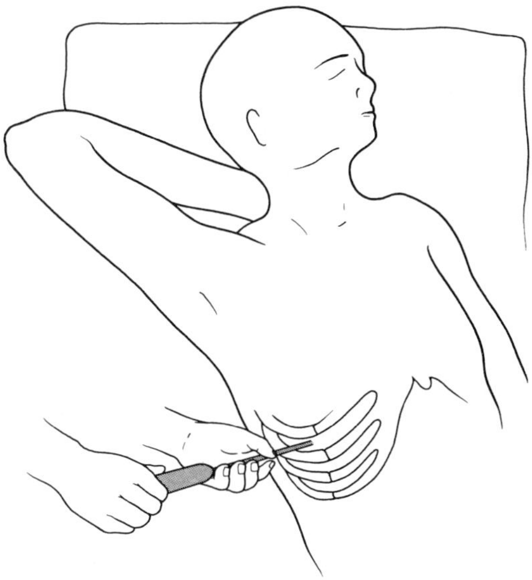

Fig. 2.2 *Position for liver biopsy.*

the pressure in the blood vessels, an aspiration may be necessary for diagnostic purposes or treatment. Prior to the procedure an x-ray will have been taken.

The procedure is carried out with the patient sitting up and leaning forward (Fig. 2.3). The doctor will withdraw fluid with a wide-bore needle. During the procedure the nurse will observe the patient carefully for any signs of respiratory or cardiac distress in the form of dyspnoea, pain, or change in the pulse rate.

Pleural biopsy

If a patient has a pleural effusion and the cause is unknown, or if carcinoma or tuberculosis is suspected, a pleural biopsy will be taken. The biopsy is of the parietal pleura and can only be taken when fluid is present because of the danger of puncturing

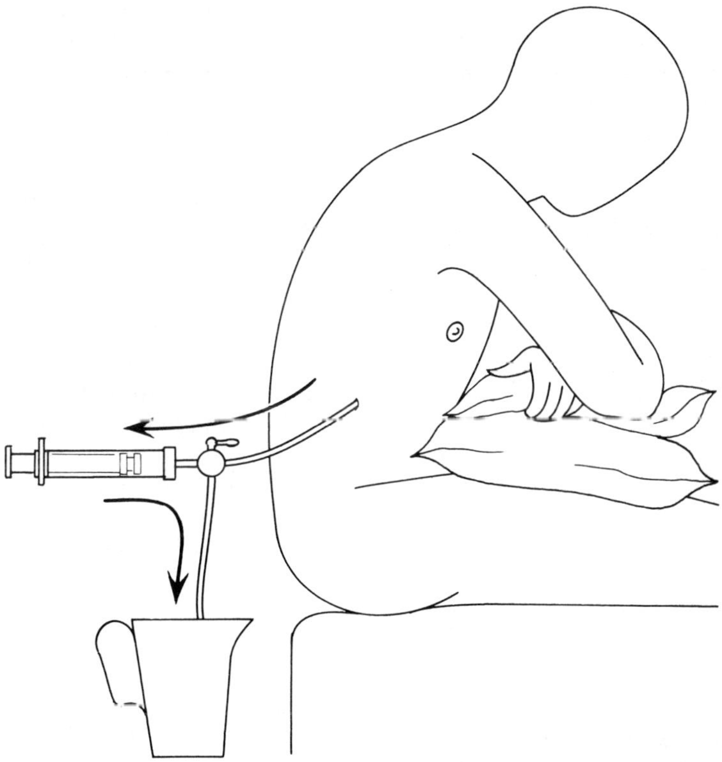

Fig. 2.3 *Chest aspiration.*

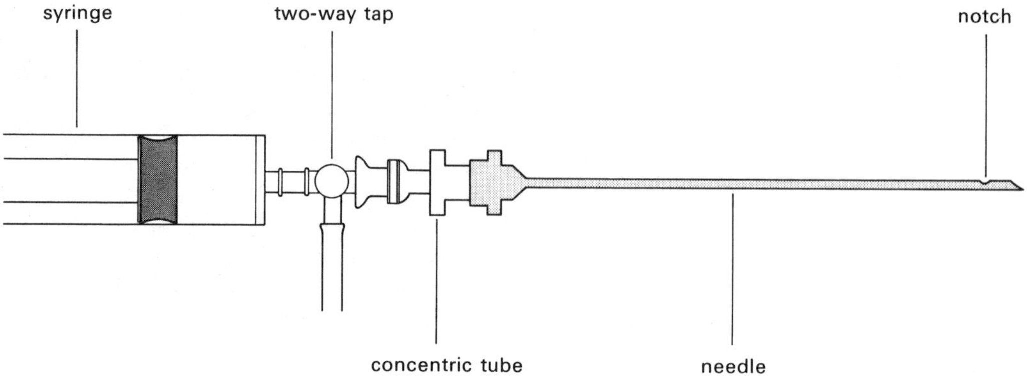

Fig. 2.4 *Abram's needle for pleural biopsy.*

the lung. An Abram's needle is used (Fig. 2.4). This has an inner cylinder with a notch in it, which when rotated will slice off the small piece of tissue drawn into the notch by suction. It also has a knob on its outer end to indicate when the notch is facing in the correct direction.

The position of the patient and the procedure from the nurse's point of view are similar to those of a chest aspiration. After cleansing the skin and injecting a local anaesthetic, the doctor will make a small incision with a scalpel, and insert the biopsy needle into the pleural space. He will then aspirate a small amount of fluid for diagnostic purposes, and withdraw the needle until he feels the notch against the parietal pleura. He will then make sure the knob is pointing downwards, and rotate the cylinder. After the biopsy needle is removed a stitch will be inserted.

OTHER PROCEDURES

Lumbar puncture

This procedure is mainly carried out to diagnose a bacterial infection or a subarachnoid haemorrhage. It may also be used in the x-ray department to diagnose a prolapsed intervertebral disc or a tumour. In this case either a radio-opaque substance or air is introduced. Spinal anaesthesia may also be introduced by this method. It is not done in the presence of raised intracranial pressure because of the danger of herniation of the brain through the foramen magnum (coning).

The procedure is usually carried out with the patient curled up on his left side with his back to the edge of the bed and his knees well up. The doctor inserts a fine needle between the second and third lumbar vertebrae. Three specimens are normally collected. The patient remains in bed for 24 hours and, if he complains of a headache, the foot of the bed is blocked.

During the procedure the pressure is measured with a glass manometer, the normal range being 75–150 mm of cerebrospinal fluid. In Queckenstedt's test, compression of both jugular veins will cause an immediate rise in this pressure, unless there is some obstruction to the flow of the cerebrospinal fluid, as with a tumour.

If it is not possible to introduce the needle in the lumbar region, a cisternal puncture may be done. This is performed by introducing a needle through the back of the neck into the cisterna magna. The area requires shaving prior to the procedure and the patient is positioned with the head bent forward.

Paracentesis abdominis

Fluid may accumulate in the peritoneal cavity due to inflammation, increased pressure in the portal vein, and abdominal tumours. The laboratory may assist diagnosis by describing its composition or demonstrating malignant cells. The patient's bladder must be emptied prior to the procedure to avoid the trocar puncturing it.

The patient is placed in a semi-reclining position. After making a small incision with a scalpel, the doctor introduces a trocar and cannula, removing the trocar and leaving the cannula in position, with tubing attached. The tubing is attached to a drainage bag, and the rate of drainage controlled by a gate clip. When the cannula is removed the puncture wound is covered with an occlusive dressing. For the first 2 hours following the procedure the blood pressure and pulse are checked every 15 minutes and the patient observed for shock.

SUGGESTED WORK

1. Look at the notes of one of the patients you are nursing and see what investigations he has had. Find out as much as you can about each of the investigations. Does every patient with the same condition have the same tests?

2. Ask if you can go with a patient who is having a special investigation. Find out if there are alternative ways of gaining the same information. What factors influence the choice of investigation?

SUGGESTED READING

Evans D. M. D. (1981). *Special Tests and Their Meanings*. London: Faber & Faber.

Jolly U. (1972). *Lumbar Puncture and Related Tests*. Nursing in Depth Series. London: Butterworths.

3

Radiological Investigations

X-rays (like light) blacken suitably sensitised photographic film. By placing the body between the x-ray source and the photographic film, the rays will be absorbed in differing amounts according to the tissue they are passing through. Bone which contains a large amount of calcium shows up white on the x-ray, while soft tissues appear grey, and air black. Straight horizontal lines on an x-ray indicate fluid levels.

The x-rays may be taken from different directions depending on which part of the body is being x-rayed. For example, the chest may be taken laterally or posterior/anteriorly. Abnormalities affecting the density of the part being x-rayed may be seen, such as tumours and abscesses in the bone.

If the function of a part needs to be observed, such as movement of the chest in breathing, or swallowing, screening may be carried out. The x-rays are directed onto a fluorescent screen, the brightness of the image being intensified so that it can be seen on a television screen.

Tomograms

These are a series of x-rays focused on different levels through the part to be x-rayed. They are taken by moving the x-ray tube and film. The shadows of structures above and below the level required are blurred out. They may reveal abnormalities deep within the tissue which would have been hidden on a straight x-ray. Lesions in the chest may be hidden by the shadow of the ribs, in which case tomograms may reveal the required information. Because they are taken at different levels, they give the exact position of any abnormality and some idea of its size.

Much more information can be gained about certain structures by using contrast agents. These are harmless radio-opaque substances, introduced into the body in order to outline particular tracts or organs.

Barium swallow and meal

Barium sulphate suspension is taken by mouth in order to outline the oesophagus, in the case of a swallow, and the stomach if a meal is given. It will demonstrate growths or ulcers if they are outlined by the barium, but not if they are on the anterior surface of the organ. The patient must be starved for at least 6 hours prior to this procedure, and any medicines containing heavy metals such as bismuth and calcium are omitted for 3 days before. Constipation is a common problem afterwards and aperients may be necessary.

Barium enema

This procedure can only be carried out with a patient able to retain the enema. Barium is run into the rectum with a catheter. Before beginning this procedure the colon must be adequately cleared. An aperient is given two nights before the x-ray; the evening before an enema, and on the morning of the x-ray, a colonic washout is conducted. The x-rays may reveal narrowing of the lumen of the gut, or a filling defect, indicating a growth. Loss of the normal indentations of the bowel will indicate ulcerative colitis.

Cholecystogram

Halogen dyes are excreted by the liver into the bile, thus enabling the gall bladder to be outlined on x-ray. The patient has a light, non-fatty meal the evening before, and is given the telepaque pills, one every 5 minutes, after the meal. He then has nothing to eat until after the x-ray the next morning. Following the x-ray, a fatty meal with eggs may be given, after which further films will be taken.

Intravenous cholecystogram

The patient is given nothing to drink for 4 hours prior to an injection of biligrafin. Non-fatty food may be eaten.

Intravenous pyelogram or renogram

Water-soluble iodine solution is injected intravenously, and this is filtered through the kidney. Films are taken at intervals to observe the passage of the dye along the urinary tract. If the blood urea is raised, the x-ray is not done, and if there is any history of allergy to iodine, the patient will be given antihistamine drugs. The day before the x-ray the patient is given a low-residue diet, and bismuth medicines are discontinued. He is given nothing to drink for 6 hours before. After the x-ray he is observed for any evidence of bronchospasm or circulatory collapse. The x-ray will demonstrate any obstructions in the tract, abnormalities in size and shape of the kidney pelvis and calyses, and the ability of the kidney to excrete the dye.

Retrograde pyelogram

For this examination a cystoscopy is first performed, usually under a general anaesthetic. Ureteric catheters are then passed into the ureters, through which the radio-opaque substance is introduced, filling the pelvis of the kidney and the ureters. The patient has been allowed to gain consciousness so that he can report any pain. Once pain occurs, no more dye is introduced. The x-rays may reveal hydronephrosis, calculi or tumours. Preparation will be that of a patient having a general anaesthetic. Aperients may be given the night before to eliminate gas. This procedure is not carried out if there is cystitis as the infection would be transferred to the kidneys. After the procedure the temperature is observed for infection of the kidney. A careful note is also made when the patient passes urine as damage to the tract may have occurred.

Cystogram

A radio-opaque dye is introduced into the bladder through a catheter until the bladder is distended. Films are then taken. The patient then micturates, which is observed on a television screen—*a micturating cystogram*—and further films are taken. This will demonstrate any ureteric reflux (a frequent cause of pyelonephritis) and urethral abnormalities.

Bronchogram

A radio-opaque substance is introduced into the bronchial tree to outline the air passages. This is done by introducing a soft rubber catheter through the nose and dripping the oil into the opening of the larynx, or by using a specially curved cannula attached to a syringe, which introduces the medium over the back of the tongue, or by injecting the medium directly through the larynx with a needle. It is useful in diagnosing bronchiectasis, emphysema, lung abscesses and atelectasis. Before the procedure is carried out there is usually a need for postural drainage for several days. Local anaesthetic lozenges or spray are given immediately prior to the procedure. Afterwards the patient must not have anything by mouth for 2 to 3 hours because of the local anaesthetic. Postural drainage will be necessary to remove the oil, and the patient will be encouraged to cough.

Arteriogram

Concentrated iodine solutions may be injected into an artery under pressure in order to outline the arteries in that area. Catheters may be introduced in order to feed the dye into the specific vessels required. This is a painful procedure and therefore the patient is sedated beforehand. If the site of the injection is hairy, it will need to be shaved. Starving for 6 hours will be necessary for some of the investigations, particularly if in the abdominal region. Stenosis and aneurysms will be revealed on the x-rays.

Lymphogram

Iodised oil is injected into a lymphatic vessel and allowed to travel to the neighbouring lymph nodes and vessels. This is carried out under a local anaesthetic and requires no special preparation.

Scanning with radioactive isotopes

A radioactive substance is one which has become unstable and therefore gives off radioactive waves. These waves can be detected by suitable apparatus. Iodine, gold and technetium are examples of substances which can be used because they are taken up by particular organs. For example, iodine is absorbed by the thyroid, gold by the liver, and technetium by the kidneys. Special apparatus sensitive to the radioactivity is used to pick up these rays. The monitoring device is passed over the part of the body to be examined. The signals it picks up will be shown in a visual form, possibly on a screen where points of light will indicate radioactivity. The closer together the points, the greater the activity. For a permanent record a series of dots may be made by the machine onto special paper. Again, the density of the dots indicates the amount of radioactivity taken up by the organ or tissue. Sometimes instead of relying on the density of the light points, different colours are used.

Tissue which has been destroyed will be unable to take up the radioactive isotope, whereas tumours and overactive glands will take up large amounts.

There is no special preparation of the patients in most cases. As with ordinary x-rays, a gown is worn. The only discomfort to the patient is that he may have to lie still in one position for a long time. If the patient is an in-patient, a card will return with him stating the name and dosage of the isotope administered.

Echoencephalography

In this procedure high-frequency sound waves are directed through the organ under examination. When they reach any structure which is different in acoustic nature from the organ, the waves will be reflected back and picked up by an amplifier. They may then be converted into an electrical current which is displayed on a cathode screen. Displacement of normal structures, abnormal lesions and enlargement of an organ can be demonstrated. It is possible to differentiate between normal and abnormal tissue by this method. There is no special preparation of the patient, unless the skull is being examined, in which case a substance is applied to the head to ensure a good acoustic contact between skull and apparatus.

Abdominal x-ray procedures should only be carried out in women of child-bearing years during the first 10 days following a period, unless the woman has been sterilised. This is to minimise the possibility of harming a developing fetus.

SUGGESTED WORK

1. Find out the type of x-ray examinations carried out on patients on your ward. Take a selection of these and investigate why they are being done, what preparation was necessary, and if the patient had any particular fears about them.
2. Look at some of these x-rays and ask the doctor if he or she will explain them.

SUGGESTED READING

Goldman M. (1978). *A Guide to the X-ray Department.* Bristol: John Wright.

4

Endoscopy

Endoscopy is a method of looking directly at the mucous membrane and contents of a body cavity or passages by means of a hollow tube with a source of light. The tube may be completely rigid, semi-rigid or flexible. The flexible tube is a fibreoptic instrument which is very expensive but which allows the doctor to reach areas which are inaccessible with the more rigid scopes. It also makes it possible to take photographs, cine films and even television films. Therefore permanent records can be made and the activity of the part can be observed, the doctor being able to study the results without prolonging the procedure. Endoscopy is complementary to barium studies, particularly where the latter give ambiguous information.

GENERAL PREPARATION OF THE PATIENT

With many of the procedures, the co-operation of the patient is necessary in order to avoid sudden movement and to change his position, therefore the procedure is avoided for very young, very old or confused patients. Patients who have other serious conditions, particularly of the heart, should have these brought under control before endoscopy is proceeded with. This method is not usually carried out in patients who are AIDS or hepatitis B antigen positive due to the possibility of infecting others.

These examinations may be done in out-patients under sedation. If this is so, the patient must be told not to drive, drink alcohol or operate machinery for 24 to 36 hours after the examination because of the effects of the premedication. This information will also be given in writing. A relative or friend should accompany the patient home. The doctor will explain exactly what the procedure consists of and what is required of him, after which the patient will sign a consent form. The nurse must make sure that the notes and x-rays are available should the doctor request them.

ENDOSCOPY OF THE UPPER GASTROINTESTINAL TRACT

This procedure is not done if an aortic aneurysm or obstruction is known to be present. A rigid oesophagoscope may be used if the oesophagus only is to be examined. Although a semi-rigid gastroscope may be used to examine the stomach, the fibreoptic instrument is more useful.

Uses

If barium meals give insufficient or ambiguous information in patients who have persistent bleeding, dysphagia or dyspepsia, this is a useful diagnostic tool, particularly as biopsies may also be taken.

Treatment of certain conditions may also be carried out by this route, such as dilatation of the oesophagus, removal of foreign bodies, gastric polypectomy, and the coagulation of leaking blood vessels by diathermy or laser beams. Removal of gall-stones from the junction of the duodenum and bile ducts can also be effected via this instrument.

Specific preparation

The patient is fasted for at least 6 hours and a premedication is given. This varies according to the doctor, but diazepam is frequently used, either intramuscularly an hour prior to the procedure or immediately before intravenously. Atropine is also given to dry up the secretions. Dentures are removed and loose teeth and crowns checked. Fifteen minutes before the procedure, anaesthetic lozenges are given, and again when the patient arrives in theatre. In some centres a topical anaesthetic is sprayed onto the throat instead. Occasionally the procedure has to be done under a general anaesthetic, in which case the patient will need to be prepared appropriately.

After the procedure

The patient is not allowed anything by mouth until sensation returns, usually in 1 or 2 hours. He should be watched carefully for any evidence of shock due to perforation of the oesophagus or stomach, haemorrhage if polyps have been removed, or cardiac arrhythmias. Observation of the respirations is also important as aspiration pneumonia or respiratory depression may occur due to the premedication.

Gastrocamera

A cheaper method of obtaining pictures of the stomach is to use a very small camera attached to the end of a tube. This is swallowed after fasting the patient and pictures are taken blind.

ENDOSCOPY OF THE LOWER GASTROINTESTINAL TRACT

Two procedures frequently carried out in the ward or out-patient department are examination of the anal canal and lower part of the rectum by *proctoscopy*, and of the rectum and sigmoid colon by *sigmoidoscopy*.

Proctoscopy

A short, wide, rigid metal tube with a blunt introducer is used (Fig. 4.1). In many of the instruments there is a light which receives its power from a battery.

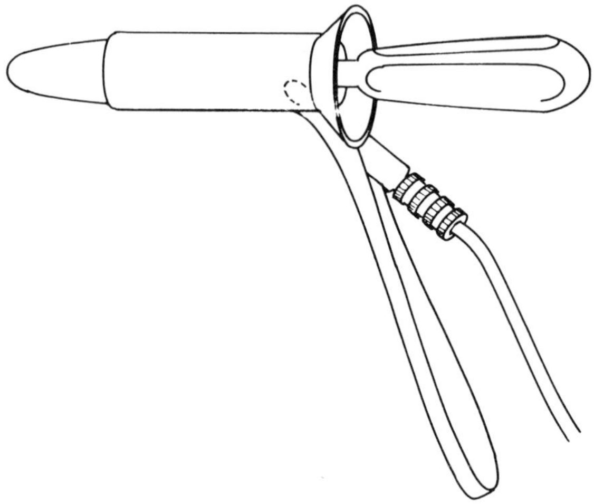

Fig. 4.1 *Proctoscope.*

Uses

This follows a rectal examination and is used to look for internal haemorrhoids, to take a biopsy of suspicious lesions, or to take a specimen of the surface cells with a swab.

Specific preparation

Normal evacuation of the bowel is sufficient. The patient is placed in the left lateral position with the buttocks to the edge of the bed. The proctoscope is warmed and lubricated. A consent form is not necessary.

Sigmoidoscopy

This procedure is also done with a rigid tube and introducer but the tube is much longer, and a light is always used (Fig. 4.2).

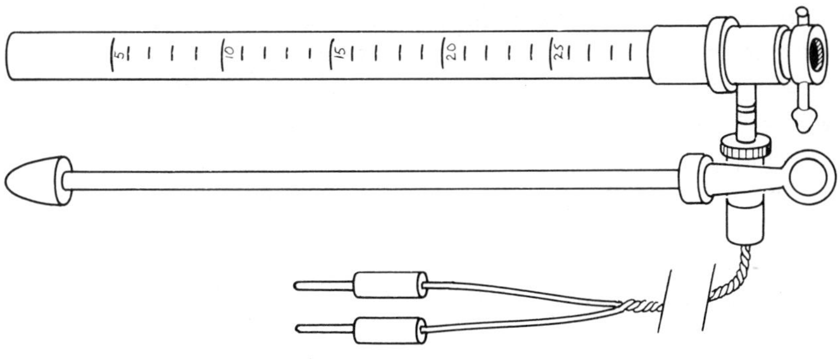

Fig. 4.2 *Sigmoidoscope.*

Uses

The procedure is used to examine inflammatory conditions of the mucosa, such as ulcerative colitis, and to take biopsies of growths.

Specific preparation

The procedure is explained to the patient and he is told that during it he will feel the need to have his bowels open, but this is a false sensation and is due to the air being pumped into the bowel. Flatus will also be passed for the same reason, and therefore he should be told not to worry about this. Preparation of the bowel depends on the condition and on the doctor's requirements. In some cases enemas and rectal washouts are used, but not if inflammation is present. Sedation is occasionally necessary.

The nurse will be responsible for positioning the patient, either in the left lateral position with the buttocks to the edge of the bed and knees drawn up, or occasionally in the knee–chest position. This latter position is better from the doctor's point of view but is much more embarrassing for the patient. The nurse also makes sure that the bulb and battery are working. The apparatus is warmed and lubricated.

After the procedure

If a biopsy has been taken, the patient will be warned that there will be slight bleeding. Perforation or haemorrhage very rarely occur. The equipment must be thoroughly cleaned.

Colonoscopy

This procedure is carried out in the x-ray department, the patient already having had a barium enema, the results of which should be available. A fibreoptic instrument which is long and flexible is used to look at the whole colon, and the progress of the instrument is monitored by x-ray. Two-metre long biopsy instruments can be used to take a biopsy. It is possible to take coloured pictures, cine film and coloured television film.

Uses

This procedure is carried out in patients suffering from polyposis or chronic ulcerative colitis to exclude malignant changes. It is also used in persistent bleeding if other examinations are inconclusive, and as a check up in patients who have had surgery on the bowel for carcinoma. It may also be used to remove polyps.

If the patient is pregnant, colonoscopy is not undertaken because of the need to x-ray. It is also avoided in patients with severe inflammation of the colon or if an aortic aneurysm is present.

Specific preparation

The preparation will vary according to the suspected condition. However, the bowel must be fully emptied. Three days before the examination the patient will be put on a low-residue diet for 2 days. The day before he will commence a fluid diet. On the morning of the examination an enema and/or washout will be given. Sedation such as diazepam will be given intramuscularly or intravenously, but if the procedure is going to take 1 to 2 hours, it will be given both intravenously and intramuscularly. The patient is asked to say if he experiences pain during the procedure.

After the procedure

The patient is heavily sedated and therefore careful observation is necessary. The patient should be warned that he may have colicky abdominal pain for some time after the examination as a result of air being pumped into the bowel.

EXAMINATION OF THE SMALL INTESTINE

A fibreoptic instrument, an enteroscope, is available to examine the small intestine for tumours, Crohn's disease, coeliac disease and gastrointestinal bleeding, but as yet it is not a commonly performed procedure.

A biopsy of the small intestine may be taken with a Crosby capsule, a spring-operated blade inside a capsule attached to a length of tubing which the patient swallows.

Specific preparation

The patient is starved from the night before. In the morning the capsule is swallowed. Once it is thought that it has reached the stomach, the patient is asked to turn on his right side. Peristalsis will move the capsule on, and its position is checked by x-ray. A biopsy is taken by attaching a syringe to the end of the tube and applying suction. This causes a small piece of mucosa to be sucked through a hole in the capsule, which the blade slices off. The capsule and tubing are then withdrawn. The patient is observed for evidence of haemorrhage and perforation, although these are rare.

LAPAROSCOPY

This procedure is carried out in theatre and may be done under either a local or general anaesthetic. A rigid tube is introduced through a small incision into the abdominal cavity, and gas is passed through this to lift the abdominal wall away from the organs.

Use

This method is mainly used for the diagnosis of gynaecological disorders, sterilisation, examination of the peritoneal cavity, and liver biopsy.

CYSTOSCOPY AND RESECTOSCOPY

A cystoscope consists of a rigid hollow tube or sheath through which a telescopic instrument is passed (Fig. 4.3). The outer sheath may contain channels through which ureteric catheters can be passed, and the head of the instrument may have valves to allow the passage of irrigating fluid. A resectoscope is a similar instrument but with a much wider bore.

Uses

The cystoscope is used to inspect the bladder for suspected growths, inflammation and stones. Ureteric catheters may be passed to collect specimens of urine from each of the kidneys or to carry out a retrograde pyelogram. A resectoscope is used for operative procedures such as transurethral prostatectomies, removal of foreign bodies, biopsy and diathermy of the bladder.

Procedure

These operations are carried out in theatre, usually under sedation, with a local anaesthetic being introduced into the urethra before the passage of the cystoscope. They can be carried out under a general anaesthetic. In order to enable the operator to see more clearly, the bladder is filled with distilled water. If diathermy is being done, glycine is substituted for water as it is a better conducting medium.

The cystoscope is a very delicate instrument and is therefore sterilised by pasteurising with water at 80°C for 10 minutes.

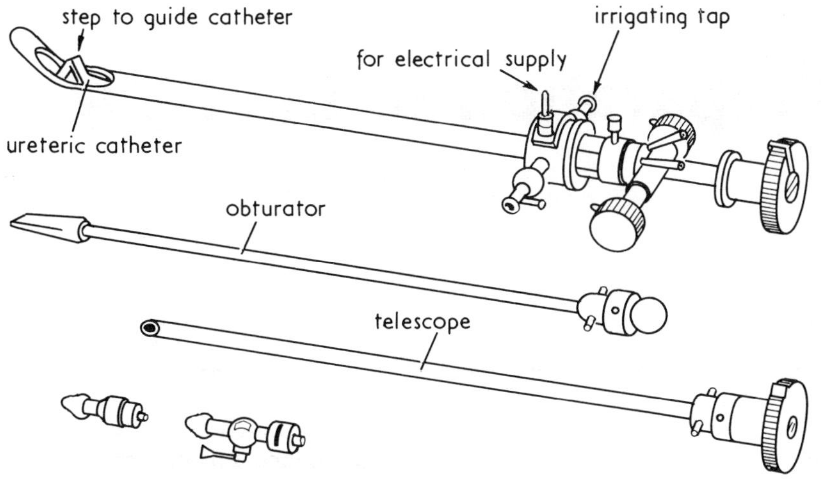

Fig. 4.3 *Cystoscope.*

BRONCHOSCOPY

Examination of the bronchi is done with a rigid bronchoscope which has a light at its end. It is most commonly carried out under a general anaesthetic but may be done after the mouth, pharynx and larynx have been sprayed with a local anaesthetic. The newer fibreoptic instrument allows a wider range of vision and may be introduced further into the bronchial tree. It also makes it possible to take a biopsy of the lung.

Uses

Inspection of the air passages, removal of secretions and foreign bodies, and taking biopsies may all be done with a bronchoscope.

Specific preparation

Any loose teeth or crowns must be noted. If there is no urgency, the procedure will not be done if there is an upper respiratory tract infection. The patient will be prepared for a general anaesthetic.

After the procedure

Observe the patient for dyspnoea and cyanosis which may indicate oedema of the glottis in children. Laryngeal spasm will cause noisy breathing. The patient will also be observed for any evidence of haemorrhage. Breathing exercises will be encouraged, and a check x-ray carried out.

THORACOSCOPY

This procedure is carried out in a specialised chest unit using a rigid thoracoscope which is inserted through the chest wall to divide adhesions or take biopsies. Before it can be done, an artificial pneumothorax must be induced. The main danger is haemorrhage.

SUGGESTED WORK

1. Ask if you can accompany a patient to the endoscopy clinic and watch the procedure.

(a) Is an anaesthetic or intravenous injection used prior to the procedure? Does every patient having this investigation have the same induction?

(b) Is the procedure unpleasant for the patient in any way? Would he be prepared to go through it again if it were necessary?

(c) What specific preparation was needed?

(d) Are there any specific observations or after-care required?

SUGGESTED READING

Hollanders D. (1979). *Gastrointestinal Endoscopy: an Introduction for Assistants*. London: Baillière Tindall.

5

Preparation of the Patient for Surgery

The preparation of a patient for surgery starts as soon as it is decided that surgery may be required. This may well be in the general practitioner's surgery. At this point the doctor will discuss with the patient the possible diagnosis and treatment, and may carry out some investigations.

The patient will then be referred to the hospital consultant in the out-patients' department, where further explanations and investigations may take place. If the patient is a smoker, the doctor will advise him to stop smoking, and if obese, to reduce weight. Contraceptive drugs may also be discontinued.

On admission to hospital, therefore, the patient may already have some idea of the surgery he is about to undergo. The nurse will ensure that a bed is prepared so that he feels expected and welcomed, as this will have a great influence on his attitudes to his stay in hospital and the surgery carried out. The nursing history will be completed during the initial period in hospital, and may be commenced during the doctor's examination, so preventing any repetition. By doing this the nurse will be able to recognise potential problems early, and alert those who will be responsible for dealing with them, particularly if they are social problems. This is a good opportunity for the nurse to build a relationship with the patient and allow him to ask about those things which are worrying him. The development of a good nurse–patient relationship can have a considerable effect on the way in which a patient is able to withstand the consequences of uncertainty and surgery. The support needed will vary according to the type of surgery carried out, the dependence of the patient, and his previous experience. His general morale and length of stay in hospital have been shown to be influenced by the attitudes of the nurses and the atmosphere in the ward.

When taking the nursing history, the nurse will first establish the details of the patient's personal information, ensuring that these are correct. She will then find out what the patient's perception and expectations about his condition are. Following this she will make a detailed assessment of his physical, mental and social states and of actual or potential needs and problems arising from these. Assessment sheets vary from hospital to hospital, but all include the following points in some way or other.

General appearance. From her observations, the nurse will note whether the patient appears well cared for and well nourished and what his general demeanour is like. Has he certain urgent needs, and is he accompanied? The patient will be weighed, and his weight will be entered in his notes.

Pain. If present, ask the patient to describe where it is, what it is like and how frequent it is. Does the patient take any analgesics to relieve it?

Sleep. Find out what the patient's normal sleeping pattern is and what he does to relieve sleeplessness, if present.

Diet. Has the patient been on a special diet and were there any problems related to this? What has the patient's appetite been like? Has he any special likes or dislikes in the way of food or fluids? Are there other factors influencing what he eats, such as difficulty in shopping, lack of money or ill-fitting dentures? Does he need help with feeding?

Bladder. Establish whether the patient has any frequency, incontinence, nocturia, dysuria or other problem. His urine will be tested for any abnormalities and the results entered in the notes.

Bowel. How often does the patient normally have his bowels opened and does he have any constipation or diarrhoea? Does he take any aperients or other related medication?

Hygiene. Is the patient able to attend to all his hygiene requirements? If not, the nurse will need to discover exactly how much he is able to do, such as his ability to manage in the bath or with the toilet. She will check on the condition of the skin and whether there are any broken or sore areas or rashes. She will note any oedema, dehydration, abnormal pigmentation or bruising.

She will also note the condition of the mouth and if there are any loose or capped teeth. Where dentures are worn, it is wise to ask the patient how well they fit.

Mobility. The patient may be completely independent, but if not, the nurse will need to assess how much he is able to do for himself. Does he require any assistance with walking, such as a tripod or prosthesis, and if so has he brought it with him? Does he need any help with dressing or special aids.

Communication. While eliciting the previous information, the nurse will be observing the responses of the patient and his ability to communicate. She will note whether he is alert or drowsy, relaxed or anxious, overexcitable or antagonistic. She will need to discover why he feels as he does in order to deal with any problem. Communication difficulties may arise due to language or dialect differences, or because the patient has a physical impediment such as deafness or blindness. If the patient is hard of hearing, find out if he has a hearing aid and whether he has brought it into hospital. Frequently the hearing aid is not working efficiently or is being used incorrectly. Impairment of vision can include loss of part of the visual field as well as partial or complete blindness. The patient may have forgotten his glasses or may not have had his eyes tested for a long time. Occasionally a patient has a false eye. Difficulty in making themselves understood because of a speech impediment may be found in the totally deaf or in someone who has had a cerebral vascular accident. Different levels of understanding can also interfere with communication, such as with the mentally handicapped. An identification band with the patient's full name, age, hospital number and consultant will be attached to the wrist.

Social. The type of accommodation that the patient lives in and the people available to support him if required may influence his discharge from hospital.

Spiritual. Find out if the patient is practising his stated religion and would appreciate a visit from the hospital chaplain or his own minister. If appropriate, would he like communion in the ward or to attend the hospital chapel?

Vital signs. The patient's temperature, pulse, respiration and blood pressure will be taken to provide a baseline against which his postoperative observations can be measured. Should there be any abnormality in these, they must be reported as the operation may have to be delayed until these abnormalities have been corrected.

This is obviously not an exhaustive list, but by looking at the specific needs of patients having particular operations it is possible to supplement it.

The patient is then asked to undress ready for the doctor's examination, during which the relatives will be asked to wait outside. The doctor will see them after he has examined the patient. A full medical examination is done, covering each system in turn. The purpose of this is to assess the patient's general health and to recognise the presence of any other disease which may hinder his progress. The doctor will also take a full medical history, noting any allergies in a prominent place on the notes. Any further investigations required will be ordered.

The nurse's role during the examination is to position the patient suitably, for example lying flat for examination of the abdomen, or in the left lateral position for a rectal examination. She is there to reassure the patient and maintain his dignity by keeping him suitably covered, and at the same time allowing the doctor easy access to those parts he wishes to examine. She will support the patient where necessary, for example when he needs to be sat up, and she will make sure that all the equipment for the examination or any tests is available. Afterwards she will make the patient comfortable.

The doctor will explain the nature of the operation and obtain the patient's written consent, or, in the case of children, the parent's or guardian's consent. In certain operations, such as sterilisation, the agreement of the spouse may also be requested, although the spouse's refusal does not mean that the patient cannot go ahead and have the operation. The doctor records in the notes any long-term drug therapy, especially steroids, anticoagulants, hypotensive agents and insulin. Where appropriate, the doctor will mark the side or area for surgery, such as a digit or eye. The anaesthetist also comes to see the patient to satisfy himself that he is fit for anaesthetic. If the patient is a diabetic or has some other medical disease, the appropriate consultant may also be requested to see him.

The physiotherapist will teach the patient breathing exercises and the necessity for moving his legs postoperatively to prevent deep vein thrombosis. With some operations she may have an even greater role.

The evening before the operation, the skin in the vicinity of the operating site will be prepared. It will be shaved to reduce infection and the patient will be asked to have a bath, but not to use talcum powder. Particular attention should be paid to the cleanliness of the navel and under the nails. Orthopaedic operations may require more extensive skin preparation.

For most operations, laxative suppositories are sufficient to clear the bowel, and for some minor operations even these will not be necessary. Some surgeons prefer the patient to have an aperient 24 hours before the operation. Specific bowel preparation will be necessary for surgery on the gastrointestinal tract (see Chapter 20).

No food or fluid is given to the patient during the 4 to 6 hours prior to the operation to prevent inhalation of the contents of the stomach while the patient is under the anaesthetic. A notice 'Nil by mouth' is placed over the bed. It is usually not advisable to starve the patient longer than this because the nitrogen from protein is necessary to repair the damaged tissue postoperatively. However, if surgery to the gastrointestinal tract is being done, there will be a longer period of starvation, and a nasogastric tube may be passed. Stomach washouts may be necessary. The patient will have been ordered a night sedation to encourage a good night's rest prior to the operation.

On the day of surgery, urine analysis is repeated and the results are recorded in the notes. The patient is prepared with a clean gown. Dentures, hairgrips, contact lenses and other prostheses are removed. Crowned teeth are noted. Jewellery and money are locked in a safe place and the patient's wedding ring covered with Elastoplast. Nail varnish and make-up are removed to enable any changes in the colour of the patient's skin to be noted by the doctor. The patient is asked to empty his bladder and is then placed on a canvas, the bed being made in such a way that the bedclothes may be easily removed in a pack. In some pelvic operations a catheter is inserted. In some hospitals a second identity band is attached to the ankle in case the anaesthetist needs to remove the wristband when giving intravenous therapy.

When all the preparations are complete, the curtains are drawn around the patient and approximately an hour before the operation a premedication is given, the time of administration being recorded on the drug chart and checklist if there is one. After this the patient should not be disturbed.

When the porter arrives for the patient he may have a slip of paper with the patient's name on it, which the nurse must check against the details of her patient. With the aid of a checklist (Fig. 5.1), she will make sure that all of the items mentioned have been dealt with. The x-rays, notes and any special equipment which may be needed will accompany the patient. The ward nurse will stay with the patient until she hands over to the anaesthetic nurse who will also check all of the above information.

Patient's notes checked with operation list for correctness
Correct identity bracelet in position
Operation form explained and signed
TPR, blood pressure and weight recorded
Allergies recorded
Urinalysis recorded
Crowns and loose teeth recorded
Jewellery removed
Wedding ring taped
Hair clips and make-up removed
Artificial eye or contact lenses removed
Dentures or braces removed
Note when patient last passed urine
Note time of last meal or drink
Surgical shave checked
Cleanliness of skin area checked
Povidine pack applied if required
Note time premedication given
X-rays and notes to accompany patient
The presence of a hearing aid
Pacemaker reported

This form should be completed by the nurse responsible for preparing the patient for theatre and signed by her. It should be checked by the nurse in charge of the ward before the patient leaves the ward and rechecked by the theatre nurse receiving the patient.

Fig. 5.1 *Example of a checklist for preoperative patients.*

THE EMERGENCY ADMISSION

This patient will have come into hospital quite unprepared. He may have been taken ill at work and may be worried about some task that has been left incomplete, or an appointment that cannot be fulfilled. No preparations will have been made for his family, in fact they may not even know that he is in hospital. He may not have brought any of the necessary toilet equipment or nightclothes with him. The nurse may therefore have to contact relatives and deal with his many other requirements.

The time allowed to prepare the patient for surgery can be very short in some emergency situations, in fact he may go to theatre directly from the accident and emergency department. This will mean that only the essential preparation of the patient for theatre is carried out. If conscious, the patient will need even greater support from the nurse than the booked admission. The consent form is signed unless the patient is too ill and there are no relatives with him. If this is the case, it is indicated on the form and the anaesthetist informed. An identification band must be attached to the patient with as much information as can be gained. If this is not available and the patient is unconscious, the date and time of admission, his admission number and the consultant's name will be used. All prostheses will be removed. If the patient has eaten within the previous 4 hours, a nasogastric tube will be passed and the stomach emptied. The advisability of carrying out the other preoperative preparations, such as shaving or the administration of preoperative drugs, will be discussed with the surgeon. If shaving is not done, the theatre must be informed.

SUGGESTED WORK

1. Do a survey of the patients on your ward and find out how much time passed from the last meal to the operation. How long did they have to wait postoperatively until they had an adequate diet? Read *Nil by Mouth* (Hamilton-Smith, 1972) and compare this with your findings.

SUGGESTED READING

Bille D. A. (1979). Pre-operative teaching—rights and responsibilities. *Todays Operating Room Nurse*; **1** (8): 9–13.
Bille D. A. (1980). The nurse's role in informed consent. *Quality Review Bulletin*; **6** (2): 25–9.
Boore J. R. P. (1978). *Prescription for Recovery*. Edinburgh: Churchill Livingstone; London: Royal College of Nursing.
Hamilton-Smith S. (1972). *Nil by Mouth*. London: Royal College of Nursing.
Mancini M. (1979). Consent to treatment; what does it entail? *American Journal of Nursing*; **6**: 1139–40.
Sloane P. J. M. (1984). Survey of patient information booklets. *British Medical Journal*; **24**: 915–19.

6

Principles of Operating Theatre Nursing

This chapter aims to open up this particular field of nursing by explaining the principles of operating theatre work in such a way that the nurse will be made aware of the part she can play, and appreciate its importance in the total management of any surgical patient. An important aspect to be appreciated by any nurse on arrival in the theatre is its complete difference from the ward area. The theatre scene and the working day of the theatre staff are geared to the number of patients requiring surgery, encompassing the preparation of the patient for surgery, the preparation of equipment, the surgical procedures, and the satisfactory recovery of the patient from the anaesthetic. A high standard of cleanliness is maintained in the preparation and disposal of equipment used in the theatre management, most particularly by the performance of a careful aseptic technique during any surgical procedure. The nurse will recognise the importance of controlling any possible source of infection, the effects of surgery on a patient (related to the management of pain), and specific nursing management which will be dependent on the type of anaesthetic given and the type of surgical procedure carried out.

There are four main areas of work within any operating theatre suite (Fig. 6.1). These are the anaesthetic room, the theatre sterile supply unit (TSSU) or instrument preparation room, the operating theatre, and the recovery room. Work in each of these areas is the responsibility of a trained member of staff and is linked to the requirements and needs of the surgical staff who work in close conjunction with the theatre team.

Prior to any series of operations, information in the form of an operating list is given to the theatre staff within each area. The list contains the number of patients requiring surgery, their names, ages, types of anaesthetic to be given, and the operative procedures to be carried out. This enables the theatre staff within each area to prepare the appropriate anaesthetic equipment, operating instruments and theatre furnishings as required within that designated area of work.

On arrival at the theatre suite, patients are received into the reception area in transit to the anaesthetic room. Here, patients are checked against the operating list, ensuring they are the correct patients for surgery. Each patient's notes are also checked for the time the premedication was given, the consent for anaesthesia form, the hospital number and any other details such as x-rays. The patient's wrist or name band is checked against the notes. (For details, see the leaflet entitled: *Safeguards Against Wrong Operations*, a joint memorandum issued by the Medical Defence Union and the Royal College of Nursing.) Patients are then transferred onto a 'clean' theatre trolley to await their transfer to the anaesthetic room.

THE ANAESTHETIC ROOM

Once within the anaesthetic room, the anaesthetist is totally responsible for the patient's well-being throughout his stay in the operating theatre suite. It is the responsibility of the anaesthetist and his assistant, who must be a trained nurse or operating

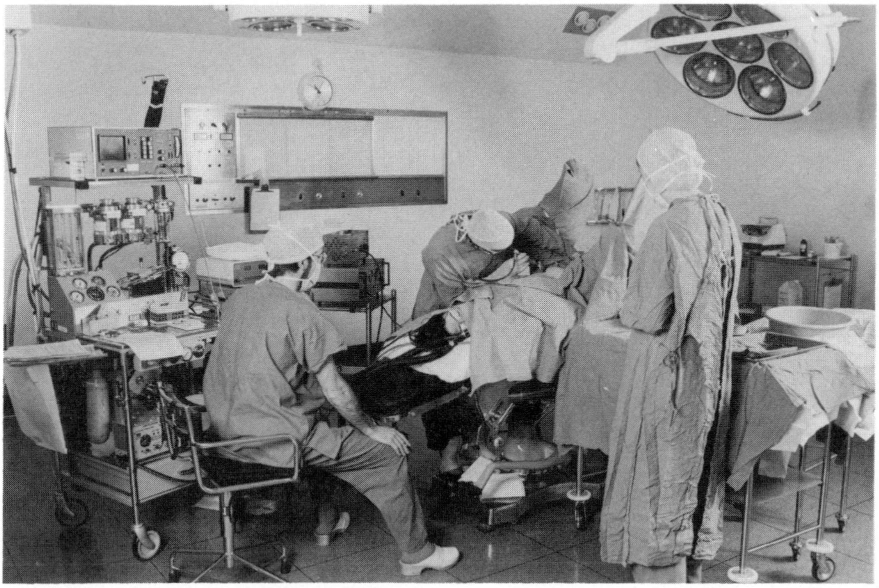

Fig. 6.1 *The operating theatre.*

department assistant, to prepare and check the appropriate equipment. This checking and double checking of each piece of equipment and drug to be used is rigorously carried out. It is vitally important in order to avoid the permanent and disabling damage that can be inflicted on patients as a result of negligence and lack of care. **Attention to detail is essential.**

On arrival in the anaesthetic room, patients will usually be sleepy from their premedication, but whatever the surgery, it is normal for them to have some form of anaesthetic, dependent on the type of surgery being carried out. This enables the operation to be performed with ease, facilitating the surgeon's role and enabling the patient to be free from pain or any discomfort.

There are three basic forms of anaesthetic: general anaesthesia, local anaesthesia, and topical anaesthesia. The majority of patients undergoing surgery invariably have a general anaesthetic as this enables the patient to be totally unaware of what is happening and therefore avoids any problems of tension or anxiety. Induction of a general anaesthetic is achieved by a combination of intravenous drugs and gases. This requires certain equipment and types of drugs and gases.

Intravenous drugs are given via a cannula inserted into a vein in the back of the hand or the antecubital fossa. The first of these drugs will be some form of 'hypnotic' agent, followed by a muscle-relaxant drug. The hypnotic, normally thiopentone, will put the patient to sleep, while the relaxant drug allows the muscles to lose their tone sufficiently for the anaesthetist to pass an endotracheal tube (Fig. 6.2) through the patient's mouth until the tip of the tube sits in the trachea. To do this he uses a laryngoscope (Fig. 6.3). An inflatable cuff at the tip of the tube is blown up, using a syringe, so that an even pressure is exerted against the tracheal wall, thus preventing any leakage of gases from around the tube and maintaining a closed circuit to the anaesthetic machine.

It is important that this manoeuvre is carried out speedily, as the patient is unable to maintain his own respirations because of the relaxant drug, therefore risking anoxia. As soon as the tube is in situ it is connected to the anaesthetic machine which carries the necessary gases for administra-

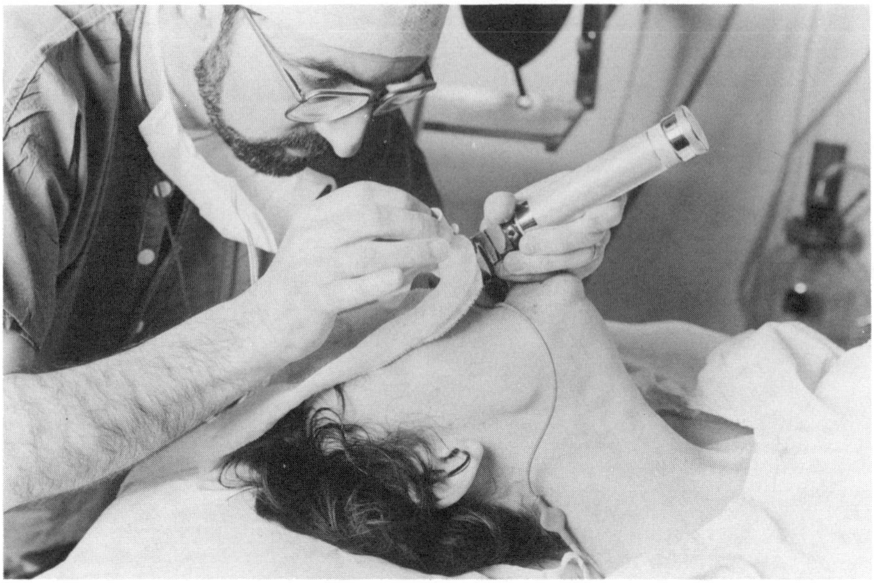

Fig. 6.2 *Passing an endotracheal tube with a laryngoscope.*

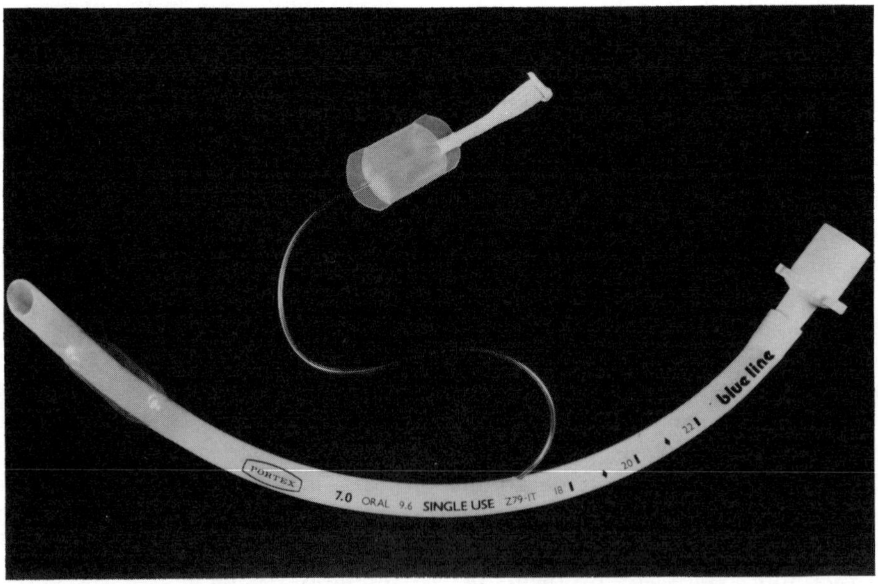

Fig. 6.3 *Endotracheal tube.*

tion to the patient. The most essential of these is oxygen and this is given immediately in 100% form, once the tube is inserted and connected to the machine. Occasionally it is given via an anaesthetic mask prior to insertion of the tube, thus avoiding the risks of anoxia. Once the patient's lungs are adequately ventilated, the oxygen level is reduced to approximately 4 litres per minute, and further intravenous drugs and anaesthetic gases are given to induce analgesia and maintain hypnosis as needed. The other gases used are mainly nitrous oxide and halothane (Fig. 6.4).

It is the responsibility of the anaesthetist and his assistant, when administering these drugs and gases, to keep a close watch on the patient's level of unconsciousness and relaxation, plus his state of analgesia. Throughout the surgical procedure their duty is to observe the patient's condition, recording the pulse and blood pressure at frequent intervals, as well as noting the colour of the patient, and any excessive fluid loss during surgery (either blood or serous fluid) which may require fluid replacement.

It is the maintenance of this 'triad' of anaesthesia, consisting of 'relaxation', 'analgesia', and 'hypnosis', that is essential in the induction and care of the patient undergoing general anaesthesia. Equipment and drugs vary from hospital to hospital, but the principles remain the same.

The other two basic forms of anaesthetic mentioned are local anaesthesia and topical anaesthesia. Local anaesthesia can be achieved in a variety of ways, by spinal or epidural anaesthesia, nerve blocks or local infiltration under the skin, each method being carried out with care and under clean or aseptic conditions. The choice of local anaesthetic is dependent on the site to be operated on, the degree of surgery to be undertaken, and the suitability of the patient for the particular type of local anaesthetic. The surgeon and the anaesthetist liaise closely in deciding what type of local anaesthetic is to be given, so that the optimum effect is achieved.

The third form of basic anaesthesia referred to is topical anaesthesia. This is less frequently seen and consists of an anaesthetic solution being directly applied to the area to be anaesthetised. The solution can be in the form of a gel, paste or drops

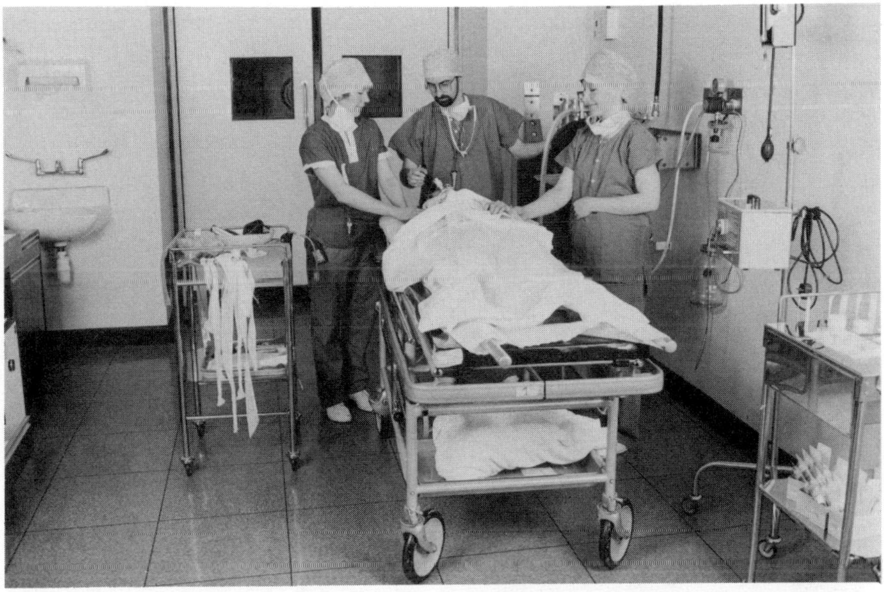

Fig. 6.4 *The anaesthetic room in which the patient is undergoing induction.*

which are applied and thus numb the surface tissue, normally mucous membrane. For example, lignocaine spray can be applied to the back of the throat prior to insertion of the endotracheal tube.

THE THEATRE STERILE SUPPLY UNIT

Theatre staff during the anaesthetic induction, or even before this, will be required to prepare the necessary equipment and materials in the other areas of theatre for the surgical procedures. One such area is the theatre sterile supply unit (TSSU). This unit has within it all the equipment for cleaning, disinfecting and sterilising a vast range of surgical instruments and sets that may be required at any time for a variety of surgical procedures. As well as this, it stores presterilised trays for emergency use plus specially made up packs of linen drapes. Other items stored are numerous boxes of ligatures, sutures and clips, presterilised and supplied by industrial firms, and a variety of prepacked and sterilised goods of rubber and plastic materials (Fig. 6.5).

In most modern theatre suites, a preset tray system is used. It is the responsibility of the TSSU staff to prepare and make up such sets as required by the surgeon. Specially prepared packs of drapes can also be made up within the unit, or they may be supplied by a central sterile supply department. Each of these packs contains the drapes and gauze swabs required for a specific operation, for example gown packs, abdominal packs and orthopaedic packs; the range is wide.

The hospital theatre suite, however, may not have such a unit. In its place will be an instrument preparation room in which similar work is carried out and which may be attached to the main body of the operating theatre. The responsibilities of the staff within these units are to supply and make up sets of instruments ready for immediate use. Some may be prepared in advance ready for use in emergencies, others can be prepared once the list of operations is known. This enables the staff to make up and sterilise the correct sets of instruments required for the particular operative procedures.

It is in this area that the nurse handles instruments, learns how to clean them thoroughly and make them up into specific sets or individual packs so that they are available on demand. Once pre-

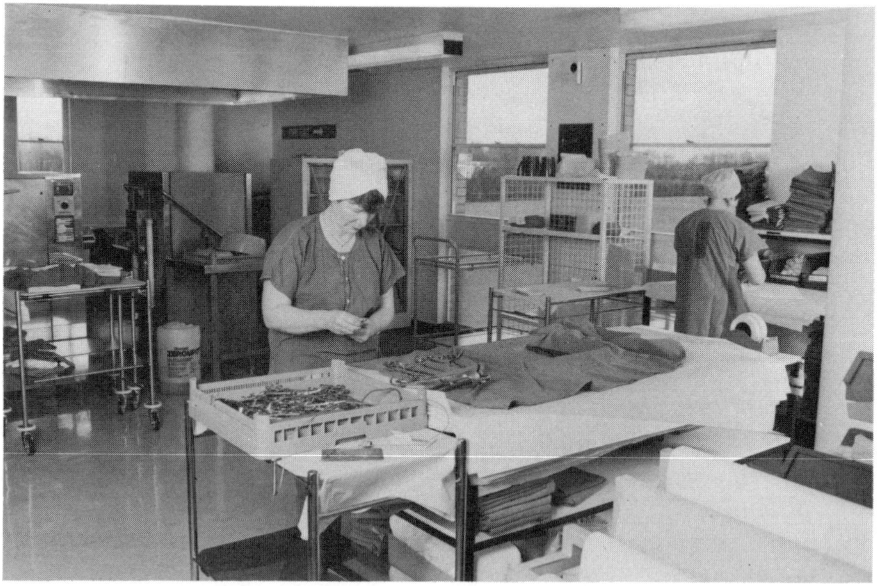

Fig. 6.5 *The theatre sterile supply unit.*

pared, these sets of instruments are then placed into caskets or trays ready for sterilisation. In some units, trays of instruments are made up containing drapes and utensils used for lotions and swabs. The range and type of instrument tray will vary from hospital to hospital, but the techniques of preparation and sterilisation are the same.

The process of sterilisation is achieved by means of autoclaves. Some autoclaves will sterilise instruments using water forced by a high temperature to form what is called a 'high steam pressure autoclave'. Other instruments can be sterilised by dry heat in what is called a 'hot air oven'. Again the variety and range of autoclaves may vary from place to place. The aim of sterilisation is to kill all spore-bearing bacteria, and so control any source of infection. This need to maintain a control over infection is an essential part of theatre work, therefore any contamination of instruments or packs by poor handling technique or faulty sterilisation is carefully avoided. Hence frequent maintenance of autoclaves, the checking of sterile goods, and a regular check on stock levels are part of the overall management of any theatre sterile supply unit or preparation room.

Once the sets are prepared and sterilised, then they, together with the correct number and type of packs that will be used during the surgical list, are transported to the main operating room. In some units, this preparation may well be carried out the night before, particularly if it is an early morning operating session. Once within the operating room, they are collected and stacked ready for use in what is called the 'lay-up room'. This is a small area which is attached to the main body of the operating theatre, like the anaesthetic room.

THE OPERATING ROOM

Preparation, meanwhile, will be taking place in the operating room itself. There are several different tasks which need to be carried out at the same time, therefore staff within the operating room are normally allocated a specific duty by a senior member of staff who will, as a rule, take overall responsibility for the management and running of the operating session, and those members of staff under her care.

These tasks can be categorised as follows: the anaesthetic nurse (who may be an operating department assistant); the circulating nurse or runner; the scrub nurse or instrument nurse; the theatre orderly; and, if there are sufficient members of staff, or if the instrument preparation room is attached to the theatre itself, then there should be a person responsible for preparing and handling the instruments and trays, as described earlier. It is (subject to staffing levels) useful to have a person responsible for the 'lay-up room' who can assist the instrument nurse in the preparation of her instruments, and at the same time gather the necessary lotions, sutures, dressings, instrument trays, and packs required for the next operation. Once each individual has been allocated a duty, they will carry out the tasks entailed within it throughout the operating session.

The anaesthetic nurse

The duty of the anaesthetic nurse or operating department assistant is to be available to assist the anaesthetist and work together with him to achieve a safe induction of anaesthesia (as described earlier), carrying out careful checks, and safe procedures as requested. The anaesthetist has absolute control over patient care, but while in this area the nurse learner will observe and gain knowledge of anaesthetic procedures, being guided and supported at all times by a trained member of staff.

The circulating nurse

The duty of the circulating nurse is one which is sometimes viewed as being very tedious or monotonous, but it is in fact a very important duty and one which requires a high sense of responsibility and a degree of common sense. The circulating nurse works initially with the theatre orderly during the early preparation of the operating area, being responsible for the cleaning of the theatre area. It is the circulating nurse who supervises the cleaning and damp dusting of all the theatre furniture and surrounds prior to any operating session, while the theatre orderly assists her in these tasks and is responsible for the cleaning of the floor area and the operating table before the list, and subsequently during the session as deemed necessary. His tasks also comprise the collection of any extra table attachments that may bĕ required, and assisting the operating department assistant in the setting up of the operating table, dependent on the position that will be adopted for the patient.

These positions vary, and are usually of four basic types: supine, prone, Trendelenberg or lithotomy (Fig. 6.6). In positioning any patient for surgery, extra equipment such as sandbags, arm-rests or other support must be available to ensure comfort for the patient, but even more importantly to protect his cardiovascular and nervous system from any permanent damage. Positioning of patients requires great care and the anaesthetist together with the theatre orderly and anaesthetic assistant are responsible for this task. Good positioning should enable easy access to the site being operated on, retain the patient's comfort and so avoid pressure problems later on.

The circulating nurse will, on completion of her cleaning tasks, be responsible for the needs of the instrument nurse. This is her prime responsibility throughout any operative procedure. She must be available to check swabs prior to surgery, be there to fetch and carry materials, lotions, swabs, or instruments as needed. Hence she 'runs' for the instrument nurse. At the same time any used swabs must be 'hung up' in preparation for checking on completion of surgery, and any specimens removed from patients must be collected from the instrument nurse and correctly labelled, as necessary. Her most important role is to check all swabs, instruments and needles used on the patient by the instrument nurse (See leaflet *Safeguards Against Failure to Remove Swabs and Instruments from Patients*, a joint memorandum issued by the Medical Defence Union and the RCN).

The instrument nurse

The instrument or scrub nurse is usually a trained member of staff and her responsibilities entail the correct handling and use of instruments prior to and during surgery; the maintenance of a strict aseptic technique throughout the procedure; and, most important, looking after the surgical team,

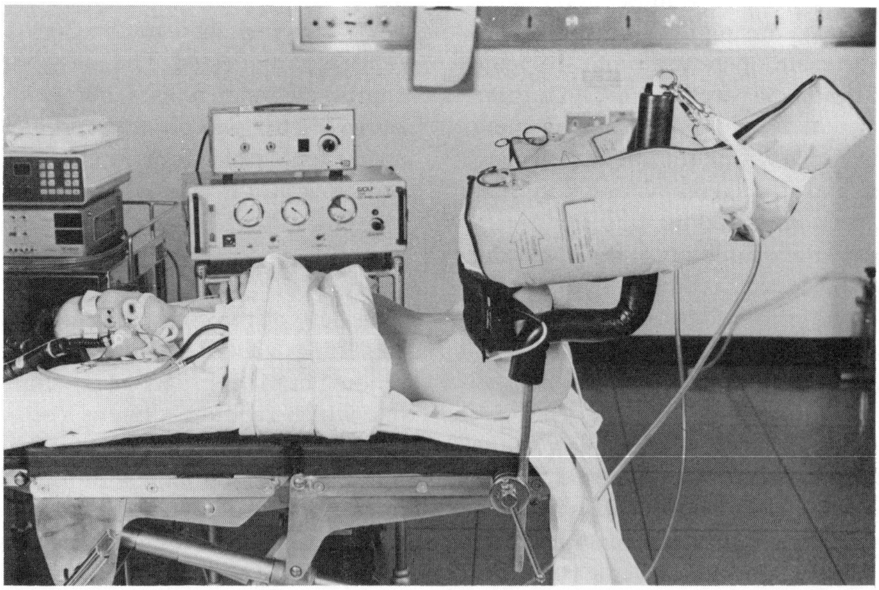

Fig. 6.6 *Patient in the lithotomy position.*

anticipating the surgeon's wishes and needs during any operative procedure. The first duty of the instrument nurse is to check that all the instruments required for the procedure are available, plus any extra items such as swabs, sutures, lotions, dressings and drains if required. She does this by liaising with the surgical team and then advising and working closely with the nurse in the lay-up room. Her next responsibility is carefully to carry out a 'scrub technique'. This is achieved by a 5-minute wash of hands and forearms with an antiseptic solution before carefully putting on gown and gloves. This hand-washing technique is referred to as 'scrubbing up' and must be carried out meticulously. The gown and gloves are put on in such a way that contamination is avoided.

Once the instrument nurse is gowned and gloved, she can then freely handle the sterilised instruments and goods, these items being passed to her by the lay-up nurse or circulating nurse, in such a way that each article is opened but not contaminated by the 'unscrubbed person'. Thus she is able to prepare and set up her instrument trolley ready for the operation. Throughout the surgical procedure, her main duty is the care of this instrument trolley, checking that she has the necessary drapes and items ready for immediate use (Fig. 6.7). Prior to the surgical incision, and preceding the closing of that incision, a strict check is made on the number of swabs, instruments and needles used on the patient. *All* instruments, swabs and needles *must* be checked whatever the surgical incision. This check is carried out with the circulating nurse or runner and is a vital part of the instrument nurse's role. During the operation she must anticipate the needs of the surgeon, being alert to any sudden change that may occur in the operative situation, such as haemorrhage from an artery, or rupture of the intestines, and even collapse of the patient requiring urgent closure of the incision site.

As the wound site is being closed, all the necessary checks must be completed, so that the instrument nurse can inform the surgeon that all the swabs, instruments and needles used on the patient are accounted for.

Once satisfied that all is well with the patient, the surgeon will inform the anaesthetist that he is completing surgery. The anaesthetist can then

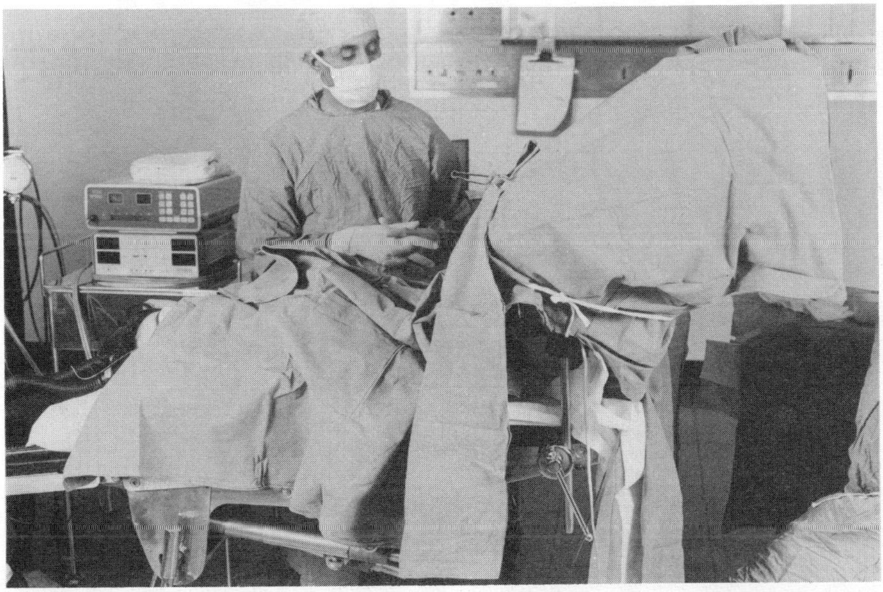

Fig. 6.7 *The operating theatre with the patient draped for surgery.*

discontinue the anaesthetic gases, apart from oxygen, if everything is in order. He may, where required, give an antidote to reverse the effects of the muscle-relaxant drug, dependent on the type used. If this is not possible, he will wait for the drug to be fully absorbed and the effects to wear off. This will be recognised by the sudden onset of spontaneous respirations by the patient. Once normal respirations are established, the endotracheal tube can be removed. A rubber Guedel airway will take its place (Fig. 6.8). This is inserted into the patient's mouth over the tongue, thus preventing occlusion of the airway by the tongue. At this stage the patient has little control over his voluntary muscles. Oxygen may continue to be given via an anaesthetic mask if felt necessary.

Meanwhile, the instrument nurse will have placed the appropriate dressing on the patient's wound, checked the drains (if present) and removed all the surgical drapes used on the patient, leaving him covered in his own theatre gown. Any blood will be cleaned from around the incision site prior to dressing the wound. Once the anaesthetist is satisfied that all is well with the patient, he will be transferred to the recovery room. The patient is carefully transferred onto the theatre trolley or his own bed. This can be done safely once all drapes and unnecessary table apparatus have been removed. It is wise to have at least three people available during the patient's transfer, one either end of the patient and the third person free to support the head or arms or the patient as required. The latter will assist in receiving the patient onto the trolley or bed. The instrument nurse, with the anaesthetist, will transport the patient to the recovery room. At the same time his assistant can inform the staff within the theatre reception to arrange collection of the next patient. This is usually done by the theatre porters who will have a slip stating the name, operation and ward from which the patient is to be collected.

THE RECOVERY ROOM

Within the immediate postoperative phase, patients are most vulnerable to complications leading to death. Therefore specially trained and

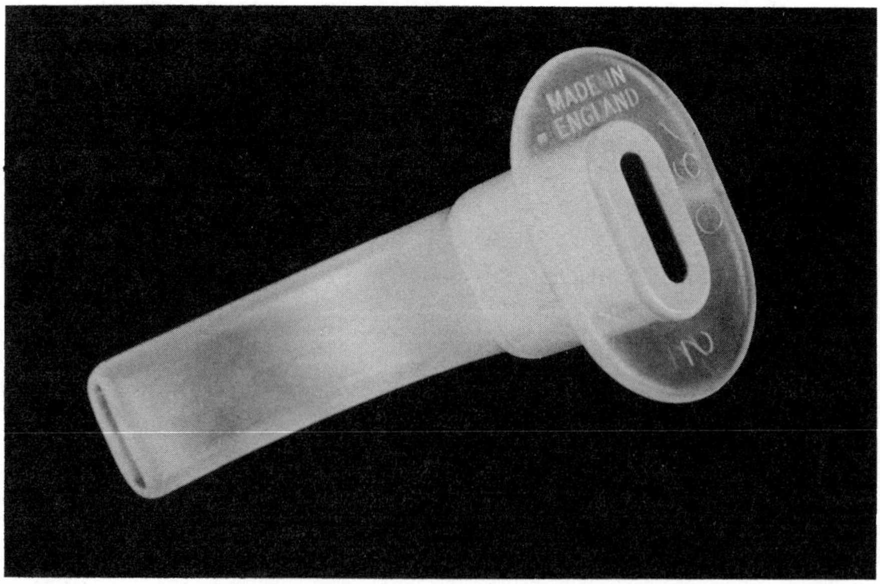

Fig. 6.8 *A Guedel airway.*

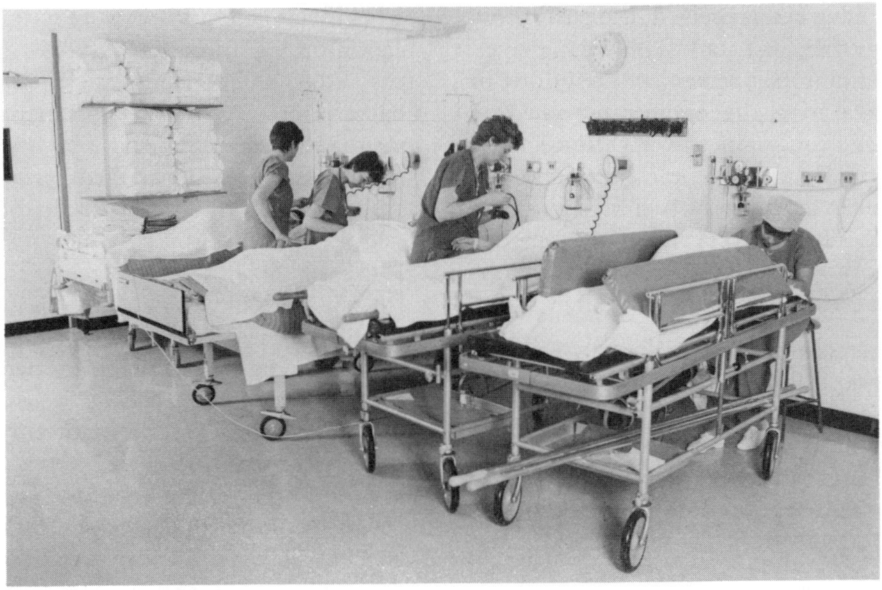

Fig. 6.9 *The recovery room.*

experienced qualified nurses, who are expert in recognising sudden changes in the patient's condition, work in this area (Fig. 6.9).

Recovery room staff will receive the patient and obtain information pertaining to the operation itself: the type of anaesthetic given, any needs such as oxygen or intravenous fluids, and finally, if in situ, what drains or intravenous infusion are present. As well as this, it is vitally important that they check the treatment card for any postoperative drugs that may be required by the patient, particularly analgesics. It is often the responsibility of the recovery room staff to give the first analgesic on the patient's recovery from anaesthetic. If there are any adverse changes in the patient's condition, the anaesthetist is informed immediately as he has the ultimate responsibility for the patient's welfare.

Duties in the recovery room comprise the checking of suction and oxygen apparatus, resuscitation equipment and anaesthetic machines (if present), plus the preparation of individual areas with gauze swabs, bowls, syringes and needles as required for each patient. Most modern recovery rooms have individual sections to accommodate each patient, each section containing all the equipment necessary for the safe recovery of the patient, such as oxygen and suction apparatus. There must be an emergency bell. A qualified nurse will remain with each patient until he is fully recovered from the anaesthetic.

Recovery from an anaesthetic can be recognised by the return of the cough and swallowing reflexes, eyelid movement (blinking), and response to verbal command. It is an important point to remember that in most patients it is the sense of hearing that is the first of the senses to return. Therefore the patient's condition should not be discussed over him.

Once the patient has regained full consciousness, although he may be sleepy, the recovery nurse will confirm with the anaesthetist that he is happy for the patient to be returned to the ward. All the completed charts and notes for the particular patient will have been received from the theatre room staff. The notes may have been delayed by the surgical team to write up all the operative details as a record of what transpired during surgery. The anaesthetist will also need to write up any details regarding the anaesthetic and any postoperative regimen required such as intravenous therapy.

Once the notes have been received, the particulars are passed on to the ward staff. The details given include the operation performed, and anything of importance concerning the operative procedure itself, the patient's condition, and any future needs that will be required for the patient, plus any drugs that may have been given to the patient during the recovery phase. The recovery room staff are responsible for notifying the ward when a patient is ready to be returned.

Obviously there are other smaller areas within a theatre suite not fully discussed, these are the changing rooms for all theatre personnel, storage rooms for anaesthetic equipment, some of which is expensive and highly technical, clean and dirty areas between the reception point, where patients are transferred to and from the wards, and a rest room.

Theatre clothing

As stated earlier, a particularly important part of theatre nursing is the control of infection. All nurses and theatre personnel visiting or working within the department are expected to change into special theatre clothing, including special footwear. A theatre hat is worn all the time and a face mask when any surgery is being performed. Shower facilities are provided to ensure good personal hygiene.

Anaesthetic gases

The use of anaesthesia is necessary if surgery is to be performed satisfactorily; however, the use of anaesthetic gases also carries a high risk. If these gases are allowed to accumulate within the operating room, they can be a danger to both patient and staff alike. Studies have been carried out demonstrating this fact. Most modern operating rooms now have a special extractor system, sometimes referred to as a 'scavenger flow system', which is able to remove these gases from source, by means of a tube passing from the expiratory system of the anaesthetic machine direct to the external environment. Another means of removing unwanted gases is by the 'laminar air-flow system'. This involves a high pressure within the operating room forcing air out into the low-pressure area of the external environment. It also reduces the bacterial content of the operating room, thus aiding the control of infection. The use of anaesthetic gases can also be a risk factor when any electrical equipment is used, particularly diathermy.

Diathermy

Diathermy is the means by which minor blood vessels can be coagulated and sealed. It necessitates the use of an electrical charge which is passed along a positive lead to a sterile diathermy probe, held by the instrument nurse, and a negative earth plate attached to the patient just prior to surgery. It is important that the instrument nurse checks whether diathermy is to be used and ensures that the earth plate is placed in position. The diathermy machine must also be checked by the circulating nurse for the correct degree of current and the secure connection of the terminal leads. It is because of the use of diathermy that patients are asked to remove jewellery and hair clips.

Administration within theatre

A senior nurse is in control of all the operating theatre rooms and their annexes as well as of the people in them. She will be responsible for off-duty rotas, staffing levels, allocation of work within the whole department and liaising with theatre colleagues in the day-to-day management of operating sessions. A particularly important aspect of the work is the control of drugs. At the end of each day the drug cupboards, usually one in each anaesthetic room and one in the recovery room, must have a thorough check on all the 'controlled' medicines contained in them, because there are a large number used.

Another part of theatre administration which is of particular importance is the maintenance of a theatre register. This is a legal requirement, as is the correct control of drugs. It requires a record of each patient as they pass through, to be kept for purposes of administration, and for referral should any patient's details be needed in cases of litigation. It must contain details of the patient's name, age, date of birth, hospital number, and address. The surgeon must write after each case information on the type of operation performed, and sign the register. Similarly, the anaesthetist is responsible for stating the type of anaesthetic given and for signing the register. Finally, the instrument nurse and the circulating nurse are responsible for noting in the register the number of swabs used on the patient, each signing the register to confirm that swab checks were correct. This fulfils the legal requirements regarding swab checks and maintains the continuous record of each patient under the care of the theatre staff. If there should be any query concerning a patient, the theatre register acts as an immediate reference point.

SUGGESTED WORK

1. Make sure you know how patients should be positioned for the most common operations you see. What equipment is needed in order to maintain them in that position?

2. What safety precautions are taken to protect the patient in the theatre in which you are working?

SUGGESTED READING

Buxton Hopkin D. A. (1970). *Anaesthetic Recovery and Intensive Care*. (Unibooks.) London: English University Press.

Graves F. T. (1981). *Seeing Theatre Nursing*. London: Heinemann Medical.

7

Postoperative Care and Complications

The care of the patient in the postoperative phase is aimed at preventing complications and ensuring as quick a recovery from the operation as is possible. Therefore observations are made in order to recognise the development of these complications at an early stage.

While the patient has been in theatre, his bed has been prepared and placed where it can easily be observed. Any equipment required for his care, such as oxygen or suction, is placed near his bed with all the charts to record the observations.

The senior nurse collects the patient from theatre, making sure that she is satisfied with his condition. She will be told what operation the patient has had and any specific instructions to be carried out on his return to the ward. The patient is normally fully conscious, but if not, he should be placed in a semi-prone position on return to his bed. Careful handling at this stage will minimise shock.

The senior nurse checks the notes for the anaesthetist's instructions regarding the patient's further care, noting any drainage tubes or catheters which require attachment to a drainage bag, or clamps to be removed. She will also note any drugs to be given and when they are next due.

The very young, the very old, and obese patients are particularly at risk for respiratory and cardiovascular disorders and must therefore be observed extra carefully. It can also be difficult to recognise cyanosis in a patient with a coloured skin.

POSTOPERATIVE CARE

Tables 7.1 to 7.3 give details of the different stages of postoperative care.

POSTOPERATIVE COMPLICATIONS

Immediately following an operation, the most likely complications are obstruction to the airway, laryngospasm or bronchospasm, respiratory depression, haemorrhage and shock. The last two have been dealt with in a separate chapter (see Chapter 8). Obstruction of the respiratory tract is more likely now to occur in the recovery room. If it does occur, suction is used to remove secretions, the patient is placed in a semi-prone position, and the foot of the bed or trolley is elevated. Laryngospasm or bronchospasm may also occur at an early stage as a result of the endotracheal tube or bad positioning of the patient. Both may be recognised by stridor or wheezing. If not dealt with promptly by repositioning the patient and giving oxygen, the anaesthetist may need to give a bronchodilator such as aminophylline. Depression of respirations due to heavy sedation will cause a build up of carbon dioxide which will result in a slow full pulse, pallor and sweating. The doctor may have to give respiratory stimulants or even ventilate the patient.

Other respiratory complications which may

Table 7.1 Immediate postoperative care

Patient's needs	Potential problems	Observations	Preventative actions	Action if problem arises
Patent airway	Partial or complete obstruction due to secretions, tongue position or vomit	Presence of noisy or shallow breathing Cyanosis	Semi-prone position keep airway in position suction if required	Place in semi-prone position Suction Elevate foot of bed or trolley Inform doctor
	Laryngo-spasm / Broncho-spasm } due to endotracheal tube or bad positioning	Stridor Wheezing	Semi-prone position	Reposition patient Give O_2 Alert anaesthetist, who may wish to give a bronchodilator
Adequate respiratory function	Respiratory depression (due to heavy sedation causing CO_2 build up)	Diminished chest movement Slow, full pulse, pallor, sweating	Avoid heavy sedation	Inform doctor, who may wish to give a respiratory stimulant Ventilation of the patient may be necessary
	Atelectasis (collapse of part or whole lobe due to plug of mucus)	Movement of chest Noisy breathing Cough, pain, temperature	Deep breathing and movement	Inform doctor Suction or bronchoscopy may be required
Adequate circulatory function	Primary haemorrhage (internal or external)	$^1/_4$-hourly pulse rising $^1/_4$-hourly blood pressure falling Check wound and drainage tubes for increased amounts of blood	Early recognition	Inform doctor Pack dressing Intravenous or blood transfusion may be commenced Patient may be returned to theatre for religaturing
	Shock	Pallor, restlessness, air hunger	Adequate analgesia careful handling	Inform doctor Raise foot of bed Intravenous infusion

follow an operation are atelectasis (collapse of a lobe or part of a lobe of the lung due to a plug of mucus), bronchopneumonia and hypostatic pneumonia. The elderly, the very young and the obese are particularly prone to develop these. Also at risk are smokers, those whose general condition is lowered, and patients having operations of the thorax or upper abdominal cavity. If the patient has not been adequately starved, as may happen in an emergency operation, he may vomit and inhale this. In order to prevent these complications, the patient is advised to stop smoking when he attends out-patients, and any chest infection is cleared before operation. Deep breathing exercises using the abdominal muscles are taught before the operation and encouraged afterwards. As soon as the patient's condition allows, he is sat up and mobilised; this also encourages adequate ventilation. If infections do occur, antibiotics and postural drainage may be necessary. Bronchoscopy may be necessary to remove a plug of mucus.

Pulmonary embolism

This may occur following the development of a deep vein thrombosis. It is due to a clot breaking off

Table 7.2 Postoperative care in the first 48 hours

Patient's needs	Care plan	Potential problems	Action
Control of pain	Adequate analgesia for level of pain	Shock Respiratory infection	Analgesia (see treatment for shock, p. 50) Antibiotics
Observations	Blood pressure and pulse readings reduced to 4-hourly if condition satisfactory	Reactionary haemorrhage Shock	Raise foot of bed Inform doctor May return to theatre for resuturing, intravenous infusion or blood
Hygiene	Wash and change patient into own nightwear Give a mouthwash Attend to pressure areas		
Adequate respiratory function	Encourage deep breathing Position pillows carefully and sit patient up as soon as condition allows	Bronchopneumonia Hypostatic pneumonia	Physiotherapy, antibiotics Inform doctor of any rise in temperature or bubbly breathing TPR 4-hourly
Wound care	Check that dressing remains dry Check that drainage tubes are patent and vacuumed if appropriate Note amount and type of drainage	Haemorrhage Excess drainage Blockage of tube	Pad with further dressings Report and record Milk tube
Diet and fluids	Sips of fluid unless contraindicated Introduce light diet gradually, if bowel sounds present	Abdominal distention Nausea and vomiting	Encourage movement; flatus tube Stop oral food and fluids Anti-emetics
	If i.v. infusion in progress, monitor and regulate carefully Maintain fluid balance chart If nasogastric tube in position, aspirate hourly and note and record amount and type of aspirate	Paralytic ileus Mechanical obstruction Peritonitis	Insert nasogastric tube and aspirate Report increase in aspirate Intravenous infusion 4-hourly temperature (see Peritonitis, p. 99)
Elimination	If no catheter, note when patient first passes urine If catheter is in position, check that it is draining and empty as required Catheter toilet	Retention of urine	Catheterisation if other means fail
Sleep	Sedation may be required the first night		
Psychological	A simple explanation of the operation is all the patient can probably take at this point He will need plenty of encouragement and support	Depression	Psychological support If persistent, antidepressants may be necessary

Table 7.2 *(Continued)*

Patient's needs	Care plan	Potential problems	Action
Mobility	Initially, sit the patient well up in bed if the blood pressure is satisfactory Sit him out of bed the first postoperative day in the morning for half an hour Later in the day, assist him to walk a short distance	Fainting	Return to lying position
Spiritual	He may feel too weak to carry out his normal observances and may need help		
Social	Visitors should be limited to close relatives until the patient is able to cope with them Next of kin may wish to see the surgeon; the operation should be explained to them	Overtired	Reduced number of visitors
Adequate cardiac function	Blood pressure 4-hourly TPR In some operations, a monitor will be required	Cardiac arrest	Resuscitation

Table 7.3 Continuing postoperative care

Patient's needs	Care plan	Potential problems	Action
Control of pain	Analgesics tailed off as need diminishes		
Adequate circulatory function	Discontinue blood pressure monitoring and reduce TPR to daily when condition satisfactory Encourage mobility Check calves for swelling or tenderness Dorsiflex foot to test for pain	Deep vein thrombosis	Inform doctor Anticoagulants
Adequate respiratory function	Continue physiotherapy and deep breathing Encourage mobilisation Note any pain in chest, difficulty in breathing or haemoptysis	Pulmonary embolism	Sit patient up Give O_2 Inform doctor Give anticoagulants
	Note any crackling sensation in skin and puffiness of the face, neck and chest	Surgical emphysema	Reassure patient that swelling will reabsorb
Hygiene	General bath or shower if wound can be kept dry Ensure bath is cleaned with disinfectant		

Table 7.3 *(Continued)*

Patient's needs	Care plan	Potential problems	Action
Wound care	Minimal handling of wound Replace dressing aseptically if disturbed	Infection Poor healing	Inform doctor Take swab, give prescribed antibiotics
	Removal of sutures, 8th to 10th day Tension sutures following this Obese patients or those on steroids may have a corset of Elastoplast and tape Teach patient to hold wound when coughing	Burst abdomen	Lay patient flat, apply firm binder or warm saline soaks if intestine exposed Inform doctor Prepare as emergency for theatre
	Remove tubes once drainage minimal (48 hours)	Fistulae and sinuses	Drainage bag, barrier cream May require operation
Diet and fluids	Restore to normal diet May require high-protein and vitamin supplements to aid healing	Poor appetite Inadequate fluid intake Lack of healing	Relatives may help Intravenous infusion
	Additional iron may also be required Encourage fluids Discontinue i.v. infusion when intake sufficient	Anaemia	Iron supplements orally or by injection Blood transfusion
Elimination	If catheter present, remove depending on operation and check patient passes urine	Retention	Intermittent catheterisation
	Note any frequency or dysuria	Urinary infection	MSU Give prescribed antibiotics
	If bowels not open by third day, give aperient	Constipation	Encourage fluids, intake of roughage and mobility
Sleep	Discontinue night sedation when adequate sleep pattern established	Altered sleep pattern	Advise on simple remedies
Mobility	Encourage patient to join in the activities of the ward Get the relatives to bring in the patient's clothes	Tiredness	Increase activities slowly
Psychological	Some patients may be linked to a relevant association	Depression	Clarify their perceptions
	A nurse therapist may be required A patient who has successfully coped with the operation may visit	Boredom Anger	Correct misunderstandings Provide support
Spiritual	A visit to the chapel may be appreciated The patient's own minister or the hospital chaplain may visit	Rejection of faith	Allow time to talk this through
Social	Relatives should be kept informed Check on home conditions and supporting relatives and friends	Rejection of support	Involve patient in all discussions

ıs and
is will
by the
ɔunt of
ıtient's
's after
s, the
ın the
ll also
blood
lence
e calf
ot is
here
ıent
ion
to a
will
in
ıse
nd
u-

ed
s.
ıt
t.
e
a
ɔ
e

a.. .... breaks off.

Abdominal complications

These are much more likely to occur following an abdominal operation, although early vomiting is usually due to the effects of the anaesthetic. A full bladder or rectum increases the tendency to vomit, and the presence of acidosis in a child will also have this effect. However, its persistence may suggest a paralytic ileus, in which case aspiration by nasogastric tube is essential with an intravenous infusion so that the intestinal tract can be rested until it recovers, and the loss of fluids and electrolytes can be replaced. Paralytic ileus occurs due to handling of the intestines during operation or following peritonitis. The latter is dealt with in a separate chapter (see Chapter 17).

Adequate preparation of the gastrointestinal tract prior to operation by starvation for at least 6 hours, and longer if the tract itself is to be operated on, is necessary. Specific preparation is described in the chapter dealing with this system (see Chapter 18). Postoperatively, the patient should not be given food until bowel sounds are heard—evidence that there is no paralytic ileus. Again, if the tract itself has been operated on, the introduction of food will be delayed for longer.

Abdominal distension is another uncomfortable complication which arises as a result of handling the intestines. Encouraging the patient to move is usually successful, but if not, a flatus tube may relieve it or peppermint water. Failing this neostigmine 0.5 mg or carbachol 0.25 mg may be given.

Burst abdomen

Obese patients, those whose nutrition has been inadequate, and patients on steroids do not heal very well. If postoperatively the patient is also unable to take in an adequate amount of nutrients, then any extra tension of the wound may cause it to break down, resulting in a burst abdomen. The wound may have looked on the surface as if it had healed when the stitches were removed, but a bout of coughing may be sufficient to open it up. The patient is laid flat to reduce the abdominal tension, and reassured. If the abdominal contents have not escaped, a tight binder or drawsheet wrapped around the abdomen will prevent this from happening. If they have escaped, sterile linen towels soaked in warm saline are applied. The patient is taken to theatre as soon as possible to be resutured. This means that he has to be prepared as an emergency operation.

Obese patients usually have tension sutures inserted to take the tension off the suture line. Any patients thought to be at risk may have a corset made of Elastoplast and tapes. Two pieces of Elastoplast are fixed to the skin beyond and parallel to the wound; pieces of tape bring together their inner edges and so support the wound. Patients with abdominal wounds are taught to hold the wound when coughing. Infection of the wound is another reason for it breaking down and this can be prevented by a good aseptic technique and minimal handling of the wound.

Fistulae and sinuses

The same factors which may hinder healing of the skin may also be operative in the internal organs. Fistulae and sinuses may occur spontaneously as a result of the breakdown of an anastomosis or may be caused by a drain being left in a long time. They are much more likely to occur if infection such as a peritonitis is present. Healing may take place spontaneously, but if intestinal contents are being discharged onto the skin, this will have to be protected or there will be excoriation. There are plastic drainage bags suitable for this on the market. Protective creams will have to be applied to protect the skin from the destructive secretions. Persistent fistulae will require operative treatment such as resection of the involved bowel segment, or a by-pass, intestinal anastomosis. By ensuring that the patient's nutritional state is satisfactory and that he is in the best condition possible for surgery, it may be possible to prevent these occurring. Drainage tubes should not be kept in position for longer than is necessary. Adequate preparation of the intestines will also help to prevent these complications from arising.

Table 7.4 Preparation for transfer home

Patient's needs	Nursing care plan
Information	Give patients the opportunity to ask questions about what has been done and how this will affect their ability to work or do other things. Tell them when they would be able to return to work, and resume sexual relationships. They may require specific teaching if they have a stoma or prosthesis. Talking to a patient with a similar condition may also be helpful
Diet	The dietitian will give advice and a diet sheet in relevant conditions
Social	Ensure that any arrangements such as structural alterations have been completed. Is the support sufficient or should convalescence be arranged? If a young mother has to avoid lifting, what arrangements have been made for the children? For some patients a home help will be required
Supplies	Items to be taken home must be ready in plenty of time before the patient's discharge. An adequate supply of dressings or appliances should be given to the patient for use until he can get a further supply. Drugs to take home will be obtained from the pharmacy in time to give an adequate explanation of what they are for and when they should be taken. The patient should be told of any side-effects that should be watched for and who these should be reported to
Mobility	Arrange for any equipment such as walking aids or a commode for night-time
Follow-up	Arrange out-patient appointment, and physiotherapy if required. The district nurse may be necessary if there are any dressings or treatments to be given. With certain patients, a clinical nurse specialist will visit. A letter is sent to the general practitioner. The patient may be linked to the appropriate patient association.
Relatives	They should be given adequate warning of the patient's discharge. They may also need to be taught how to assist the patient by lifting or carrying out a simple treatment
Safety measures	If the patient is on steroids or anticoagulants, he will need either a card or a medic alert bracelet or necklet
Transport	If the patient cannot provide his own transport, a hospital car may be arranged. Some patients will require an ambulance

Surgical emphysema

This is due to air which has escaped into the tissues of the chest wall and may enter the tissues of the neck and face. It most commonly occurs following operations on the neck and nearby, after tracheostomy and after chest operations. On touching the skin over the area, a crackling sensation is felt. If it reaches the face, it may be sufficient to close the eyes and therefore the patient may be very distressed by it. He can be reassured that it will be gradually reabsorbed. It may also be caused by the *Clostridium welchii* which causes gas gangrene in wounds, so its presence must always be reported.

Gas gangrene

In severely injured tissue in which there has already been some necrosis, if the *Clostridium welchii* is able to enter, gas gangrene will develop. In this particular type of gangrene the patient rapidly becomes ill, with a raised temperature and rapid pulse. The tissues become tense and discoloured and crepitation is felt under the skin due to the formation of gas. There is also a characteristic smell like acetylene gas. The gas may show up on x-ray. The treatment is to excise the damaged tissue, give anti-gas gangrene serum and antibiotics. Hyperbaric oxygen may also be used and a blood transfusion may be necessary because of the destruction of the red blood cells.

Subphrenic abscess is discussed in Chapter 17.

Urinary complications are dealt with in Chapter 38.

SUGGESTED WORK

1. Find out what elements of care are common to most surgical patients postoperatively. Take one of these elements and see how it has to be adapted in different ways from one patient to another.

2. Find out all the arrangements which have to be made for one of your patients on discharge.

SUGGESTED READING

Edmondson E. (1971). *Care of the Unconscious.* Nursing in Depth Series. London: Butterworths.

Gay P., Pitkeathley J. (1979). *When I Went Home.* Oxford: King's Fund, Oxford University Press.

Roberts I. (1975). *Discharged from Hospital.* RCN Research Project, Series 2, No. 6. London: Royal College of Nursing.

Robusto N. (1980). Advising patients on sex after surgery. *Association of Operating Room Nurses Journal*; **32** (1): 55–61.

Vance J. P., Corrigan A. (1983). *Postoperative Care.* London: Heinemann Medical.

8

Blood Clotting, Anticoagulants, Haemorrhage and Shock

BLOOD CLOTTING

Blood takes 3 to 5 minutes to coagulate and this is called the clotting time. It requires the presence of thrombocytes, fibrinogen, prothrombin and calcium salts which are normally present in the blood.

In small wounds such as a pin prick, the bleeding is stopped as a result of the contraction of the capillaries and sealing by a platelet plug. In large wounds, where the bleeding is from arterioles and small arteries, the haemorrhage is stopped as a result of vascular contraction and a blood clot sealing the blood vessel (Fig. 8.1).

ANTICOAGULANTS

In patients having some forms of surgery, such as those involving the chest, where there is a high risk of deep vein thrombosis occurring, anticoagulants may be given. Warfarin and phenindione (Dindevan) act on the liver reducing some of the factors required for clotting and, in particular, prothrombin. Because they act in an early stage of the clotting process, they take some time to be effective. They are therefore usually given in conjunction with heparin to start with. The dosage is regulated according to the prothrombin index.

Heparin inactivates thrombin so that it does not convert fibrinogen into fibrin. It is destroyed by the gastrointestinal tract and must therefore be given by injection. The usual route is intravenously, a loading dose of 5000 units being given and then either repeated doses of 10 000 units 6-hourly or an infusion controlled by mechanical means. It may also be given subcutaneously into the loose tissue of the abdomen.

Some drugs prevent the absorption of vitamin K from the intestine, or interfere with its action. As vitamin K is necessary for the production of prothrombin in the body, the blood will be less likely to clot, and therefore the amount of anticoagulants required will be reduced. Salicylates, some antibiotics and chlorpromazine have this effect. Certain drugs speed up the metabolism of the anticoagulants and therefore the dose will need to be increased. A number of tranquillisers have this effect.

HAEMORRHAGE

Site of haemorrhage

Bleeding may occur from the capillaries, as with an abrasion of the surface of the skin, in which case blood will ooze from the wound. It may occur due to damage to a vein, particularly when varicosed veins are damaged by trauma. In this type of bleeding the blood wells out persistently and is dark red or blue in colour. Blood from a severed artery spurts out with each beat of the heart and is bright red in colour.

The bleeding may be external, from the surface of the body where it can be seen easily. It may be internal but reveal itself by escaping from one of the orifices of the body such as the vagina or rectum. When there is no free flow of blood

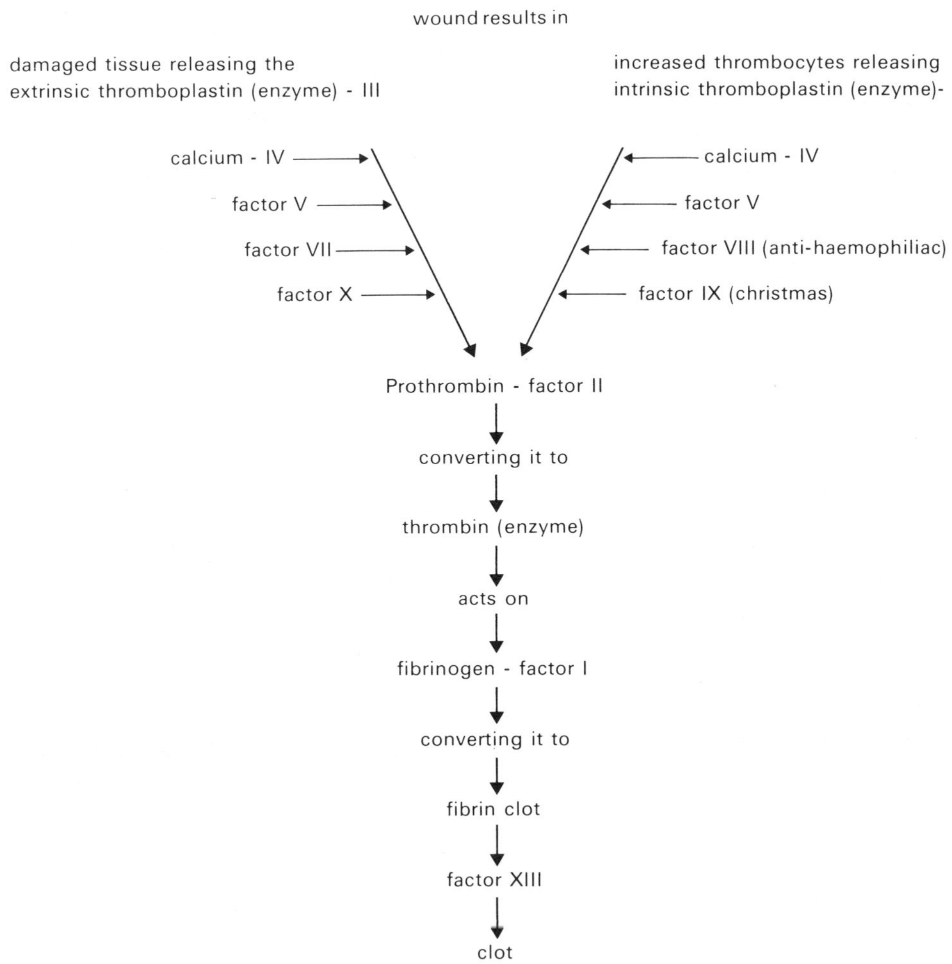

Fig. 8.1 *Blood clotting process in a large wound.*

externally, it is called a concealed haemorrhage. This would happen if the liver or spleen were ruptured, when the bleeding is into the peritoneal cavity. Another important form of internal bleeding is that from a closed fracture into the surrounding muscles. There may be as much as 2.5 litres of blood lost following a fracture of the femur.

Arterial bleeding may be classified according to the time when it occurs. A *primary* haemorrhage occurs at the time of injury, or during an operation. A *reactionary* haemorrhage occurs within 24 hours of the injury or operation and is due to the rise in blood pressure as the shock produced by the operation subsides. This rise in pressure may force out clots which have formed at the end of the small blood vessels which have not been ligated, or may dislodge insecure ligatures off the larger vessels. *Secondary* haemorrhage is caused by infection. This most commonly occurs 8 to 14 days after the operation. There is usually a slightly blood-stained discharge before this type of haemorrhage, and a raised temperature.

Results of haemorrhage

As a result of the haemorrhage, the circulating blood volume and therefore the blood pressure are low. If more than 1.5–2 litres are lost, there will be irreversible damage to the kidneys. In order to overcome this loss of fluid volume the body responds initially by constricting blood vessels. During the following 1 to 2 days, plasma fluid is replaced from the tissues. The more severe the loss and shocked the patient, the longer it takes to restore the fluid volume. Red blood cells are restored by the red bone marrow within 2 to 6 weeks.

Clinical manifestations of haemorrhage

Weak, rapid pulse.
Pale, cold, clammy skin.
Blood pressure and temperature fall.
Restlessness.
Sighing, or gasping respiration (air hunger).
Thirst.
Blurred vision, giddiness and fainting.

Management

Immediate arrest of haemorrhage

Direct pressure should be applied over the part with a firm dressing and bandage or, if this is not immediately available, with the fingers, unless there is a foreign body in the wound. In the latter case a ring bandage may be applied until the foreign body can be removed. If a limb is affected, it should be elevated. Pressure points, where the artery supplying the part crosses a bone, may be used, but usually direct pressure is the most effective.

Tourniquets are rarely used because of the danger of gangrene if left on too long or damage to nerves and blood vessels. They may occasionally be necessary following amputation of a limb, if a ligature slips on a large blood vessel. In this case a Samway's anchor tourniquet is used, which consists of a stout rubber tube with a metal anchor catch at one end to hold the rubber tubing. An Esmarch's rubber bandage may be applied in theatre if a lower limb has to be operated on. The rubber bandage is applied tightly from toe to thigh; it is then unwound from the toes, so emptying out the veins. To control haemorrhage from the upper limb during operations on it, a pneumatic tourniquet (e.g. sphygmomanometer cuff) is used to avoid the possibility of injury to the nerves and vessels of the arm; it may also be used on the leg. *The exact time a tourniquet was applied must always be recorded* by one of the theatre staff; and although the length of time it can safely be left on varies with the circumstances, in general the maximum periods are 45 minutes for the upper arm and 90 minutes for the lower limbs.

Surgical arrest of haemorrhage

During operation, minor blood vessels are sealed by coagulation with diathermy, and the larger ones are ligated with catgut thread or silk. Clips may be used to seal off vessels. Wounds may be packed with sterile gauze or with substances which encourage clotting such as gelatine sponge, fibrin foam or a type of cellulose. Thrombin, adrenaline or snake venom may also be used to encourage coagulation. Heat in the form of hot lotions (up to 48°C) is useful in large bleeding cavities such as the uterus, when it is given as a hot douche. Cold, in the form of ice packs, also reduces bleeding. Drugs such as aminocaproic acid (Epsikapron), ergometrine or oxytocin (pitocin) may be used in certain forms of haemorrhage.

Special forms of haemorrhage

If bright, red, frothy blood is coughed up, this is called a haemoptysis. The bleeding has occurred from somewhere in the respiratory tract, at or below the level of the larynx. An epistaxis is a nose bleed. Vomiting of blood from the upper gastrointestinal tract is called haematemesis, and is usually mixed with acid gastric contents in a semi-digested state. It is therefore brown or black in colour, like coffee grounds. The presence of digested blood in the faeces from the intestinal tract results in melaena, a black tarry stool. If blood is present in the stool but not visible, it is called occult blood and can only be detected by chemical tests. Haematuria is the presence of blood in the urine due to haemorrhages from some part of the urinary tract. Bleeding into the thorax is called a haemothorax. Extradural, subdural, intracranial and subarachnoid haemorrhages occur either on the surface of the brain or within the substance of it and may rapidly cause death, unconsciousness or paralysis. Menorrhagia and metrorrhagia are different forms of vaginal bleeding.

Haemorrhagic diseases

Any absence of the factors necessary for clotting will lead to abnormal bleeding from wounds or into tissues. Thrombocytopenia, haemophilia and Christmas disease are such conditions. Although these will be treated on a medical ward, they may require surgery for some other condition, however, an operation will be avoided if at all possible. If it is unavoidable, sufficient blood must be grouped and cross-matched in readiness. In thrombocytopenia a platelet-rich infusion may be given, and in haemophilia, cryoprecipitate or freeze-dried factor VIII.

SHOCK

Shock occurs when the output from the heart is insufficient to maintain the circulation to the tissues and there is a low blood pressure.

Causes of surgical shock

Reduction in the blood volume (oligaemia)

This is the most potent cause of surgical shock and may occur due to the following.

1. Severe or prolonged haemorrhage.
2. Loss of plasma as a result of severe burns, severe soft tissue injury (as in a crush injury), or severe infection such as peritonitis, pancreatitis and septicaemia. This is because the plasma escapes through the walls of the capillaries, which have become unusually permeable, and collects in the tissues.
3. Loss of water and electrolytes from vomiting and diarrhoea, intestinal fistulae, acute intestinal obstruction and paralytic ileus. It may also occur due to severe sweating, and excessive loss of urine as in diabetes insipidus, which will occur following a hypophysectomy.

Dilatation of blood vessels

This occurs in the following.

1. Patients who have had steroids withdrawn, or who are given insufficient coverage during the stress of an operation.
2. Anaesthetics such as ganglion-blocking agents, epidural anaesthetics or spinal anaesthetics, although the anaesthetist controls the situation by giving increased amounts of oxygen.
3. Urethral shock when catheterisation is carried out in some patients with an enlarged prostate.

Effects of shock within the body

The severity of the shock is always directly proportional to the extent and duration of the reduction in the blood volume, or dilatation of blood vessels. These two factors result in a diminished amount of blood returning to the heart, and therefore a reduced cardiac output and low blood pressure. There is vasoconstriction of the peripheral blood vessels in an effort to compensate and this leads to a lack of oxygen in the tissues (tissue anoxia). The heart rate increases in an attempt to supply the tissues with sufficient oxygen. There may also be vasoconstriction of the veins, which is why there may be difficulties in setting up a transfusion or getting it to run satisfactorily. If severe shock (systolic pressure below 60 mmHg) persists for more than 45 minutes, irreversible damage occurs to the kidneys, and toxic substances are released which keep the vessels dilated and lead to heart failure and death.

Clinical picture

1. A low blood pressure. In slight shock the systolic blood pressure is lower than normal but

not below 100 mmHg, the pulse rate is 100–110 beats per minute, and the extremities are warm. In moderate shock the systolic blood pressure may fall to 70 mmHg, the pulse rate is 120–140 beats per minute, and the extremities are cold. In severe shock the systolic blood pressure may be 60 mmHg or even lower, the pulse is imperceptible (rate 140–160 beats per minute, counted with a stethoscope over the heart), and the extremities are cold.

2. The pulse is rapid, weak and thready and often irregular.
3. Respirations are shallow and sighing.
4. Temperature is subnormal.
5. The skin is cold and clammy, with pallor and a grey tinge to it, especially of the nose and ears.
6. The patient will become very thirsty.
7. The patient becomes very restless and apathetic and may become unconscious.
8. Vomiting, diminished urinary output and frequently incontinence of urine and faeces are present.
9. The pupils become dilated but react to light.

Management of surgical shock

The treatment will depend on the cause. If fluid has been lost from the circulation, then it will have to be replaced either by blood or plasma. Synthetic plasma expanders may also be used. Normal saline will not be retained in the blood vessels and is therefore unsuitable. Moderately shocked patients require 1 litre by intravenous infusion, and those with severe shock 3 to 4 litres, the first litre of which will be given in 10 minutes. If the patient is allowed fluids by mouth, these should be encouraged and may include glucose drinks.

The best way of monitoring shock is by the central venous pressure (this is dealt with more fully in Chapter 12). It is an accurate guide to the circulating blood volume.

In order to increase the blood supply to the brain, the foot of the bed should be elevated; this also aids the venous return to the heart.

Pain is a significant factor in the development of shock and should therefore be adequately controlled by sufficiently strong analgesia. If the patient is very shocked, the drug may not be absorbed immediately if given subcutaneously; it will therefore need to be given intravenously.

The patient must not be overheated as this will cause vasodilatation of the skin vessels, so diverting the blood away from the essential centres.

Oxygen should be given in a high concentration, but if there is respiratory depression, respiratory stimulants such as nikethamide will be given, and if this is insufficient, positive pressure inflation of the lungs using a closed anaesthetic circuit to inflate the lungs rhythmically with oxygen.

Cardiac stimulants and peripheral vasoconstrictors may be given to increase the efficiency of the cardiac output and to overcome vasodilatation of blood vessels. However, treatment with vasoconstrictors such as metaraminol (Aramine) is only a temporary measure and is usually avoided. Intramuscular and intravenous steroids are used more frequently.

SUGGESTED WORK

1. Find out which patients on your ward have suffered either from shock or haemorrhage following surgery.

(a) Was this due to the type of operation, because the patient was a high risk for some reason, or to other factors?

(b) How was it treated?

SUGGESTED READING

Thal A. P. (1971). *Shock, A Physiological Basis for Treatment*. Chicago: Year Book Medical.

9

Blood Grouping and Blood Transfusion

BLOOD GROUPING

Everybody's blood contains certain factors which can be classified into two main systems, the ABO system and the Rhesus system.

The ABO groups

The antigens (agglutinogens) A and B are found on the surface of the red blood cells. Some people have both A and B; some either A or B; and others do not have either of these antigens. If an antigen is absent, antibodies (agglutinins) to it will be found in the plasma. The individual's blood is grouped according to which antigen he possesses, which is discovered by testing his blood against group A and B sera (Fig. 9.1). Details of the blood groups are shown in Table 9.1.

When giving a blood transfusion, it is the compatibility of the donor's cells with the plasma of the recipient which is important. Figure 9.2 shows which blood may be given to which patient. From this it can be seen that a recipient with group AB blood may receive blood from any one of the other groups, and therefore group AB is called the *universal recipient*. Group O blood, on the other hand, may be given to any patient and therefore it is called the *universal donor*.

Blood tested (red blood cells)	Serum A (anti B serum)	Serum B (anti A serum)
AB	agglutination	agglutination
A	no agglutination	agglutination
B	agglutination	no agglutination
O	no agglutination	no agglutination

Fig. 9.1 *Details of blood groups.*

Table 9.1 ABO blood groups

Group	Percentage of population	Phenotype	Antigen on cell (agglutinogen)	Antibody in plasma (agglutinin)
AB } may be subgroups	3	AB	A and B	None
A } may be subgroups	42	AA/AO	A	Anti-B
B	9	BB/BO	B	Anti-A
O	46	OO	None	Anti-A/Anti-B

recipient	donor AB	donor A	donor B	donor O
AB	✓	✓	✓	✓
A (anti B)	X	✓	X	✓
B (anti A)	X	X	✓	✓
O (anti A, anti B)	X	X	X	✓

Fig. 9.2 *Blood compatibility.*

Cross-matching

It is not sufficient to know the individual's blood group to avoid incompatibility. Blood from the donor must be tested against that of the recipient to see if they are compatible and do not clot together (agglutination) (Fig. 9.2).

The Rhesus factor

Although there are three possible antigens involved in the Rhesus factor, the commonest and therefore the most important is the D antigen. Those who possess it are known as Rhesus positive (D positive) and about 85% of the population falls into this group. In the remaining 15% the D antigen is absent and they are therefore classified as Rhesus negative (D negative).

There are not normally any antibodies in the blood, but if an individual is Rh −ve and receives Rh +ve blood, antibodies will be formed causing agglutination of the blood. This will also happen in a fetus which is Rh +ve, if the woman bearing it is Rh −ve. If Rh −ve blood is given to a person who is Rh +ve, there will be no reaction. Therefore in an emergency Rh −ve blood is always given.

Other groups

There are some other blood groups which do not have antibodies circulating in the blood except after a blood transfusion or pregnancy. These have to be specifically tested for if there is incompatibility which is not explained by the ABO and Rhesus groups.

Blood donors

Only those people who are in good health may offer themselves to become a blood donor. If they are suffering from any one of a number of diseases, from hay fever to diabetes or cancer, they will not be accepted. Any history of jaundice or recent contact with it will prevent them from being donors. Homosexuals will be tested for the AIDS virus. Blood is taken from the potential donor to test for syphilis and the level of the haemoglobin. If the latter is below 13 g/100 ml in a man and 12.5 g/100 ml in a woman, they will be rejected.

Plasmaphaeresis

Normally blood cannot be taken from a donor more than four times a year, to enable him to replace blood cells. More frequent donations would result in anaemia. With plasmaphaeresis the blood is taken from the donor in the normal manner. The cells are then extracted from the plasma and returned to the donor. Because the donor no longer has to replace the cells, he is able to donate blood much more frequently without detriment to himself. From the plasma extracted it is possible to remove the anti-haemophiliac factor, platelets and antibodies which can then be used for different recipients.

Fresh blood, whole blood and packed cells

Whole blood is blood as it was taken from the donor, with nothing removed, which has been citrated to prevent clotting. In the average adult, 1 unit will raise the level of the haemoglobin by about 7%.

Fresh blood is used within a few hours of donation. It is whole blood containing the factors which deteriorate rapidly. However, now that it is possible to separate out and store these vital factors, there is less need for this type of blood.

Packed cells contain the cells of 2 units of blood in some plasma. They will be used in anaemia where there is no loss of blood and danger of overloading the circulation if too much fluid is infused.

Leucocytes may also be separated out from the blood and used separately if required.

Plasma can be kept for a year or more, much longer than blood. The group of the person donating it is not important as incompatibility does not arise; it may therefore be collected from numerous donors. It is usually dried and stored in the form of powder which has to be reconstituted with pyrogen-free, triple-distilled water before use. (Pyrogen is a name for small quantities of protein present in water which, unless removed, cause pyrexia and other forms of reaction.) The distilled water must be added under strictly aseptic conditions. It should be shaken well to dissolve the dried plasma completely, and if it becomes an opaque brown, should be discarded. Occasionally serum hepatitis arises from within a few weeks to 6 months after the transfusion. The risk is minimised if the plasma is stored at room temperature for 6 months before use.

Plasma is frequently given when whole blood is not available, and is particularly useful if the patient has had extensive burns. Its large molecular size means that it is retained in the circulation and so restores the blood volume.

Dextran is a plasma substitute composed of large molecules which are too large to pass through the capillary walls. It is therefore also used to restore blood volume. It does interfere with the blood grouping reactions, so blood should be taken for testing before the infusion. Rheomacrodex 10% in normal saline is used at the same time as blood to inhibit the aggregation of the blood cells within the blood vessels.

BLOOD TRANSFUSION

Reasons for blood transfusion

The main reason for a patient receiving a blood transfusion is to restore blood volume following haemorrhage. This may have occurred due to trauma, surgery or conditions such as a peptic ulcer or oesophageal varices. In severe anaemia it may also be necessary to give a blood transfusion, although it is usually given in the form of packed cells.

Care of a patient receiving a blood transfusion

Before the transfusion is started, the patient should be told what to expect, and be made comfortable. He may wish to empty his bladder. If more than 1 unit is to run through, his garment may need to be removed from the arm to be used. The prepared trolley and intravenous infusion stand will be placed on the opposite side of the patient to the hand which he uses, unless the transfusion is being resited.

In order not to waste blood, the infusion is started with normal saline. The blood is collected from the blood bank (where it is stored at 4 °C) about half an hour before it is required. When collecting it the following details must be checked with the notes: the patient's surname and first names, date of birth, hospital number, blood group, blood transfusion service number and expiry date. Any discrepancy should be checked with the pathological laboratory supplying the blood. Before the blood is given to the patient, it is checked by two people, one of whom is a registered nurse or doctor. Great care must be taken when checking the blood. After checking it, a slip is torn off the label on the bag and entered in the patient's notes. (See Chapter 10 on intravenous infusions regarding general care of the infusion while running.)

Observations related to possible complications

Pyrexia with rigors may occur due to contamination, the recipient's antibodies reacting to some substance in the blood, or because the blood has deteriorated. The patient's temperature, therefore, should be taken at least 4-hourly during the blood transfusion and for some time afterwards. Should the temperature rise, the rate of the transfusion is reduced and the doctor informed. He will decide whether to continue the transfusion or not.

A rising pulse rate (recorded half-hourly) laboured breathing, cough, pain in the chest, oedema or increase in the jugular venous pressure will indicate overloading of the circulation. This will occur if large volumes are given quickly or the patient is elderly, anaemic or already has a weak heart. Slow the infusion, unless the symptoms are severe when it should be stopped, and inform the doctor. He will usually administer intravenous diuretics.

Severe pain in the loins, flushing of the face, rigors and pyrexia, falling blood pressure, jaundice and diminished output of urine indicate some degree of incompatibility. If suspected, the transfusion should be stopped immediately, because the smaller the amount of blood transfused the greater the chance of recovery. The greatest danger is renal damage due to the fall in the blood pressure, which will lead to all the effects of renal failure with retention of waste products and electrolyte disturbance. The patient will be given compatible blood or plasma in order to raise the blood pressure and treated as renal failure. This means that the fluid intake will be restricted to 500 ml plus the output each day, a low-protein, high-carbohydrate diet will be given and the electrolytes monitored carefully.

Oedema of the face and bronchospasm may result from an allergic reaction to the blood.

Hypothermia may arise if large amounts of cold blood are given in anaesthetised patients, and this can cause ventricular fibrillation.

An air embolism will cause death if as little as 10 ml of air enters the heart in a very ill patient. Therefore care must be taken not to allow air to enter the system.

Some diseases such as serum hepatitis, AIDS, syphilis and malaria can be transmitted by a blood transfusion, although with all the stringent precautions taken in screening donors this rarely happens.

Tetany, cardiac arrest and a tendency to bleed may all occur if very large, rapid transfusions are given. The blood calcium and the platelets will be reduced and need to be replaced.

When the blood transfusion is discontinued, the blood bag is returned to the pathological laboratory with the residue of the blood still in it.

SUGGESTED WORK

1. Find out the procedures in your hospital for storing, collecting and disposing of blood.

SUGGESTED READING

Department of Health and Social Security (1973). *Notes on Transfusion*. Edinburgh: DHSS.

Dodd E. B., Lincoln P. J. (1975). *Blood Group Topics*. London: Edward Arnold.

10

Fluid and Electrolyte Balance; Intravenous Infusions

FLUID AND ELECTROLYTE BALANCE

Approximately 70% of the weight of an average adult consists of water: 50% is within the cells (intracellular) and 20% extracellular. In an average adult of 70 kg, the total body water will be in the region of 50 litres: 35 litres of this will be intracellular and 15 litres extracellular. Of this extracellular 15 litres, 3–4 litres will be within the blood vessels (intravascular) and 11–12 litres within the tissues between the cells and the capillaries (interstitial fluid).

Fluid in the lymph vessels, synovial joints, cerebrospinal fluid, the aqueous and vitreous humours of the eye, and from the serous membranes such as the peritoneum, pericardium and pleura, and the gastrointestinal secretions form part of the extracellular fluid. The body water moves freely between each compartment (Fig. 10.1).

The way in which the fluid is distributed in the body is dependent upon the concentration of substances (called electrolytes) within the compartment, and in particular on potassium and sodium. Electrolytes are substances which, when dissolved in fluid, separate into ions. Half of these ions in the body have a positive charge (cations)

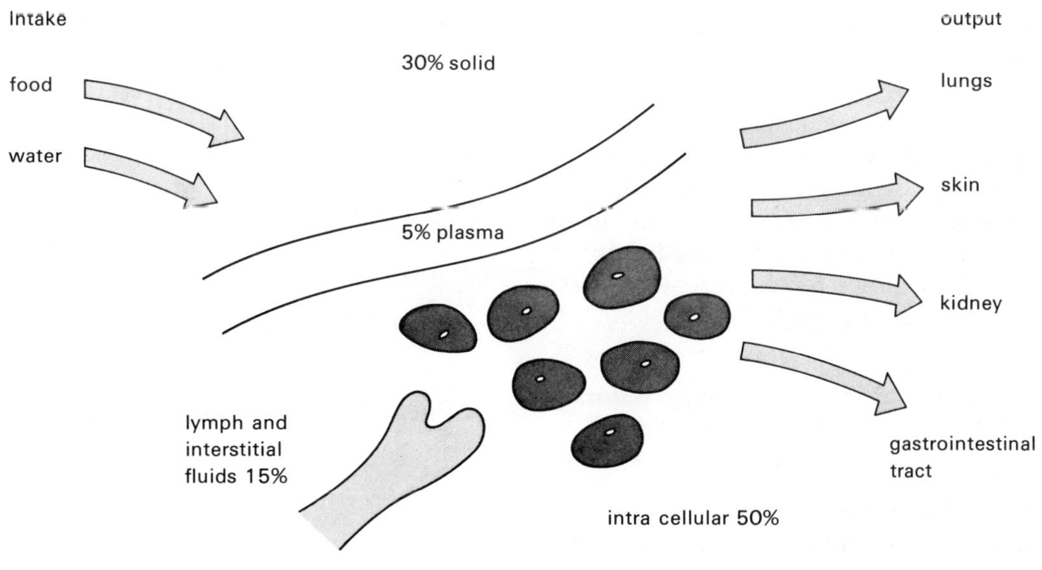

Fig. 10.1 *Distribution of body fluid.*

and half a negative charge (anions). There is therefore always a balance between the two—that is, homoeostasis. Within the cells the main ions are potassium (K^+) and phosphate (HPO_4^-). The quantity of potassium determines the volume of intracellular fluid. In the extracellular fluid, sodium (Na^+), chloride (Cl^-), and bicarbonate (HCO_3^-) are the chief ions, and in the plasma there is also protein (Fig. 10.2).

The fluid and electrolytes are taken into the body in the food that we eat and the fluids we drink. Food contains both electrolytes and a large amount of water, and the activity of metabolising the food in the body also produces water. There are several routes by which water and electrolytes are excreted from the body, although the most important route is via the kidneys. Fluid, sodium, potassium and hydrogen ions are excreted by this route. The output of fluid is controlled by the antidiuretic hormone secreted by the posterior lobe of the pituitary gland. The excretion of sodium is also controlled by aldosterone which is secreted by the adrenal cortex. The lungs excrete water and carbon dioxide, therefore lowering the level of carbonic acid in the body. Fluid and a small amount of sodium are excreted through the skin, although the amount will increase in sweating. Some fluid is lost in the faeces.

The parathyroid glands control the level of calcium within the body, and the central nervous system has an overall control of fluid and electrolyte balance by the mechanisms of thirst and hunger, and its functions of controlling the respiratory rate and depth, and temperature. The average individual will excrete 1000–1500 ml of urine in 24 hours, but this will vary according to the intake. Loss from other routes (insensible loss) amounts to 1–1.5 litres in 24 hours.

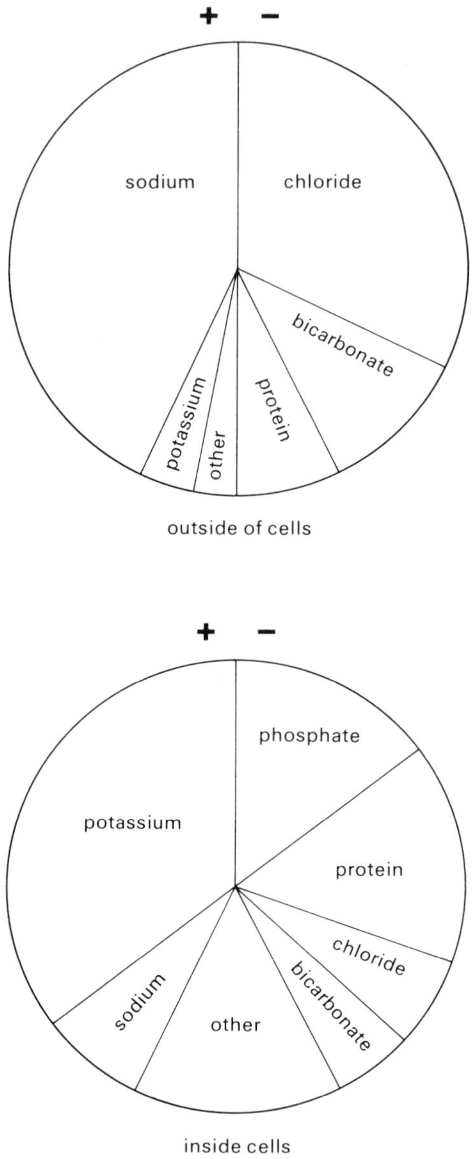

Fig. 10.2 *Distribution of electrolytes in the body.*

Disturbances of fluid and electrolyte balance

Insufficient intake of fluids

This may occur in the person who is too weak to make the effort to drink, because of severe illness, age, or following major surgery. An unconscious patient is dependent upon the nurse to supply sufficient fluids. A painful mouth or an obstruction in the oesophagus may also lead to insufficient fluid intake.

Excessive output

This is present in diabetes insipidus and if a

hypophysectomy is performed, which will cause a polyuria. Uncontrolled diabetes mellitus will also result in polyuria. Fluid may be lost from the body as a result of vomiting or diarrhoea.

Adequate intake but insufficient output

This may arise if the kidneys are not functioning efficiently, as in renal failure, or because the circulation to the kidneys is diminished, as in congestive cardiac failure.

Loss of potassium

Loss of potassium from the gastrointestinal tract may occur as a result of diarrhoea, ileostomy, gastric or intestinal drainage, vomiting or fistulae. Loss may also occur from burns, sweating, severe tissue injury and starvation. Uncontrolled diabetes and renal disease will also cause loss of potassium, and it is removed by some diuretics. A reduction in the level of potassium will lead to weakness and alkalosis; too much will lead to a cardiac arrest. The latter may occur if potassium is added to an infusion.

Alteration in sodium levels

This may occur if salt is lost from the body in gastrointestinal disorders such as diarrhoea, vomiting, ileostomy, gastric or intestinal drainage or fistulae. Some diuretics, sweating, Addison's disease, diabetes insipidus and an intestinal obstruction may also cause loss of sodium. Loss of sodium in the body leads to a reduction in the osmotic pressure in the tissues, dehydration, and an increase of urinary output.

Acid–base balance

Acids are substances which give up hydrogen ions; bases take up hydrogen ions. The acidity of a substance is measured by the concentration of free ions, and this is called the pH. The pH range is from 0 to 14; 7 is neutral, 0–7 is acid and 7–14 alkaline. The most extreme ranges of the blood which are compatible with life are 7.0–7.8; beyond these limits the cells die. The normal pH range of the blood is 7.35–7.45 (Fig. 10.3). If it is lower than this, we say a person is acidotic; and if it is higher, alkalotic. The level of the pH is controlled by the ratio of carbonic acid to bicarbonate, which is normally 1 : 20. So in acidosis there is an increased amount of carbonic acid to bicarbonate, and in alkalosis there is an increased amount of bicarbonate to carbonic acid.

Some foods, drinks and drugs we take in increase the acidity of the body, whereas others increase the alkalinity. In order to maintain the balance in the body there are three mechanisms. *Buffers* act immediately neutralising acids and alkalis. Examples are haemoglobin, protein and the carbonic acid/bicarbonate system. *The lungs* are able to neutralise acids quickly by excreting carbon

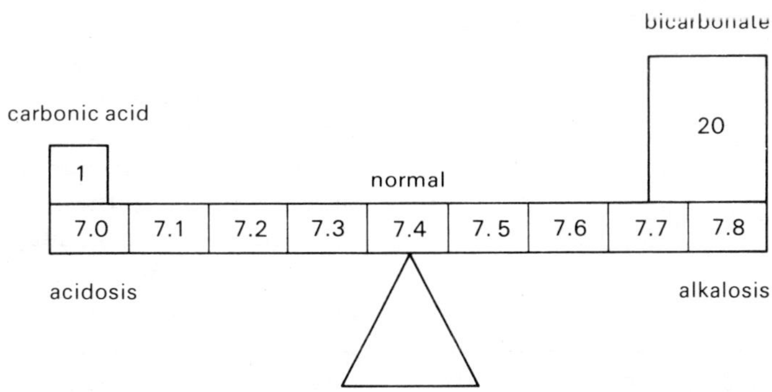

Fig. 10.3 *Limits of pH of blood.*

dioxide. Hydrogen ions are absorbed by the water which is produced by this process:

$$H + HCO_3^- = H_2CO_3 = CO_2 + H_2O$$

The kidneys are important for the more permanent excretion of acids and bases, excreting hydrogen ions and ammonia.

Acidosis will occur in patients who have lost alkaline substances in severe diarrhoea or where the excretion of acid is diminished due to shallow breathing as a result of depression of the respiratory centre from drugs or anaesthetics, or renal failure. An increase in the breakdown of acid substances in the body, which happens in diabetic ketosis and cardiac arrest, will also cause an acidosis. Other causes are the intake of acid poisons, such as aspirin, and the reabsorption of chloride which takes place if the ureters are transplanted into the colon (see Chapter 38). Acidosis leads to deep, rapid respirations in an effort to remove carbon dioxide from the body. The urine smells of ammonia.

Alkalosis will occur if hydrochloric acid is removed from the body by vomiting, especially when it occurs as a result of pyloric stenosis. For the same reason, excessive gastric aspiration will also remove acid. Overbreathing and overventilation with a respirator will cause alkalosis because of the increased amount of carbon dioxide lost, and therefore of hydrogen ions in the accompanying water produced. Overmedication with alkalis also causes alkalosis. Alkalosis will cause tetany.

The terms acidosis and alkalosis have been used to describe these conditions, but definitions of these terms vary to such an extent that it is much better to specify the individual changes which occur.

INTRAVENOUS INFUSIONS

Reasons for their use

1. Maintenance of electrolyte and fluid balance in patients following surgery, disorders of the alimentary tract and renal tract, injury, overwhelming infection, metabolic disorders such as diabetic coma and dehydration. There are a variety of intravenous solutions which may be used in these conditions such as sodium chloride 0.9%, dextrose 5% in sodium chloride 0.9% or 0.45%, specific electrolyte solutions such as Darrow's, Hartmann's, and Ringer's solution. Sodium bicarbonate and sodium lactate may be used to correct acidosis.

2. Restoration of fluid volume following haemorrhage, shock or extensive burns. Sodium chloride may be given but it is not so effective as plasma, dextran or blood as these are not lost to the tissues through the capillary membrane.

3. As a vehicle for drugs such as antibiotics, heparin, potassium and lignocaine. Dextrose 5%, sodium chloride 0.9% or a mixture will be used to carry the drug according to its stability in the solution and the needs of the patient.

4. Feeding the patient when it is not possible to do this via the gastrointestinal tract due to disease or surgery. Proprietary substances containing emulsified fats and specially treated amino acids are given.

5. Forced diuresis to remove drugs such as aspirin and barbiturates which are excreted by the kidney. Mannitol 10% and 20% may be used for this.

6. Reduction of cerebral oedema with substances such as glycerol in sodium chloride 0.9%.

7. Replacement of carbohydrates by dextrose 5% or sorbitol 30%.

Equipment used (Figs. 10.4 and 10.5)

There are various types of needles and cannulae which the doctor may use. These range from the tiny scalp vein needle which was originally produced for babies, to a wide variety of polythene catheters and cannulae introduced with a metal needle. Some of these have an additional port through which drugs may be added. The Gordh needle has a rubber diaphragm through which drugs may be introduced. The nurse should be familiar with those currently available in her hospital, and should find out the preferences of the doctor.

There are also many different types of plastic

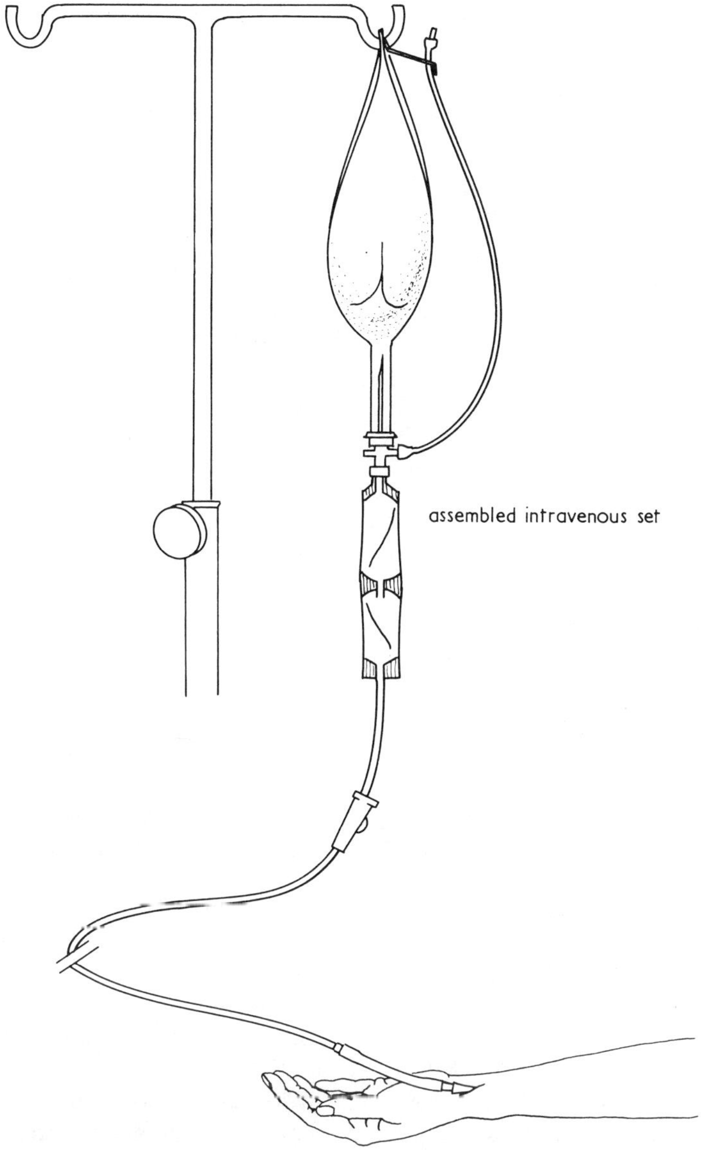

Fig. 10.4 *Assembled intravenous set.*

giving-sets. They may have a metal or plastic cannula for introducing into the container of intravenous solution. The plastic one is usually preferable if a PVC bag is being used, to minimise the possibility of it being punctured. Filter chambers vary in size, and it is important that an adequate one is used if blood is being given. Those sets suitable for use with blood may have a pressure pump. There will be a drip chamber and a flow control mechanism to control the rate of the infusion. Near the needle adaptor there is usually a latex flashball where drugs may be injected.

A paediatric giving-set may be used if a greater degree of accuracy is required. As well as the parts

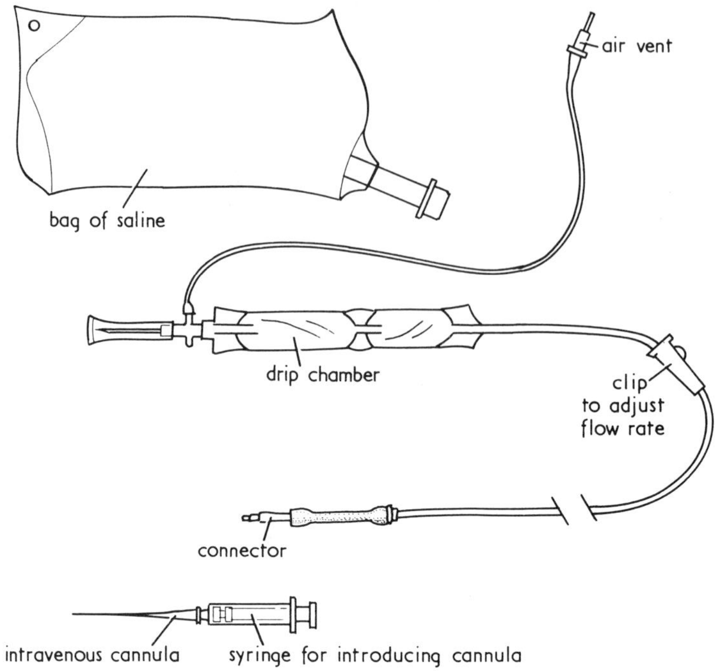

Fig. 10.5 *Equipment for intravenous infusion.*

already mentioned, this also has a 100-ml chamber. At the bottom of this chamber there is a rubber float, a safety device which seals off the outlet when the chamber is empty. The drip chamber is calibrated so that when it is running at 60 drops a minute the patient will receive 60 ml in 1 hour. There are various points at which drugs may be introduced, according to the strength required.

The fluid may come in PVC bags, polyprop-ramide pods or polyfusors, or bottles. Some substances cannot be put in the PVC bags because they leach out plastisers. There are various types of plastic bag, some of which have a pull-back entry port for the giving-set, whereas others have a tear-off seal with a protected entry port. The pods usually have an entry port which requires swabbing with an alcohol preparation. The entry port to the polyfusor requires twisting off. Bottles have rubber bungs protected by a metal cap and it may be necessary to swab the rubber bung with an alcohol solution. Many of the bags are inside a plastic outer wrapping, which should be inspected for damage or fluid on its inside, and if present the bag should be discarded.

All fluids are checked against the prescription sheet, which is separate from other medicines, to ensure that the correct fluid is being given to the correct patient and at the correct rate. The expiry date of the fluid is also checked and the fluid itself inspected for any abnormality. Preferably, any additives will have been already added in pharmacy, but if not, only a suitably qualified nurse who has undergone instruction may add them to the infusion. She will be meticulous in the way in which she checks them with another nurse. Any additives will be marked on the infusion bag. The infusion fluid will be entered on a fluid balance chart.

The protective sheath is removed from the end of the cannula by a gentle push and twist. The cannula of the giving-set is inserted into the outlet port, taking care not to contaminate it with the fingers. If it is being inserted into a plastic bag, the bag should not be held horizontally or there is danger of piercing it with the cannula. The infusion is suspended on a stand and the giving-set primed with fluid by squeezing the filter chamber gently so that the drip chamber is half-filled, and there are no air bubbles present. The infusion is now ready for the doctor to attach it to the intravenous cannula or needle.

Care of a patient receiving an intravenous infusion

Before the infusion is commenced, the patient should be told what to expect, and asked if he requires to empty his bladder. He should have a suitable garment on to enable bags to be changed if required. The infusion is usually put into the opposite arm to that which the patient uses.

After the doctor has inserted the cannula into a vein and attached it to the giving-set, the nurse may need to apply a bandage and possibly a splint. The point at which the cannula enters the skin should be visible, and care should be taken not to apply the bandage too tightly. Having checked the rate of the infusion, the patient should be made comfortable and anything he requires placed at hand.

The nurse should check regularly to see that the infusion is taking place at the correct rate. As a shocked patient recovers, so his blood vessels become less collapsed and an infusion will speed up. If the infusion stops, the nurse should check to see if the tube is kinked or the bandage too tight. Should the needle be against the side of the vein, moving the arm slightly will help to release it. Warmth may help if the infusion has slowed down due to a spasm of the vein. A clot in the needle, air bubble or venous thrombosis may be the cause of the infusion stopping. The last-mentioned is most likely to occur if dextrose solutions are being used. Should the cannula or needle become dislodged, the fluid will run into the tissues causing local oedema and pain. The infusion must be stopped. If a bottle is being used, it is particularly important that it does not empty and allow air to enter the system. As little as 10 ml of air can be sufficient to kill a patient.

If the patient has not lost fluid from the circulation, and intravenous fluids are introduced, it is possible to overload the circulation, particularly if sodium chloride is being used in the elderly or very young. A rising pulse, dyspnoea, cough, pain in the chest, pulmonary oedema and a raised jugular venous pressure would indicate this. Irregularities of the pulse may indicate the approach of a cardiac arrest in too rapid an infusion of sodium chloride, or overdosage with potassium. The latter may occur if potassium is added to an infusion and is not adequately mixed with it. Too much potassium causes mental confusion, listlessness, hypotension, and weakness in the legs. The infusion should be stopped and the doctor informed.

While the patient is on an intravenous infusion he will require help with washing, using a bedpan and eating his food. The food should be given to the patient in such a form that he can manage it with one arm.

When the infusion is to be discontinued, the puncture wound is covered by a sterile dressing, firmly applied. The intravenous cannula and giving-set are disposed of in such a way that they are not a danger to other people.

SUGGESTED WORK

1. For what reasons are the different patients on your ward having an intravenous infusion?

(a) What substances are being given?

(b) How will the doctor decide when the infusion should be discontinued?

SUGGESTED READING

Hinwood B. (1981). *Integrated Science Applied for Nurses*. London: Baillière Tindall.

Miller M. J. (1983). *Pathophysiology: Principles of Disease*. London: Baillière Tindall.

Roberts A. (1978). *Body Fluids*. London: Macmillan.

11

The Nutrition of the Surgical Patient

The nutrition of an individual depends upon many different factors, such as the availability of food in a suitable form; the ability and desire to eat it; absorption of the nutrients; metabolism of those nutrients; and the rate of excretion. An individual's requirements will change according to his environment, activity and disease.

Patient's coming into hospital for surgery fall into certain groups, each with their own particular problems. The booked patient is generally in a good nutritional state, but there are some patients who, because of their disease, have developed certain deficiencies which are best corrected before the operation. This may be done before admission to hospital. Many patients come into hospital for emergency surgery and their nutritional state is variable. Obesity can cause just as many problems for the surgeon as a deficiency.

Preparation of the patient for surgery varies, but most surgeons consider that 6 hours is sufficient length of time to starve the patient prior to operation to ensure an empty stomach, and to prevent vomiting. Emergency operations may only have 4 hours, whereas those being prepared for surgery on the gastrointestinal tract may be starved for 24–48 hours. Remembering that protein is necessary for repair of the body and that starvation increases the patient's anxiety, the nurse should ensure that he is not starved for longer than is necessary. Initially, postoperatively the patient will be unable to eat, therefore when food is given it should be appropriate to his needs.

The average patient is in a good nutritional state before arriving in hospital and it is often this patient's diet which is most neglected. He should have a well-balanced diet containing an adequate amount of all the essential nutrients. This will include protein, fat, carbohydrate, vitamins, minerals, roughage and water.

ESSENTIAL NUTRIENTS

Protein

Protein should form 10–15% of the calorific intake and is particularly important in the surgical patient because of the inevitable loss following the operation. It is necessary for the replacement of cells and the building of new tissue including such substances as haemoglobin and the plasma proteins. There must also be an adequate supply of the other nutrients to ensure that protein is spared for its primary use and not used up for energy. If there is insufficient intake, the body's own store of protein in the liver and the muscles will be used, the patient becoming listless and lacking energy. Eventually the plasma protein will be reduced and oedema will occur. A person is said to be in nitrogen balance if the nitrogen intake in the diet equals the amount excreted. Sources such as meat, fish, eggs and cheese contain all the eight essential amino acids, but second-class proteins do not. Therefore great care needs to be taken if the patient is a vegetarian to ensure that he does not lack one or more of these.

Following operation there is an increase in the excretion of nitrogen due to the breakdown of cells in the body. Normally this continues for 2 or 3 days postoperatively, but it may go on longer. It does not appear to be possible to stop this process, but obviously in the postoperative phase it is important to replace the protein as soon as possible.

Fat

Fat is a concentrated source of energy. It insulates the body from environmental temperatures, protects organs and is a vehicle for the absorption of fat-soluble vitamins A, D, E and K. It also slows down the activity of the stomach and therefore makes a meal more satisfying. Fat is contained in butter, margarine, cream, eggs, meat, milk and nuts. Stores of fat are easily available if the intake falls. The greater the amount of hydrogen in the fat, the more saturated it is. Animal fats are saturated, whereas most vegetable fats are unsaturated. It is thought by many that the latter are less likely to cause the deposition of atheroma. Fat is emulsified and absorbed by the action of bile salts on it. Patients who have disease of the gall bladder or liver may not tolerate fats very well.

Carbohydrate

Carbohydrate provides heat and energy and allows protein to be used for its main purpose. The brain only uses glucose, an end-product of carbohydrate digestion. A small amount is stored as glycogen in the liver and muscles but most of the excess is converted to fat. Food in this category tends to be cheaper, for example bread, potatoes, cakes, biscuits and sugar. Because of this, and their palatability, these food may easily be taken in excess, with a decrease in the amount of other nutrients taken, resulting in malnutrition.

Within the carbohydrate group are those substances which contain fibre or cellulose. These include bran, cereals, vegetables, fruit and nuts. These are not absorbed and retain fluid, therefore they aid the passage of the food residue in the intestine, preventing constipation.

Vitamins

Vitamins are essential in small amounts for certain chemical activities to take place in the body. They include vitamins A and D from dairy produce and oily fish, vitamin B from cereals, and vitamin C from fruit and vegetables. Following surgery there is a reduction in the amount of vitamin C. As this is necessary for wound healing, tissue formation and iron absorption, the postoperative patient should be given plenty of fruit and vegetables and may require supplements. Folic acid, one of the B group, may also be reduced, causing a megaloblastic anaemia. This is found in green vegetables, egg and liver. Some antibiotics, such as tetracycline, destroy the normal flora of the intestines, so interfering with the synthesis of vitamin B and causing sore mouth and tongue. It is often necessary to administer extra vitamin B with these drugs, or yoghurt which alters the flora in the gut and enables the organisms to synthesise vitamin B.

Minerals

Minerals are also substances required to control various activities in the body. Some of these are found in large quantities in the body, such as calcium, potassium and sodium, whereas others are present in much smaller amounts, for example iron and iodine. Nevertheless, these trace elements may be just as important for the efficient functioning of the body.

Iron deficiency is frequently present in women during the child-bearing years due to the menstrual loss. Any chronic or acute bleeding disorder will also lead to low levels. Lack of vitamin C and malabsorption from other causes will also lead to anaemia, and patients with malignant disease or renal disease will have an associated anaemia. It is preferable to correct this prior to operation, so that the haemoglobin is able to carry a full amount of oxygen to the tissues following operation. If there is time, the patient will be given oral preparations of ferrous iron and possibly vitamin C as well. If appropriate, he will be advised that liver and green vegetables are a good source of iron. It may be necessary to give him iron intramuscularly or even in the form of an intravenous infusion. If the anaemia is due to blood loss, a blood transfusion may be given. Patients on iron preparations frequently suffer from constipation or occasionally diarrhoea.

Calcium requires vitamin D for its absorption and is found in milk, cheese and eggs. It is required for bone formation and repair, teeth, blood clotting, action of muscle, the heart and the nerves. In patients remaining in bed for a long time, such as those on traction or with major debilitating illness, calcium is lost from the bones to the blood, and is excreted via the urinary tract. There is therefore the danger of renal and bladder calculi, unless plenty of fluids are given. In certain forms of malignancy the bones become more porous, so leading to pathological fractures. If the parathyroids, which control the levels of calcium in the body, become diseased or are removed during a thyroidectomy, the level of circulating calcium becomes less and tetany occurs. Major blood transfusions containing sodium citrate will lead to continuous bleeding because of the lack of calcium.

Potassium and *sodium* are important in fluid and electrolyte balance and are dealt with in Chapter 10. Some fruit drinks are high in potassium and have to be avoided in patients with a high blood level, whereas many diuretics cause large amounts of potassium to be excreted.

Water is very important for the maintenance of health and this is dealt with in Chapter 10.

OTHER FACTORS AFFECTING THE NUTRITION OF THE PATIENT

There are many other factors which influence what the patient eats. Availability of the food does not just mean that it is supplied on a tray in front of the patient. It may be unavailable for other reasons; for instance, when sandwiches have been wrapped in cling foil and the patient has one arm in a plaster; or when an unpeeled orange or salad is given to the patient who has an intravenous infusion in one arm. Occasionally it is the thoughtless positioning of a tray which makes the food 'unavailable'. Certain types of food are quite unsuitable if the patient is lying on his back or is blind, for example spaghetti or kippers.

Ensuring that the patient has an empty bladder, is sat up comfortably, and has his water at hand are all part of the nurse's preparation for the meal. If he wears false teeth, they may need to be cleaned and given to him. It is unpleasant for any patient to eat a meal if someone else is on a bedpan. If bedpans are offered prior to the meal being served, this situation should not arise.

The patient's diet should have been ordered according to his needs. An overweight patient requires a reduction in the amount of carbohydrate and calories, whereas the underweight may require more. A patient may have cultural or religious taboos which rule out certain types of food. There will be some foods he just dislikes or has never had before. The availability of sauces and condiments may help to make the meal more acceptable. A meal heated in the oven during doctor's examination is never as appetising as it was initially. Meal times in hospital are usually quite different from those at home, leaving a long interval between an early evening meal and breakfast, unless the patient supplements these himself.

Appetite is associated with hunger, but not necessarily so. The bored patient will nibble at biscuits, sweets and fruit even if he has had sufficient. Conversely, the patient may have been given bad news about his prognosis or be worried about his job or events at home and so lose his appetite. Surgery, anaesthesia and drugs all have an adverse effect on the appetite. The palatability of food is an important factor. A meal soaked in gravy or custard may not appeal to one patient whereas another may find difficulty in eating a dry meal. If all courses, including the cup of tea, are presented together, this can discourage a patient, just as big helpings will. Fruit juice makes a good appetiser.

Meal times are often social events, and more is usually eaten in company with other people. Most patients enjoy their meal better sitting in the dining room or at a table with others, but smoking should not be allowed in the eating area as many patients are put off their food by the fumes.

Feeding the patient unable to help himself

Many people feel a loss of dignity in being fed; they feel reduced to the status of a child. They may also feel they are a burden, particularly if the nurses appear in a hurry. Where the patient can manage on his own without becoming too tired, the nurse should look for ways of making it easier. Heat-retaining plates, special cutlery and crockery and non-slip mats will help. Polythene tubing or flexible straws and sloping mugs may enable the patient to drink unaided. If food has to be cut up, it is better to do this before bringing it to the patient so that he is not made conscious of it. The food should look appetising and be the correct heat, and the patient should be asked how he prefers to eat it. Some prefer to have a mix of flavours in their mouth at one time, others prefer one food at a time. Extra salt and sauces may also be required. The nurse should feed the patient at the rate he finds comfortable. After the meal, a drink of water will help to make the mouth feel fresher. Oral toilet may be necessary.

Feeding with a nasogastric tube

Some patients are unable to take in sufficient nutrients, even with help, and may need a nasogastric tube to be passed. There are a variety of tubes which may be passed into the stomach or duodenum via the nose or mouth. The most common are the Levin's tube and the Ryle's tube which have a medium-sized lumen and are suitable either for aspiration or for the introduction of nutrients. Sometimes they have a radio-opaque end to enable the position of the tube to be checked. A very fine-bore tube with an introducer is available for feeding the patient, and this is particularly suitable if it is to be in position for a long period of time or the patient is unable to tolerate the other tubes. The Maurice Lee tube has a double lumen which enables the stomach to be kept empty by aspiration, but at the same time allowing nutrients to be introduced into the duodenum. The Miller–Abbott's tube is also a double tube, but in this case there is also a balloon which is inflated via one of the channels. The inflated balloon will travel down the intestine until stopped by an obstruction. The tip of the tube goes beyond the balloon and is used for aspiration.

The nasogastric tube has two main purposes in surgery. It is used in operations on the gastro-intestinal tract to keep it empty and prevent distension due to either gas or fluid. It may therefore be aspirated at regular intervals, attached to a suction pump, or left on free drainage attached to a drainage bag, which allows gases to escape. The second use of the tube is to feed the patient who is unable to take nutrients by mouth. It is preferred to the intravenous route in the majority of patients, although occasionally diarrhoea is a problem and cellulose has to be added to the feed. Liquidised meals or artificially produced liquid diets containing the correct proportion of nutrients may be given via this route, but care must be taken that they are at the correct temperature.

When introducing a nasogastric tube, the tip of the patient's nose is slightly tilted and the tube is passed along its floor, **not** in an upward direction. As the tube reaches the back of the throat, the patient is asked to swallow. In the average patient, when the first ring on the tube is level with the nostril, the tube has reached the cardiac sphincter, and the pyloric sphincter of the stomach when the second ring is in this position. When the tube is in the stomach its position is checked by aspirating or by introducing air down it while a second person listens over the stomach with a stethoscope. If there is any doubt, a senior person must be consulted.

The fine-bore nasogastric tube is issued with a guide wire which is passed through the metal end of the tube as far as the 'stop' ring on the guide wire. The tube is then passed in the same manner as a normal nasogastric tube. Once in position, the guide wire is removed. If this causes any difficulty, the tube is in the wrong position and should be taken out. After the guide wire has been removed it is possible to check its position by using a three-way adapter on the tube and aspirating, but it is not suitable for regular aspiration. If considered necessary, its position can be checked by x-ray. This tube can remain in position for long periods of time without being changed. Special proprietary feeds are provided, although the diet kitchen can produce a suitable mixture.

SUGGESTED WORK

1. Find out what the daily nutritional requirements are and then check the following diets to see if they meet these.

(a) Normal diet of a patient on the second postoperative day.

(b) Fluid diet.

What could be done to correct any deficiencies?

SUGGESTED READING

Ministry of Agriculture, Fisheries and Food. *Manual of Nutrition*. London: HMSO.

12

Central Venous Pressure and Total Parenteral Nutrition

CENTRAL VENOUS PRESSURE

As the blood leaves the heart and passes through the arteries, capillaries and veins, the pressure in it is continuously dropping, although gravity does increase the pressure in the capillaries of the lower limbs. In order to overcome the effect of gravity and return the blood to the right side of the heart, several factors come into play. The pumping action of the muscles, one-way valves in the veins, and the suction effect of a negative pressure in the chest and positive pressure in the abdomen all help to ensure an adequate return to the heart. The control of the diameter of blood vessels is responsible for varying the venous return according to the body's need. The amount of blood returning to the heart via the veins is an important factor in controlling the heart's output.

The higher arterial pressure can be measured with a sphygmomanometer, but sometimes we need a more sensitive measure of the activity of the circulatory system. The introduction of a manometer into the right atrium to measure the central venous pressure (CVP) is a way of monitoring the function of the heart and the vascular system. The central venous pressure is the result of the pressures in the thorax, activity of the heart, the diameter of the veins and the amount of blood in the circulation. If the first three are normal, it is an accurate means of monitoring the fluid requirements of a patient on intravenous therapy.

Clinical reasons for inserting a central venous pressure line

If fluid is to be introduced into the cardiovascular system by means of an intravenous infusion or blood transfusion and there is any danger of overloading the circulation, then a central venous pressure line will be necessary. Therefore any patients who are elderly, or who have a history of heart failure, myocardial infarction or severe anaemia, and those undergoing cardiac surgery are candidates for this procedure.

Any condition which decreases the amount of circulating fluid, such as blood loss, severe dehydration, shock and severe infection such as peritonitis, can be controlled more efficiently if a CVP line is in position.

It is also useful to detect the presence of continuing haemorrhage when this is hidden and a sudden rapid loss may occur. The CVP is a much more sensitive, and therefore quicker, indicator of change than the pulse or blood pressure.

Method of setting up a central venous pressure line

The doctor will insert a catheter or cannula (under strict aseptic conditions) directly into a vein or by cutting down the vein. This is normally done under a local anaesthetic. In order to increase the size of the vein and reduce the possibility of an air embolus entering, the patient may be placed in a head-down position. The position of the catheter is checked by x-ray, which also indicates if a pneumothorax has been induced. One of the following routes may be used.

1. Femoral vein in the leg. There is a high risk of thrombosis and infection.
2. Antecubital vein in the arm. This requires a long catheter to be threaded up to the right atrium.
3. Subclavian vein near the clavicle.
4. Jugular veins in the neck. These are mainly used by anaesthetists in theatre.

Either subclavian vein is frequently used because, being large veins and having a fast blood flow, there is less likelihood of a thrombosis forming. These veins arise from the jugular veins and drain into the innominate veins and so into the superior vena cava and the right atrium. Occasionally, because of this vein's proximity to the lung, a pneumothorax may be caused. The catheter is usually held in position with a suture.

The central venous pressure apparatus (Fig. 12.1)

This consists of an intravenous line with a side arm. At the junction where this side arm joins the main intravenous line there is a three-way stopcock to control the direction of the fluid. Behind the stopcock is a plate to fix the manometer to the infusion stand. Also supplied will be the measurement scale which will be fixed to the infusion stand. A levelling tube will be used to place the measurement scale and manometer in the correct position. Once the patient is comfortably positioned, preferably in a semirecumbent position, one end of the levelling tube is placed on the reference point of the patient, usually the manubriosternal angle, and the other on the zero point of the manometer (see Fig. 12.1). The latter is adjusted until the fluid level or air bubble is in a central position. The pressure being read is that of the right atrium.

The trolley is prepared as for an intravenous infusion plus the above equipment. The set should be primed with fluid before it is attached to the patient and the stopcock placed in a position to allow fluid to run from the infusion to the patient (see Fig. 12.1). The tap is then turned to allow fluid to enter the manometer tube and then returned to the previous position. The doctor then attaches the end of the intravenous tubing to the catheter in the patient. The flow rate is then adjusted, and may be just fast enough to keep the line open.

Reading the central venous pressure

The zero point is set using the levelling tube. The tap is then turned to connect the patient to the manometer (Fig. 12.2). At first there is a slight rise and fall in the level of the fluid due to respiration. When the fluid level is stable it should be read against the manometer. The stopcock should then be returned to the position allowing intravenous fluid to enter the patient. Measurement of the CVP should be done as quickly as possible to prevent clots forming in the patient's catheter. The reading is recorded and compared with the previous results. If the intravenous infusion has slowed or stopped, the medical staff should be informed.

The nurse will have asked the doctor the levels above and below which he wishes to be informed. Usually this is ± 5 cm H_2O. If it is above this level, overtransfusion is indicated, and if below, hidden bleeding. A steady rise or fall may be just as significant. Three successive observations in a continuing upward or downward direction should be reported. These observations are usually made 1/2–1-hourly, depending on the reason for the observation and the state of the patient. A venous pressure monitor charged with batteries makes the nurse's task much easier.

Observations which may be carried out immediately after the CVP line has been inserted are those of the blood pressure and pulse for any indication of cardiovascular disorder, and the respirations to recognise a pneumothorax or pulmonary oedema. Wound infection, phlebitis and, rarely, septicaemia may arise and therefore the patient's temperature will be taken.

TOTAL PARENTERAL NUTRITION

This is a method of supplying all of the body's nutritional needs by means of the intravenous

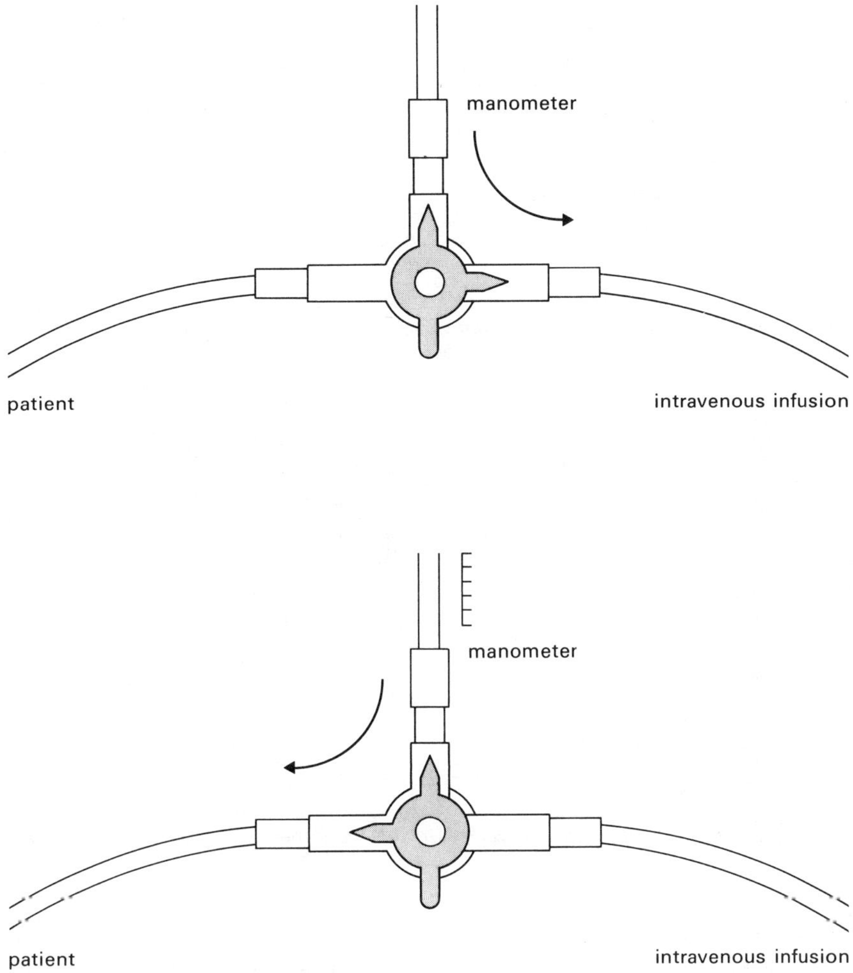

Fig. 12.1 *Central venous pressure apparatus.*

route. It can be used for any patient who is unable to receive sufficient nutrients by means of the gastrointestinal route, either orally or by nasogastric tube. The subclavian vein is usually used, although a Broviac catheter, a fine flexible silastic catheter, may be introduced through the skin into the superior vena cava and from there to the right atrium of the heart. This is usually inserted under strict aseptic conditions in theatre.

In any patient undergoing starvation and trauma to the body, including surgery, there is loss of nitrogen from the body. If the patient was previously healthy, he will lose some weight, but given extra protein he will soon recover. However, with some patients their general condition before surgery is very poor and as a result of this healing of wounds and internal anastomosis may be slow and there may even be a breakdown with the formation of fistulae. Patients suffering from malignant conditions, and in particular carcinoma of the oesophagus where the patient may have had dysphagia for some time, are poor operative risks for this reason. If surgery is to be carried out, the general condition of the patient must be built up if there is to be a reasonable chance of success. In a patient with severe ulcerative colitis there will have been

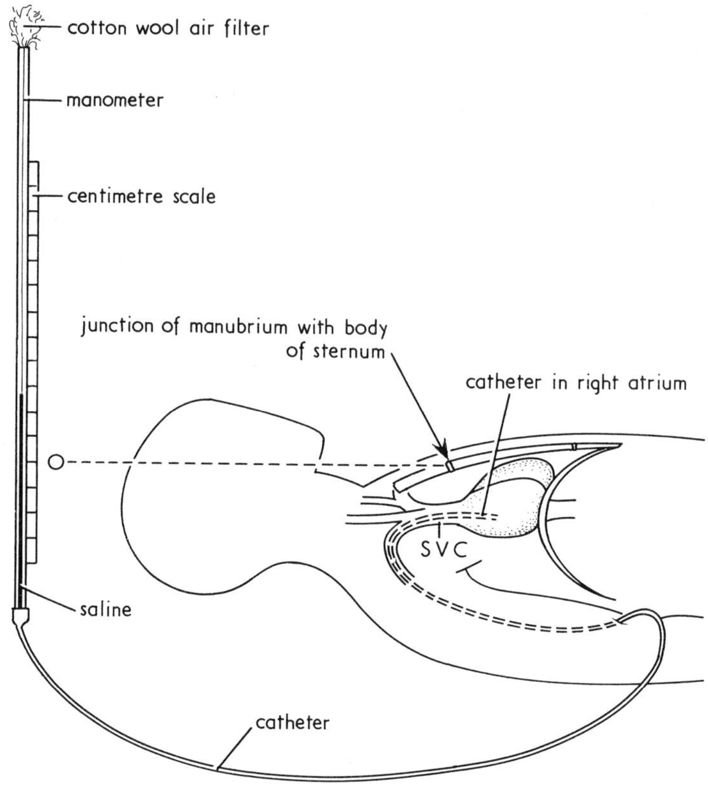

Fig. 12.2 *Connecting the patient to the manometer.*

severe loss of protein and salts from the body and possibly little time to make this up before surgery; thus parenteral nutrition may be lifesaving. Severe multiple injuries, surgery of the head and neck, and resection of a large part of the gastrointestinal tract are other surgical reasons for parenteral feeding.

All the nutrients can be supplied in this way so long as they are sterile and non-toxic, which means that they are expensive to produce. In order to provide sufficient calories without too much fluid, an emulsified fat solution is used. This is either 10% or 20%, usually the latter. Some calories have to be given in the form of glucose or fructose, the former requiring insulin to metabolise it. The practice has been to give this in a 5% solution because of the problem of thrombophlebitis with stronger solutions. However, some doctors are now giving 20% or even 50% solutions. The protein is given as a 10% amino acid solution and may be mixed with fructose and ethanol. Trace elements may need to be added. All three solutions may be given at the same time for the best effect. Fat protects the veins and so will prevent thrombophlebitis occurring from the administration of the other two substances. In order to supply sufficient calories and proteins, 1 litre of fat emulsion, 1 litre of amino acid solution, and 1–2 litres of glucose 20% in 24 hours may be prescribed by the doctor.

During the administration of the nutrients the patient must be observed carefully. Four-hourly temperature, pulse and blood pressure should be taken for evidence of infection or effect on the cardiovascular system. A fluid balance chart must be strictly kept and a note made of the consistency of the stools. Daily or twice-daily weight is recorded. The blood is tested with a Dextrostix and the glucose level assessed with a glucometer every 4–6 hours. The lower and upper limits will be set by the doctor, and intravenous glucose or insulin given according to the readings. At the point where the catheter is inserted there will be a dressing which will need changing at least every 48 hours, and a new giving-set may be necessary every 24 hours. Any rashes, nausea, vomiting, or jaundice must be reported. The doctor will take blood for haemoglobin, serum electrolytes, blood urea and serum protein. If the patient is on intravenous fat, the laboratory must be informed as this may affect the equipment and alter results. A 24-hour collection of urine may be sent to the laboratory for estimation of protein loss.

SUGGESTED WORK

1. Ask a doctor if he would explain to you the reasons for using central venous pressure, how it is set up and how it should be measured.

2. Find a patient who is on parenteral feeding and discover the regime being used to feed him. Are there any particular precautions or care that have to be taken of the intravenous line?

SUGGESTED READING

Grant A., Todd E., Eds. (1982). *Enteral and Parenteral Nutrition.* London: Blackwell Scientific.

Moghissi K., Boore J. R. P. (1983). *Parenteral and Enteral Nutrition for Nurses.* London: Heinemann Medical.

Russell W. J. (1974). *Central Venous Pressure.* London: Butterworths.

13

Aspects of Wound Repair

TISSUE REPAIR AND REPLACEMENT

The following process applies to all types of tissue damage whether it is in the skin, the intestines or some other part of the body. Repair takes place partly as a result of the original cells being replaced and partly by growth of connective tissue. The balance of these two processes depends on the tissue which has been damaged and its ability to regenerate cells, as well as on the degree of damage. Nerve cells do not regenerate, although if the cell has not been damaged, the nerve fibre will grow again. Bone and skin are particularly good at replacing damaged tissue. If the original tissue is replaced by a large amount of connective tissue, scarring will be present and the function may be impaired.

Healing by first intention (Fig. 13.1)

This is said to occur in wounds which are clean and the edges have been brought close together, such as in a surgical operation. These wounds heal quickly and leave very little scar. The following processes take place.

1. As a result of the incision the wound bleeds in the small space between the wound edges, forming a clot of fibrin, blood cells and debris.
2. Fibroblasts from the surrounding tissue enter into this clot and multiply rapidly, gradually converting it into granulation tissue.
3. At the same time the capillaries at the edge of the wound send out buds which grow into the blood clot so that the granulation tissue becomes very vascular and bleeds easily.
4. White blood cells (polymorphs) escape from the blood vessels by a process of *diapedesis*, in which they insert pseudopodia into the junction between the epithelial cells and then flow through it. These white cells, with other cells from the reticuloendothelial system, macrophages and histiocytes, remove the remains of the blood clot and any dead tissue by a process of phagocytosis in which they engulf the debris and dissolve it by the release of enzymes.
5. The fibroblasts lay down collagen fibres, so forming fibrous tissue. As it is formed it contracts, so reducing the amount of capillaries in the scar tissue formed. The macrophages disappear.
6. At the same time as these processes are occurring, the epithelial cells on the surface of the surrounding skin multiply, gradually growing across the surface of the gap.

Healing by second intention

Although this is essentially the same process as that already described, it takes much longer and produces more scarring because the wound either covers a large surface area (as in a burn) or is infected (as in a bedsore or abscess).

1. A larger clot is present in the wound, there is more dead tissue for the reticuloendothelial cells to remove and, if infection is present, they will have to destroy the bacteria as well.
2. As with first intention healing, the fibroblasts

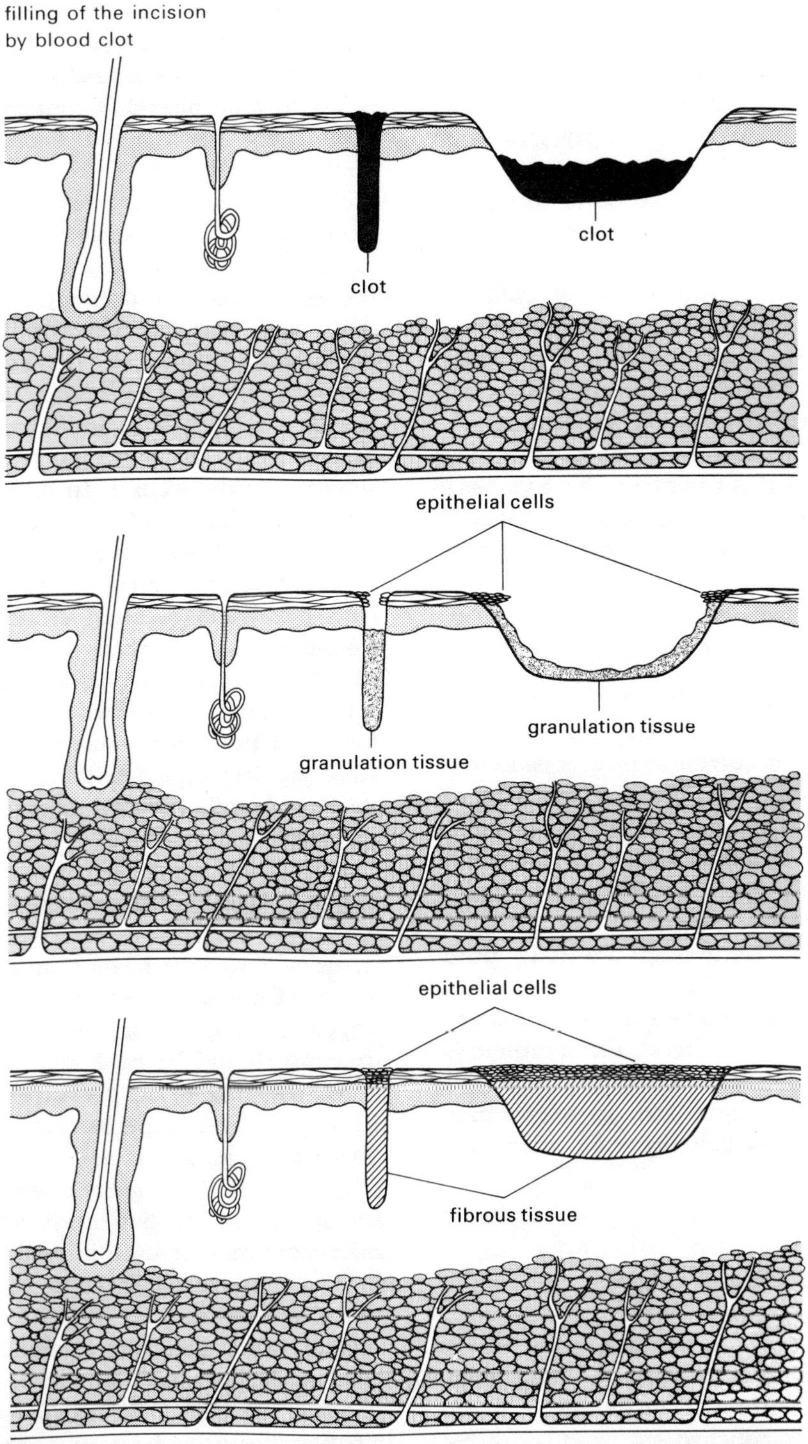

Fig. 13.1 *Healing by first intention.*

and capillary loops infiltrate the clot, starting in the base of the wound and gradually filling the defect, so forming the vascular granulation.

3. At the same time the epithelial cells on the surface of the surrounding skin multiply, gradually spreading across the surface of the wound, but as they have a large surface area to cover this takes some time.

4. As the granulation tissue is converted into fibrous tissue by the laying down of collagen threads, the blood supply decreases. Therefore less oxygen and nutrients reach the surface epithelial cells. If the wound is too extensive, the centre of it may not heal. Therefore in very large wounds skin grafting is done. The scar formed appears thinner and more shiny as well as paler than skin as it has a poorer blood supply and no pigment cells. Special structures such as hair, sebaceous and sweat glands are not reformed.

Speeding up the healing process

The aim is to encourage healing by first intention and therefore an incision is sometimes made to prevent a jagged tear occurring as in an episiotomy. Contamination is avoided and any serous fluid or debris is allowed to escape via a drainage tube. Some wounds have debris removed surgically, which is the quickest way (debridement), others are cleaned with cleansing agents such as eusol or hydrogen peroxide. Antibiotics are only used against specific infection after a wound swab has been taken. Wounds should be kept clean and dry to prevent bacteria gaining access. Extra protein is required for the healing process, particularly if very much tissue has been lost, in which case increased amounts of carbohydrate and vitamin C are also required.

ASEPSIS AND WOUND CARE

The definition of asepsis is freedom from pathogenic organisms. In order to apply a dressing in an aseptic manner, a non-touch technique is used. The dressing is not touched by hand, only by forceps. The purpose of a dressing is to protect the wound from infection, to absorb any discharge from it and, if necessary, to fill any dead space that is present so preventing abscess formation.

To prevent the risk of contamination, dressings should not be changed unnecessarily. If they become wet through discharge, micro-organisms are able to enter the wound and therefore the dressing requires renewing. The presence of pain or infection will indicate a need for the wound to be redressed, and if the dressing becomes displaced it will have to be replaced, otherwise it may remain in position until the clips or sutures (Fig. 13.2) require removing. Dry wounds and stitches should not be swabbed with lotion as this also allows organisms to enter. The dressing should be suitable for the wound. In most cases gauze or a plastic dressing is sufficient. If discharge is present or drainage tubes are in position (Fig. 13.3), a more absorbent wool and gauze dressing may be used, with a keyhole dressing around the tube. If a wound needs to be lightly packed, ribbon gauze is suitable. Where an occlusive dressing is required, Vaseline gauze is the dressing of choice, although for small puncture wounds flexible collodion is suitable. Care should be taken to replace the lid of the flexible collodion container firmly or the substance will thicken.

Antibiotics are not used on wounds unless a swab has been taken and the infective organism and its sensitivity are known. Foreign bodies and dead tissue will impede healing and are therefore removed. Constant movement of the part will also impede healing, so splinting may be necessary. The dressing should be held securely in place either with strapping or, if pressure is required, with Elastoplast or a crepe bandage. Cotton and conforming bandages may be used and can be disposed of after use. Tubular gauze or elasticised net is used for speed. If the patient is allergic to plaster, micropore may be used instead.

Dressings are best done in an area kept for this purpose, but if they are done in the ward, bedmaking and other disturbances should not have taken place in the previous hour to allow organisms time to settle. Infected dressings are left until last, and if a patient has several dressings, the cleanest is done first. Any explanations should take place prior to

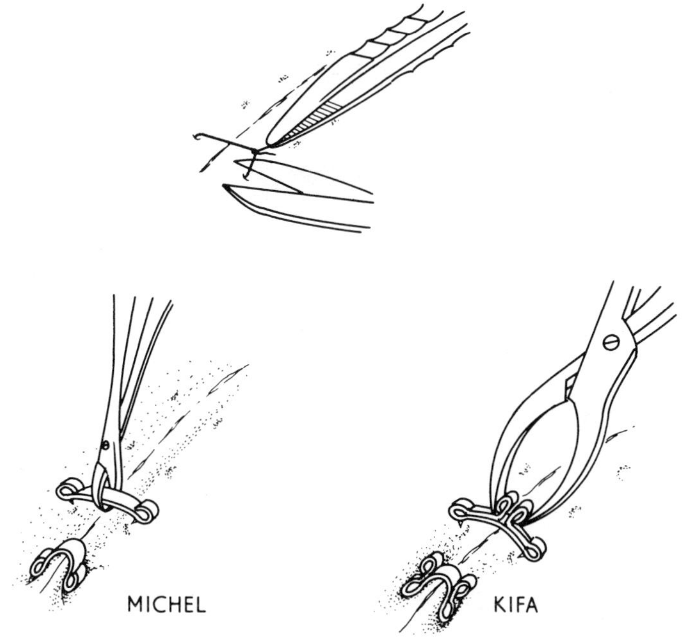

Fig. 13.2 *Removal of sutures and clips.*

the procedure, and there should be no unnecessary talking during it, nor should the wound be exposed for longer than is necessary.

After the trolley has been cleaned from top to bottom with soap and water it must be dried thoroughly. Sterile dressings and forceps, which are supplied from CSSD, must be checked prior to use to ensure that they are sterile and have not been contaminated. On the packet there may be a coloured strip which will undergo a colour change when sterilisation has taken place. A solution for cleansing the wound may be supplied in an individual sachet.

The patient should be positioned in such a way that the nurse has good access to the wound and the patient is comfortable. A good light is essential. Care should be taken not to contaminate the sterile field by touching with the hands, contaminated forceps or dressings. Therefore the nurse should not reach across the sterile field or spill lotion. If any sterile item is contaminated; it should be discarded. The wound should be cleaned from its centre to the edge—from the clean to the dirty area.

Before the nurse leaves the bedside the patient will be made comfortable and the bags with dirty dressings and forceps closed. Dressings and forceps are disposed of in the appropriate containers. If any sharp objects have been used, such as stitch cutters, these must be disposed of in a suitable container.

INFLAMMATION

This is the reaction of living tissues to the invasion of micro-organisms, injury, chemicals, extremes of temperature, foreign bodies, radiotherapy, ultraviolet light and x-rays. The cardinal signs of inflammation are redness, heat, swelling, pain and loss of function.

Following the injury there is a transient constriction of arterioles which is followed by an increased blood flow to the area due to the dilatation of the capillaries and smaller arterioles. If this is on the surface of the body, it will appear red and warm.

The walls of the capillaries and smaller venules

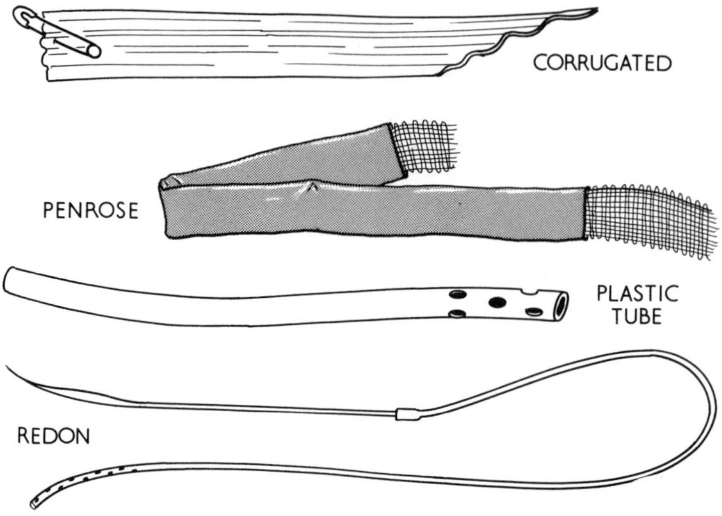

Fig. 13.3 *Drainage tubes.*

become more permeable, so allowing plasma proteins to escape. This fact, coupled with the increased pressure in the vessels, leads to an escape of fluid with salts and plasma into the surrounding tissues (exudate), which will be seen as oedema if the inflammation is on the surface of the body.

Leucocytes gather against the walls of the blood vessels and migrate through the junctions of the epithelial cells by the process of diapedesis already mentioned. In the earlier stages these are mainly polymorphs and later monocytes. These, with the large macrophage cells or histiocytes from the local tissues, engulf and destroy invading organisms by the process of phagocytosis.

The healing process may then take place normally and restore full function with normal tissue, replace it with fibrotic, scar tissue, form an abscess, or continue as chronic inflammation. The inflammation may spread locally into the lymph vessels causing a lymphangitis, or into the bloodstream causing septicaemia. If the inflammation occurs in a serous membrane such as the pleura, peritoneum or pericardium, or into a synovial joint, an increase of serous fluid is produced with a high protein content (exudate), for example a pleural effusion. A collection of pus may form in the tissue due to the destruction of large numbers of white blood cells and bacteria with the breakdown of tissue. This forms an *abscess* and is surrounded by an area of inflammation. Because the abscess enlarges and spreads along the line of least resistance, it may burrow for a long distance before reaching the surface and bursting. Abscesses are drained in order to prevent their spread and the damage of further tissue. Abscesses not only occur in the subcutaneous tissue, but also in other organs such as those of the gastrointestinal tract. Pus occurring in a cavity such as the gall bladder or pleural space is called *empyema*.

Boils are the result of infection in a hair follicle, sweat gland or sebaceous gland due to *Staphylococcus pyogenes*. Styes are boils on the eyelids. A carbuncle is a localised infection of the subcutaneous tissues, which has been carried there by the bloodstream. It may break down to form many sinuses and is much larger than a boil, and will therefore take longer to heal. Carbuncles of the face are especially dangerous because the infection may spread to the intracranial veins. The patient should be warned not to squeeze them, neither are they incised. Cellulitis is spread of inflammation in tissues such as skin as a result of infection by such organisms as the β-haemolytic *Streptococcus* or *Staphylococcus*.

Paronychia is an infection of the nail fold. It starts as an infection of the skin in the region of the nail cuticle. Pus forms under the horny layer and spreads under the nail to the nail bed, causing necrosis of the root. *Acute suppurative tenosynovitis* is caused by infection of the tendon sheath in the hand by *Streptococcus pyogenes*. It causes severe pain, flexion of the finger affected, and swelling. An incision is required to release the tension or severe damage may occur. Palmar, web and pulp infections may occur in the hand and may require incision to release the tension to avoid damage to tissue.

Toxaemia occurs in all conditions of inflammation and produces constitutional signs and symptoms. The toxins from the bacteria are absorbed into the bloodstream while the organisms themselves remain in or near the site of their entrance. It causes a rise in the temperature, pulse and respiration rates. The white cell count is raised (leucocytosis) and the patient feels unwell with a headache, dry mouth, furred tongue and loss of appetite.

Management of inflammation

1. Rest the affected part, for example a hand may be put in a sling.
2. Heat by means of kaolin poultices, fomentations, hot baths and electric pads.
3. Incision and drainage.
4. Irrigation of the wound with a cleansing agent.
5. Chemotherapy to kill the organism (bactericidal) or to prevent its multiplication and so allow the leucocytes a chance to overcome it (bacteriostatic).
6. Rest the individual while the temperature is raised.
7. Analgesics, such as codeine, may be required.

SUGGESTED WORK

1. Find out how the care of different wounds varies.
   (a) Which types of operation require a wound drain?
   (b) How long does the original dressing stay on?
   (c) What type of stitches are used?
   (d) When are the stitches removed?
   What reason is given for these variations?
2. What is the incidence of wound infection on your ward?
   (a) Where are infections recorded?
   (b) What organism is most commonly implicated?
   (c) What responsibility does the cross-infection sister have for these infections?

SUGGESTED READING

Bickerton J., Small J. (1982). *Bandaging*. London: Heinemann Medical.

Broome W. E. (1971). *Dressing Techniques*. Nursing in Depth Series. London: Butterworths.

Winner H. I. (1983). *Microbiology in Patient Care*, 2nd edn. London: Hodder & Stoughton.

14

Surgical Pain and its Relief

Pain is something that the majority of people have suffered, and yet it is one of the most difficult experiences to judge in another person. The amount of pain experienced does not necessarily vary according to the extent of the injury. The same damage may cause different degrees of pain in different people, just as minor surgery may be just as painful, or even more so, than major surgery. Although pain appears to be a physical sensation which acts as a protective mechanism, there is a large psychological component.

Receptors in the skin are sensitive to the sensation of pain, and nerves in the smooth muscle of hollow tubes such as the gastrointestinal, biliary and renal tracts are sensitive to distension. This information is transmitted via the peripheral and autonomic nerves, respectively, to the spinal cord, where it is relayed to the sensory cortex of the brain. It may also form part of a reflex arc. In the brain it is interpreted in the light of previous experience. Certain parts of the body are more sensitive than others because they have a larger area of representation in the brain.

Pain in the surgical patient may be due to the condition which has brought him into hospital. It will vary according to the organ affected. The patient may be able to point to the specific spot where the pain is, or it may be much more vague. Occasionally it may be bilateral. With some conditions, such as appendicitis, the pain will move; more usually it remains in one place. The pain may have gradually increased in intensity or have occurred suddenly without any warning, and in some cases it will come and go. Its character will vary according to the part of the body affected; for example, if it occurs in the gastrointestinal tract, the ureters or biliary tract, it may be spasmodic and colicky. There may be factors which aggravate or relieve the pain such as food or activity, and there may be associated symptoms. The nurse's observations of the pain will help the doctor in his diagnosis.

Pain invariably occurs following surgery and this is due more to the amount of retraction required during the operation than to the incision, because of the amount of tissue damaged. Retraction in a cholecystectomy involves the diaphragm, which makes breathing painful postoperatively. Breathing and coughing may not only cause pain following thoracic surgery, but also in abdominal surgery, if breathing is deep involving abdominal muscles. Muscle spasm is particularly likely to occur after abdominal surgery.

Pain of varying degrees may occur due to complications of the operation or the treatment, and the nurse must be alert for this. Intestinal obstruction, peritonitis, cystitis, bronchopneumonia, wound infection, haematoma, pressure sores, allergy to plaster and venous thrombosis will all cause pain. Therefore, when the patient complains of pain or, from her observations of his general appearance, facial expression, colour, lack of movement, pulse, respirations and blood pressure, the nurse recognises that he is suffering pain, she should be able to recognise whether it is what might be normally expected or indicates some complication. If it is the latter, the nurse must be able to describe its nature, position, duration and intensity to assist the doctor in his diagnosis.

The reduction of postoperative pain will reduce complications such as shock, vomiting, deep vein thrombosis, pulmonary embolus or bronchopneumonia. Pain stimulates the release of steroid hormones from the adrenal cortex, so causing an increase in the amount of protein broken down; this delays healing of wounds. The increase in steroids also depresses the immune response giving greater opportunity for infection to occur. It is therefore of great importance in the recovery of the patient to control postoperative pain.

We do know that there are many factors that influence an individual's sensitivity to pain. The attitudes towards pain of the culture in which a person has been raised may teach him to accept a certain level of pain without complaining, or, conversely, he may expect to express his emotions freely. Nurses coming from a different culture may have different attitudes. Individuals within a culture also vary in their reaction to pain due to varying personalities and family background. But even more important from the nurse's point of view is the fact that research has shown that the more anxious a person is the more sensitive he is to pain. If the individual is also suffering from lack of sleep or is generally debilitated, his ability to tolerate pain is reduced still further. If this is so, it follows that the more the nurse can do to reduce those anxieties, the more she will also reduce the level of pain, and this will in turn reduce the length of the recovery period.

These anxieties arise as a result of the patient's condition, the proposed treatment, and the effects of its outcome on his life and that of his family. Some anxiety is inevitable, but a great deal can be reduced by effective communication at the right time. Lack of information allows the patient's imagination to work overtime and prevents him from making logical decisions. If the general practitioner has taken time to explain what may be wrong and the possible treatment in hospital, it will help the patient to be in the right frame of mind for what he is to face. He may be anxious about the actual admission to hospital, investigations to be carried out, the operation or the anaesthetic. The nurse admitting the patient should have built up a relationship with him that enables him to feel free to ask questions without fear of feeling foolish. Because of his anxiety he may find it difficult to ask the right questions, and to assimilate the information given to him. He may therefore ask different people the same question, getting a slightly different answer each time, so adding to his anxiety.

It is important that the doctor or the sister explains to the patient exactly what is going to be done and its effects both in the short term and long term. The language used should not be technical, nor should too much information be given at once, but rather small amounts as they become appropriate. The previous knowledge of the patient will influence how much he remembers. It is therefore essential to find this out first of all.

If the patient knows what to expect, he can prepare himself mentally for it. Patients are often surprised at the amount of pain experienced after operation and are therefore not ready to face it. They need to be told what drainage tubes etc. may be in position on their return from theatre, so that on seeing them they do not think that the outcome of the operation was more serious that was expected. The reasons for early mobilisation should be explained to enable the patient to see the positive benefits and to co-operate.

Any important information or instructions to be followed after the operation should be given in writing for the patient to refer to as necessary. He should be shown how to turn himself with the minimum of discomfort, how to effect relaxation of abdominal muscles, deep breathing using the diaphragm, and exercises of the feet and legs. If he knows what is expected of him and why it is done, he will want to take an active part in his recovery.

Lessening anxiety and early mobilisation are a major part of reducing pain, but they are not usually sufficient to reduce the postoperative pain. Strong analgesics such as pethidine, papaveretum and morphine are usually prescribed by the doctor, with antiemetics to prevent nausea and vomiting. Respiratory depression is another unwanted effect of these drugs, particularly in patients with previous respiratory disease, in which case a respiratory stimulant such as doxapram will have been prescribed. The analgesic should be given according to the need of the patient, which is usually 6- to 8-hourly, remembering that analgesics take 20 to 40 minutes to act.

The patient should not be forced to have drugs he does not want, nor should they be withheld. If the analgesic is not given until the pain is severe, it will not be as effective and a larger amount will be required. The way in which an analgesic is given will enhance its effect; patients usually think that an intramuscular injection is more potent than oral administration.

Pain is always worse if there is nothing to distract the individual's mind from it. Therefore the patient may be much more aware of pain at night than during the day. Night sedation, a quiet ward, empty bladder and a warm drink may enhance the effectiveness of analgesia. Counter pain or changing the sensory input will also assist in the relief of the patient's discomfort. This can be done by massaging the affected part, by the application of heat or cold, vibration or electrical stimulation.

If the patient is to undergo a particularly painful procedure which will not last for long, such as removal of a chest drain, dressing of a large wound or physiotherapy, Entonox, a mixture of 50% nitrous oxide (laughing gas) and 50% oxygen, may be given. This is given via a face mask or a mouthpiece, whichever is preferred by the patient. The patient administers the gas himself so there is no danger of too much being given, because the mask is released if the patient becomes drowsy. Two to three minutes inhalation is necessary to allow an adequate concentration to build up.

SUGGESTED WORK

1. Find out how soon after returning from theatre most patients receive their first postoperative analgesic. Is this the same on other surgical wards? If not, what is the reason?
2. Does the frequency with which analgesics are given vary with the type of operation, the age of the patient, or some other factor?

SUGGESTED READING

British National Formulary. London: BMA and The Pharmaceutical Society of Great Britain.

15

Microbiology: Cross-infection and the Surgical Patient

Infection in the surgical patient may lead to chronic debilitating conditions such as fistulae or even death. At the least it will keep the patient in hospital for a longer time, so delaying his return to work. It is therefore of importance to reduce the possibility of this occurring as much as is feasible.

The skin normally acts as a barrier to infection, and surgery immediately opens up this defence. The more extensive the operation, the more susceptible the patient will be to infection. If there is extensive damage to tissue following crush injuries or gangrene, then infection is almost certain to be present. The nutritional state of the patient will determine how effectively his body will be able to fight against infection. The patient who has been unable to eat sufficiently prior to operation, or who is generally debilitated due to chronic illness, will be much more likely to become infected, even from organisms which normally would not cause infection in a healthy person. If the patient's ability to fight infection is reduced due to drugs such as steroids or cytotoxic drugs, micro-organisms will rapidly grow.

Many patients coming into hospital for surgery also have other diseases, such as diabetes, which make them much more vulnerable to infection. Drug addicts and alcoholics also have less resistance to infection. Apart from the physical state of the patient, his psychological state also has an effect on his resistance, and if he is depressed about the long-term effects of the operation, his resistance will be lowered.

In surgery there are many sources of infection, but the main routes are by direct contact or indirectly through contaminated equipment such as suction apparatus, nebulisers, humidifiers, catheters, thermometers, baths, bedpans, crockery, blankets etc. Any procedure which bypasses the normal defence mechanisms of the body, such as catheterisation, or which introduces a foreign substance, such as a prosthesis, makes it easier for organisms to grow. Warmth and moisture provide ideal conditions for organisms and therefore the area around a tracheostomy may easily become infected, and urinary infection will occur if the bladder is not fully emptied.

Direct contact may come from members of the staff who are infected and are still working, or from those who are unknown carriers of infective organisms. Hospital staff frequently carry resistant forms of staphylococci or streptococci around moist areas of the skin. The longer a patient stays in hospital preoperatively, the higher the risk of infection.

MICRO-ORGANISMS MOST COMMONLY FOUND IN SURGICAL PATIENTS

Staphylococcus aureus

This is a Gram-positive coccus which, when looked at under a microscope, is present in clusters. It causes a large number of hospital infections, most commonly wound infections, but may also cause septicaemia, osteomyelitis and meningitis. It may infect tracheostomy wounds, and colonise on replaced heart valves. Spread is by direct contact from another patient or member of staff. Skin conditions such as eczema or psoriasis, if infected, may harbour the organism, and therefore such patients, if on a surgical ward, should be isolated, and staff with these conditions should not work on a surgical ward. Particular care should be taken when shaving a patient preoperatively not to cause nicks in the skin—surgeons often prefer electric razors for this reason. Skin disinfection is always carried out prior to surgery or the introduction of a needle.

Streptococcus pyogenes

This is a Gram-positive coccus which, when looked at under the microscope, is present in chains. It may cause wound infections such as cellulitis and often interferes with the healing of skin grafts. The organism is found in the throats and noses of carriers.

Streptococcus viridans

This is commonly present in the mouth and has an affinity for damaged heart valves, it is therefore a particular problem if the valves are replaced.

Escherichia coli

A Gram-negative rod normally found in the gastrointestinal tract, this bacteria will grow anywhere there are moist conditions. It is spread by contaminating the hands by faeces. The patient may infect himself, or he may be infected by staff, causing wound, respiratory tract or urinary tract infections.

Klebsiella

A Gram-negative rod also found in the gastrointestinal tract, this bacteria also causes wound, respiratory and urinary infection.

Proteus

This is another Gram-negative rod found in the gastrointestinal tract which frequently causes urinary infection but may also affect wounds.

Enterobacter

A Gram-negative rod found in the gastrointestinal tract and causing urinary infection, this bacteria is sometimes found in anaesthetic machines, eyedrops or antiseptic solutions.

Pseudomonas aeruginosa

This Gram-negative rod is also found in the gastrointestinal tract. It thrives in moist conditions such as tracheostomy wounds, nebulisers, or even vases of flowers. Infections from this organism produce a typically green pus with a characteristic smell.

Salmonella species

These Gram-negative rods are present in contaminated food, water and animals such as poultry. This group includes the organisms causing typhoid, paratyphoid and food poisoning. They may also settle in the gall bladder causing cholecystitis.

Clostridia

Gram-positive rods which form spores protecting them from adverse conditions, these organisms are found in conditions where there is a reduced supply of oxygen (anaerobes), such as in deep wounds in damaged tissue, particularly if the blood supply is reduced. They are normally present in the gastrointestinal tract and in soil.

Cl. welchii causes gas gangrene in wounds. The person infected is toxic and complains of pain in the affected area. Cellulitis is present with an unpleasant, smelly discharge.

Cl. tetani causes tetanus or lockjaw and is a potential danger in accidents which have occurred in contaminated soil.

Aspergillus

This is a common fungus which normally does not attack man, but if a patient is on prolonged steroid therapy, then it may infect the lungs.

Candida albicans

A yeast-like fungus this is also an opportunist pathogen and most likely to grow where the normal organisms have been destroyed due to antibiotics. It also attacks patients with a lowered ability to fight infection, such as diabetics. It causes thrush in the mouth and vagina and may cause an intestinal infection.

METHODS TO REDUCE SPREAD OF INFECTION

One of the main approaches to this problem is to reduce the number of organisms available to infect the patient. Standard procedures and a safe code of practice, for example with hepatitis, help to ensure that everyone knows what should be done. A high standard of personal hygiene, both of staff and patients, will help to reduce the bacterial population, particularly if showers are used instead of baths. No infected member of staff should be on duty in a surgical ward, and infected patients should be isolated. Carriers may require specific treatment.

Equipment used for any invasive procedure is sterilised, but in procedures not requiring sterile equipment the terminal disinfection unit may be used instead. The sterilising or cleansing lotions used are tested at intervals for their effectiveness and, if necessary, changed. Where possible, the lotion is supplied in single-use sachets.

Wounds are not touched unnecessarily and may be covered by a plastic spray. When dressing a wound, a non-touch aseptic technique is used; if there is damaged tissue, this is removed by debridement. Patients due to undergo surgery to the gastrointestinal tract not only have a thorough clearance of the bowel, but are also given non-absorbable antibiotics to reduce the number of bacteria. Prior to an amputation the patient will have the skin prepared with povidine compresses or some similar antiseptic.

Any patient who is considered to be particularly at risk of developing an infection will be reversed barrier nursed. He may also be put on antibiotic cover or even given parenteral nutrition. Antitetanus toxoid is given to casualties if it is thought that they are at risk and they have not had a dose in the past year.

All infection should be recorded, the cause found, and further outbreaks prevented.

Destruction of bacteria

The aim is to remove or destroy all pathogenic micro-organisms. In order to be effective, all pus and organic matter should have been removed.

Dry heat

This is an effective and reliable method. Most vegetative bacteria are killed in 10 minutes at a temperature of 65°C. However, staphylococci, tubercle bacillus, and spores may be resistant, and some equipment is damaged by heat.

Moist heat

Although boiling and steam under atmospheric pressure can be used, the most effective is steam under pressure. The time taken and the temperature employed will depend upon the pressure used. Pasteurisation can be used for some fluids which would be damaged by sterilisation.

Irradiation

Infra-red, ultra-violet light and gamma-rays may be used to sterilise items of equipment which would be spoilt by heat. Many commercial packets employ these methods.

Gases

Ethylene oxide 12%, an explosive gas, or formalin and steam may be used for delicate materials where penetration is difficult.

Chemicals

The effectiveness of these is dependent upon the removal of organic matter, the correct strength applied, and sufficient contact time. Hypochlorite solutions, alcohol, iodine and chlorhexidine are amongst those frequently used particularly for cleansing of the skin.

SUGGESTED WORK

1. Find out how the suction apparatus is cleaned and sterilised between patients.

2. If it is possible, visit the laundry and find out if it has any problems regarding the linen sent to it from the wards.

3. See if you can visit the CSSD or terminal disinfection unit, and find out:

(a) which type of equipment is dealt with by each of these departments;

(b) whether any sterile equipment is bought from outside firms;

(c) what methods are used for sterilising equipment.

SUGGESTED READING

Burk E. J. F., Hildick-Smith G. Y. (1978). *The Infection Prone Patient*. Boston: Little Brown.

Campbell Smith, S. (1984). *Infection Nursing*, 1st series 2, 9, 2nd series 7, 8.

Editorial (1980). Hospital infection—the past 10 years and the future. *Journal of Hospital Infection*; **1**: 179–81.

Williams R. E. D. (1978). Infection and the injured patient: lessons and opportunities. *Injury*; p. 9.

16

Tumours and the Role of Radiotherapy in Surgery

Neoplasms (or new growths) arise as a result of a change in any one of the types of cell in the body. The increase in the number of cells is greater than that required for normal replacement, and although they may retain some of the functions of the tissue they are not beneficial to the body. Some are very slow growing but others may be extremely rapid.

Although the word tumour is often applied to such growths it has a much wider meaning. The literal translation is 'swelling' and therefore it can be applied to temporary swellings such as occur with inflammation, cysts or in a pyloric stenosis.

Neoplasms can arise from any tissue in the body, although they are much more likely to do so in, for example, epithelium, than in nervous or muscle tissue, a factor which appears to be related to the ability of the tissue to replace itself. Although a neoplastic growth usually consists of one type of cell, at times there are more. It usually starts to grow in one particular site but may spread to other parts. However, there are some neoplasms, such as lymphosarcoma, which may develop in several places at the same time.

In most cases we do not know why neoplasms occur. Several members in a family may develop the same type of growth, suggesting that there is a genetic predisposition to the condition, or, conversely, a resistance in those who do not develop the disease. Certain substances such as nicotine are known to cause the development of malignant tumours.

Neoplasms can be divided into two broad groups (benign and malignant) according to certain characteristics. Figure 16.1 and Table 16.1 show the main differences between these two groups of neoplasms.

Gastric ulcers, ulcerative colitis, polyps of the large bowel and skin damaged by ultra-violet rays are premalignant conditions which, if they persist over a number of years, are liable to undergo malignant change.

Tumours are classified according to the tissue in which they arise (Table 16.2). Tumours of the nervous system are called *neuromas* (these are rare) and those of the nerve sheath *neuroblastomas*. The latter occur mainly in children. Tumours of the brain and spinal cord (*gliomas*) are unencapsulated and tend to infiltrate. Malignant proliferation of the white blood cells is called *leukaemia*, and of the lymphatic tissue *malignant lymphoma*, *lymphosarcoma* or *reticulum cell sarcoma* (e.g. Hodgkin's disease).

SPREAD OF MALIGNANT TUMOURS

Local spread

This occurs directly into those organs or structures which are in direct contact with the tumour. It may be into the skin overlying the tumour, as in carcinoma of the breast, or, as in the case of carcinoma of the uterus, to the bladder and rectum.

Lymphatic spread

Malignant cells may grow down into the lymphatic vessels or break off and travel as emboli to the

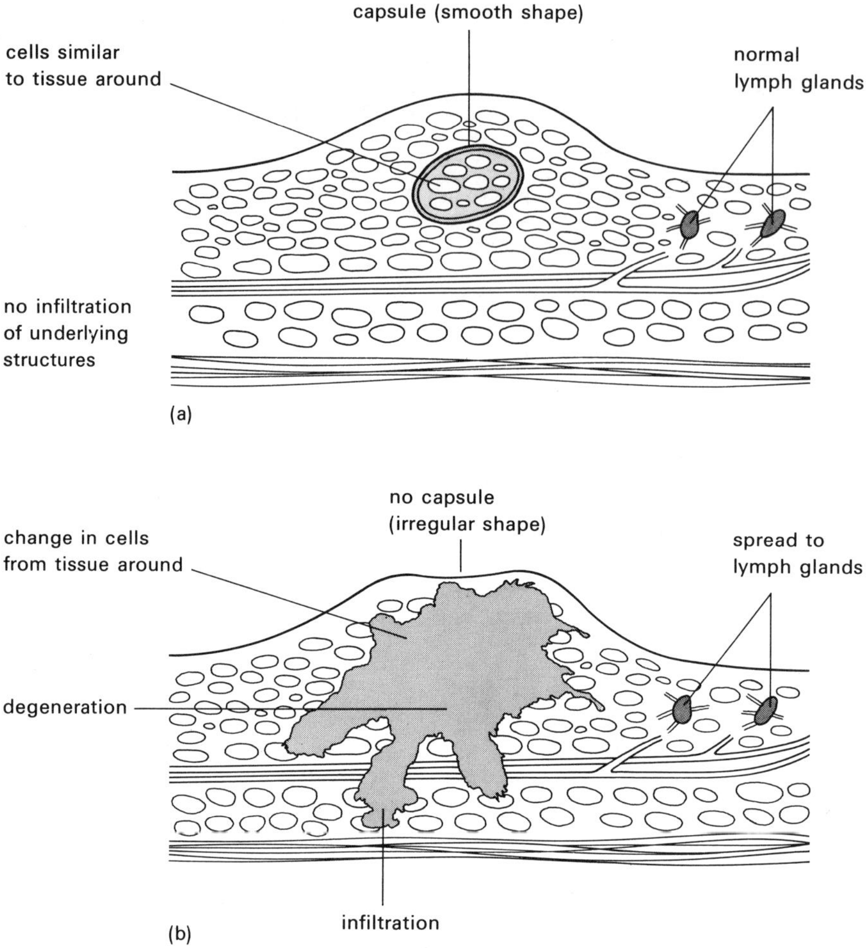

Fig. 16.1 *(a) Benign tumour. (b) Malignant tumour.*

nearest lymph nodes, and from there on to other organs of the body. They are particularly likely to travel to the bones, and the peritoneal and pleural cavities.

Through the bloodstream

The venous drainage of an affected organ may carry malignant cells on to the next organ in its path. Carcinoma of the intestinal tract can travel via the mesenteric veins to the portal vein and so carry malignant cells to the liver.

Implantation

This most commonly occurs in the peritoneal cavity where malignant cells, having reached the upper part of the abdominal cavity through the lymphatics, spread to the lower organs and peritoneum. This type of spread may also occur during operation, however careful the surgeon may be.

THE ROLE OF RADIOTHERAPY IN SURGERY

Radiotherapy is a treatment in its own right for many conditions such as a rodent ulcer and at

Table 16.1 Characteristics of benign and malignant neoplasms

Benign	Malignant
Cells are similar to those of the tissue in which they arise	The shape and appearance of the cells change rapidly from those of the tissue in which they arise
Growth is usually slow	Growth is rapid
Surrounded by a fibrous capsule	No capsule
Do not usually degenerate	Degeneration occurs at the centre due to lack of blood supply
May press on other structures or displace them, but do not infiltrate them	Destroy the tissue in which they arise and infiltrate into the surrounding organs along the line of least resistance
Remain at the site in which they arise and do not spready by metastasis	Spread to other organs via the lymphatics, bloodstream, and into serous cavities
May be oversecretion of a gland	Loss of function or inappropriate function of gland.
	Sometimes take on the function of the tissue in which they arise
	May be hormone dependent
	May be cachexia (loss of weight)

certain stages of carcinoma of the cervix. It may also be used palliatively to reduce the side-effects of inoperable malignant conditions, such as the pain in bone metastases, ulceration in breast cancer, or dysphagia in carcinoma of the oesophagus. However, radiotherapy may also be used in conjunction with surgery in malignant conditions to reduce the size of a tumour, so making it possible to operate. Spread may be prevented by irradiating the regional lymph nodes and, in certain types of cancer which have a tendency to recur, radiotherapy may help to prevent this. In cases where it is not possible to remove the growth totally, the remaining tissue may be destroyed by radiotherapy.

In 1895 Röntgen discovered x-rays while passing a high-voltage current through a vacuum tube, and in 1902 Marie and Pierre Curie produced radium. These discoveries opened up the way for new methods of diagnosis and treatment.

All substances are made up of millions of atoms, each of which consists of neutrons, protons and electrons. At the centre of each atom is the nucleus which contains the neutral neutrons and the positively charged protons. Arranged in orbits around the nucleus are the negatively charged electrons. The number of these component parts varies according to the substance. Sometimes the combination of neutrons and protons is unstable and may break up into a more stable form. Unstable substances undergoing this break up are said to be radioactive. In radiotherapy, artificially produced radioactive substances are also used.

Radiation may be used as x-rays from a machine, such as cobalt or caesium beams; the source may be *sealed* in solid containers such as tubes, needles, grains or wires; or the radioactive material may be unsealed in a liquid which may be drunk or injected.

The curie, millicurie and microcurie indicate how much radioactivity is present. The rad, röntgen, and rem are comparable terms, the measurement used depending on the type of radiation involved. (The rem is the amount of radiation absorbed in rads adjusted according to its effectiveness on the tissue receiving it. For practical purposes it can be taken to be equal to a rad or röntgen.) The dose of radiotherapy required by the different malignant tumours varies, but the most rapidly dividing are the most effectively treated. As the substance destroys itself, the time taken to reach half its original activity is said to be its *half-life.*

The further away one is from the source of radiation, the smaller the dose received. For example, if the distance is doubled, a quarter of the dose is received; and it is trebled, a ninth of the dose is received. For radioactivity to be fully effective the tissues must be well oxygenated, which is often not true of malignant tumours. In this case hyperbaric oxygen (oxygen under pressure) aids the efficiency of the radiotherapy.

Treatment by external beams of radiation

The aim of the treatment is to concentrate as much of the energy on the tumour as possible and spare

Table 16.2 Classification of tumours

	Benign		Malignant	
Tissue	Tumour	Examples	Tumour	Examples
Epithelium	Papilloma	Bladder, rectum, skin warts	Carcinoma	Gastrointestinal tract, respiratory tract, bladder, skin (rodent ulcers)
Glandular	Adenoma	Breast, pancreas, thyroid	Adenocarcinoma	Gastrointestinal tract
Connective			Sarcoma	
Fibrous	Fibroma	Gums, skin,	Fibrosarcoma	Developing from fibroma
Fatty	Lipoma	Neck, shoulders	Liposarcoma	
Bone	Osteoma	Ends of long bones	Osteosarcoma	
Cartilage	Chondroma	Ends of long bones, fingers	Chondrosarcoma	
Muscle	Myoma	Uterus (fibroids)	Myosarcoma	
smooth	Leiomyoma			
striated	Rhabdomyoma			
Lymphatic vessels	Lymphangioma	Neck, tongue	Lymphangiosarcoma	
Blood vessels	Haemangioma	Birth mark, abdomen, brain, skin	Haemangiosarcoma	

the normal tissues. In order to do this the physicist must measure the landmarks of the body meticulously. He has to take into consideration the amount of radiation other tissues may suffer without damage, avoiding as much as possible vulnerable areas such as the spinal cord or eyes. With the radiographer, he will calculate the dosage required and how much is to be given at what interval (Figs. 16.2 and 16.3).

The patient is positioned on a treatment table and the machine, (which is very large) is positioned over him. Because of the danger of repeated radiation to the staff, the patient is left alone and the machine operated from outside the room. There is an observation window and the patient has some means of contacting the staff. Although there is no discomfort from the treatment itself, anymore than with an x-ray, it can be very frightening for the patient. The procedure takes only a few minutes, and may be repeated three times in a week for 4 to 6 weeks. If the patient is fit enough, the treatments can be carried out on an out-patient basis.

Frequently a combination of beam radiation and a sealed source (Table 16.3) is used at different times. Surgeons may insert metal clips when operating in order to show where the tumour is and therefore enable the radiotherapy to be focused on it.

Great care has to be taken by the doctor when inserting these sealed sources of radiation (Fig. 16.4) in order to limit the contact time of himself and other members of staff. Some of them have to be introduced under a general anaesthetic. In order to reduce the contact time for staff, a non-radioactive container may be introduced, and when in the correct position the radioactive substance placed in it. Unsealed sources are also used (see Table 16.4).

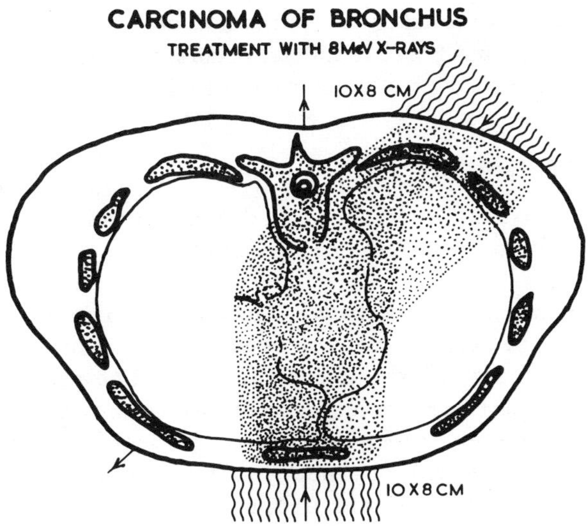

Fig. 16.2 *Carcinoma of the bronchus. Treatment with x-rays.*

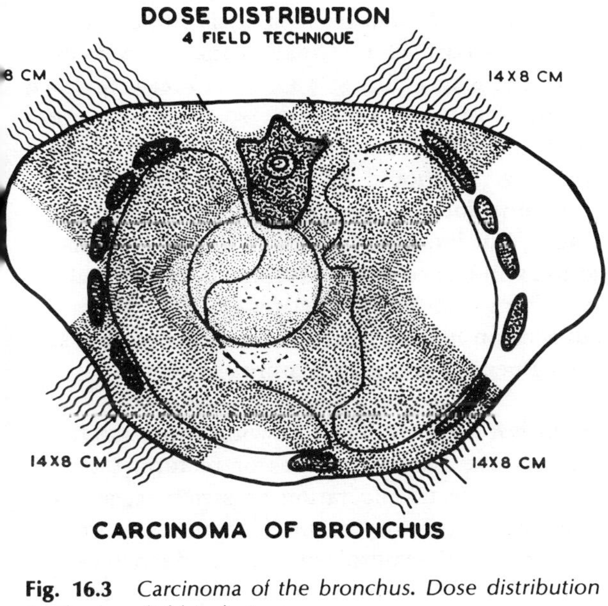

Fig. 16.3 *Carcinoma of the bronchus. Dose distribution by the four-field technique.*

Table 16.3 Sealed sources

Substance	Container	Use	Half-life
Cobalt-60	Tubes, needles	External	5.3 years
Gold-198	Grains	Implanted, e.g. bladder	2.7 days
Iridium-192	Grains, wires	Lymph nodes, breast lumps	74 days
Caesium-137	Needles, tubes	Tongue, mouth, cervix	30 years
Yttrium Y-90	Rods	Pituitary gland	2.5 days
Strontium-90	Plaques	For surface application, particularly to the eye	
Radium (used less nowadays)	Needles, tubes	Cervix, body of uterus, tongue, some skin	1620 years

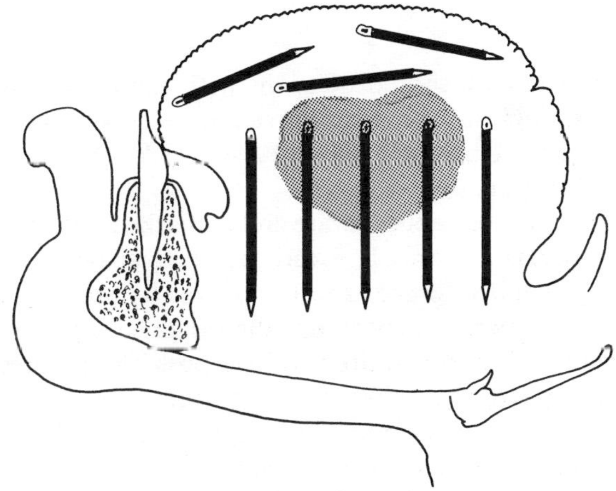

Fig. 16.4 *Needles implanted into the tongue.*

Responsibilities of the nurse caring for patients undergoing radiotherapy

All staff in frequent contact with radioactive material should wear a film to measure the amount of radiation received. The maximum permissible dose is 3 rem in 13 weeks or 5 rem in 1 year. (For further information see *The Safe Use of Ionizing Radiations* (1973), London: HMSO.)

Table 16.4 Unsealed sources

Substance	Method of administration	Use	Half-life (days)
Iodine-131 (colourless, tasteless liquid)	Oral	Cancer of thyroid, thyrotoxicosis	8
Gold-198	Instillation	Peritoneum, pleura	2.7
Phosphorus-32	Injection	Polycythaemia	14

External beams

Although great care has to be taken not to stay with the patient when he is receiving his dose of radiation, the patient himself is not radioactive and is therefore not a source of danger to others. He may remain in close contact with other people without any risk to them. The nurse's main responsibility will be to ensure that the patient has received an adequate explanation of what to expect, to reassure him, and to deal with any side-effects.

Sealed sources

As little time should be spent with the patient as possible, just sufficient to give the necessary nursing care. Obviously he will have to be given an explanation.

The bed is kept separate and is marked with the appropriate symbol. Lead protective barriers, long-handled forceps and lead boxes for transport of the radioactive substance should all be available and used where required. Where possible, needles etc. should be checked 4-hourly at least. A note is kept of the time of insertion or application and care is taken to remove the source at the correct time and in the correct manner. Loss is reported at once and nothing removed from the ward until the radioactive substance has been found.

Unsealed sources

In this case there is risk both from radiation and from contamination as a result of spillage.

As before, the patient is isolated. Special precautions are taken in the method of disposing of excreta and linen. If spillage occurs, there are very strict procedures which must be adhered to.

Adverse reactions to radiation

The effects of radiation will depend on which part of the body is being treated and the dosage used.

In the region of the mouth The mucous membrane may become dry with an associated inflammation which may allow infection to enter. The patient will therefore lose his sense of taste and with this his appetite. If *Monilia albicans* is present, nystatin will be prescribed by the doctor. Oral care will be of great importance, with frequent mouth washes and a soft tooth brush. The patient should be encouraged to drink plenty and a soft diet provided.

In the thoracic region The care described here applies following treatment of the breasts, lungs or oesophagus. Dermatitis, dysphagia and pneumonitis can occur. The dermatitis may vary from a mild erythema (redness) to a moist breaking down of the skin. To avoid this, soap or any other unprescribed substances, should not be used on the area. It should be patted not rubbed dry. Calamine lotion may be sufficient in the early stages, but later gentian violet or hydrocortisone lotion will be necessary. Dysphagia may be helped by giving aluminium hydroxide gel (Mucaine) suspension half an hour before meals, with a soft diet. Pneumonitis may require antibiotics.

In the pelvic region The following applies to treatment of the bladder, uterus or rectum. Cystitis, diarrhoea, rectal ulceration or stricture, and vaginal discharges may occur. Kaolin and morphine mixture or other antidiarrhoeal medicines can be used to control the diarrhoea. Nystatin pessaries may be required if a *Monilia albicans* infection is present in the vagina. Fluids should be encouraged and roughage reduced. Potassium citrate mixture may help the bladder irritation.

The brain Headaches, vomiting, visual disturbances and possibly fits may be present due to cerebral oedema. Anticonvulsants, analgesics and antiemetics may be ordered. To reduce cerebral oedema the doctor may prescribe dexamethasone or another steroid.

The blood Anaemia and leukaemia may arise as a result of radiation and may necessitate a blood transfusion.

SUGGESTED WORK

1. Find out if any of the patients on your ward having surgery for a malignant condition will be having any form of radiotherapy.

(a) For what reason are they having it?

(b) What special precautions and care will be required?

Section II

17

Appendicitis and Peritonitis

The emphasis in the nursing care of these conditions is on the very careful observation of the patient that is necessary, any changes being reported to the doctor promptly, as immediate attention may be life saving. They frequently present as surgical emergencies and therefore the nurse must recognise those aspects of the preoperative preparation which are essential and those which may be omitted.

The vermiform appendix is a blind-ended tube about 7.5 cm long, although it can vary from this considerably. It is attached to the caecum, but the actual position varies from being tucked up behind the caecum (retrocaecal) to hanging down over the pelvic brim (Fig. 17.1). It is similar in structure to the caecum, with a lining of mucous membrane and two layers of muscle, although, unlike the caecum, the outer longitudinal coat is complete. Peritoneum covers it. A large amount of lymphoid tissue in the walls helps to localise infection.

The peritoneum is a thin, smooth, slippery membrane which lines the abdominal cavity and covers all the organs within it. It is a serous membrane and is therefore capable of absorbing and secreting large amounts of fluid. It is also a double membrane, the layer in contact with the abdominal wall being called the parietal layer, and that which covers the organs, the visceral layer. The parietal layer has a very extensive sensory nerve supply and is therefore sensitive to reflex and inflammatory irritation.

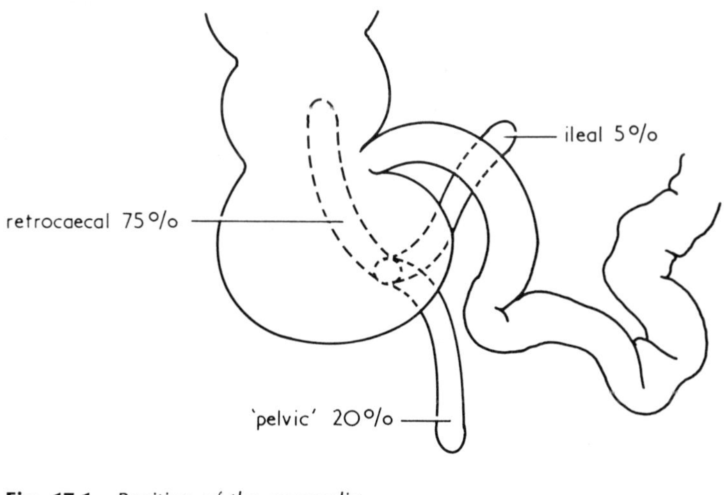

Fig. 17.1 *Position of the appendix.*

Specific emphasis in the nursing history

Elimination. Find out from the patient whether he has any disturbance of bowel function.

Vomiting. Note the presence of nausea or vomiting, its character, the amount, and how long it has been present.

Nutrition. Find out what the patient's appetite has been like.

Vital signs. Note any increase in temperature and pulse rate.

Pain. Find out where the pain is and if it has altered its position. Note the type of pain and any changes in its character.

General appearance. Is the abdomen distended or the patient frightened to move because of pain?

APPENDICITIS

The actual cause of appendicitis is not known, but it is much more common in the West than in the poorer countries, which suggests that diet is a contributory factor. It occurs most commonly between the ages of 10 and 25 years. The appendix becomes blocked due to an inflammatory swelling of the mucosa or a bolus of food, and infection arises from the presence of *Esch. coli* and *Streptococcus faecalis.* The organ tries to expel its contents, which causes the typical colicky pain. Following this the inflammation spreads to the peritoneum around the appendix and this causes the localised pain in the right iliac fossa. If a blockage has occurred from a bolus of food, the blood supply to that section of the intestine will be cut off and the part will become gangrenous. This may then rupture, causing a localised abscess or generalised peritonitis.

Clinical picture

The patient may have been aware of vague abdominal discomfort, indigestion, or alternating constipation and diarrhoea, or the attack may have begun without any warning. Initially the patient complains of a generalised colicky abdominal pain which increases in intensity and is mainly in the umbilical region. This later becomes a persistent, sharp pain localised to the right iliac fossa. When the doctor examines the abdomen, particularly if this is after 12 or more hours, rigidity is present. Tenderness will occur especially in the right iliac fossa at McBurney's point (Fig. 17.2). If the doctor removes his examining hand suddenly from the right iliac fossa, the patient will complain of a sudden sharp pain (rebound tenderness). Pressure on the left iliac fossa may cause pain on the right side due to the transmission of pressure by the gas-filled intestines (Rovsing's sign). If the appendix is in the pelvis, there will also be tenderness on rectal examination.

There will be a loss of appetite with nausea which may be accompanied by vomiting, breath that smells and a furred tongue. Initially the

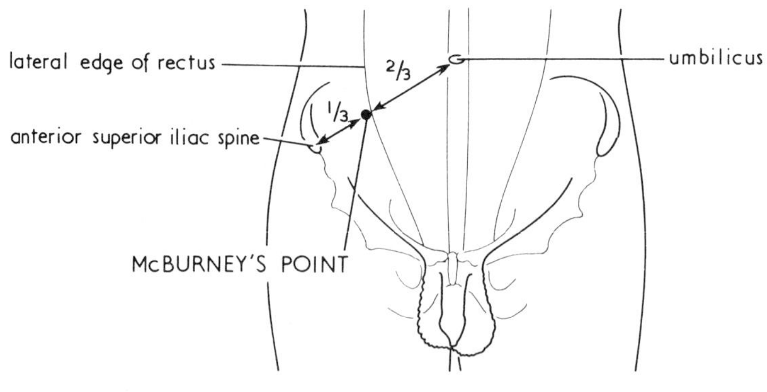

Fig. 17.2 *Main area of tenderness in appendicitis.*

temperature rises slightly, increasing later up to 39°C. At the same time the rate of the pulse will also increase up to 100 beats per minute. Although constipation is most likely to occur, diarrhoea may be present.

Management

These patients are treated by an appendicectomy unless there is an abscess, which would be indicated by a high swinging temperature, raised pulse rate and sweating. On examination the blood will show a marked increase in the number of white blood cells (leucocytosis).

Specific preoperative preparation

This is usually an emergency operation and so the nurse must check if the patient has eaten in the last 4 hours or if he has been vomiting. If he has eaten or vomiting is present, a nasogastric tube will be passed and aspirated. If there are urinary symptoms indicating that the appendix is near the bladder, the patient will also be catheterised. The nasogastric tube will be kept in position if there is any suggestion of peritonitis, and an intravenous infusion set up.

The operation

A skin incision is made by the surgeon in the right iliac fossa (Lanz incision) to produce a good cosmetic effect when it heals. After ligating or using diathermy on the superficial blood vessels, the muscles are divided in the same direction as their fibres. The peritoneum is then incised and the caecum and appendix brought to the surface. The mesentery to the appendix is cut and the base of the appendix crushed and tied with a ligature. Around the base of the appendix a purse-string suture is inserted; the appendix is then cut away and its stump inverted into the caecum by means of the purse-string suture. The abdomen is then closed without drainage, unless the appendix was perforated. In this case the intraperitoneal drain is usually brought out to the surface by a separate incision.

Specific postoperative care

If the removal of the appendix was straightforward, without any drainage, the usual postoperative care will be given, the stitches being removed on the fifth to seventh day. No solids are allowed until bowel sounds return, which is usually within 12 to 24 hours of the operation. Sips of fluids may be given if vomiting is not present. If the patient complains of distension, movement should be encouraged, and a flatus tube or enema may be required. Oral laxatives or suppositories will be given to stimulate the action of the bowel on the third day. If a drain is in position, this will need the usual attention and observations. The patient should be observed for any evidence of complications.

Complications

Peritonitis

This will be indicated by a raised temperature, pain which persists on or after the second postoperative day, and slight tenderness at a site away from the wound. There may be vomiting or, if a nasogastric tube is in position, a large amount of aspirate, and the abdomen may be distended. With all patients following an abdominal operation there will be some pain and pyrexia and with the administration of analgesics and hypnotics the symptoms may be masked. (See the section on peritonitis for the care and observations, p. 99.)

Abscesses

Abscesses, which are most commonly in the right iliac fossa or the pelvis, give rise to symptoms between the third and sixth day after the operation (Fig. 17.3). A subphrenic abscess less commonly occurs, and may be associated with a paralysed diaphragm and pneumonia. There is a swinging temperature, raised pulse and the passage of mucus *per rectum*. Antibiotics will be prescribed and a drainage tube may need to be inserted by the surgeon. X-rays will have been taken to confirm the diagnosis.

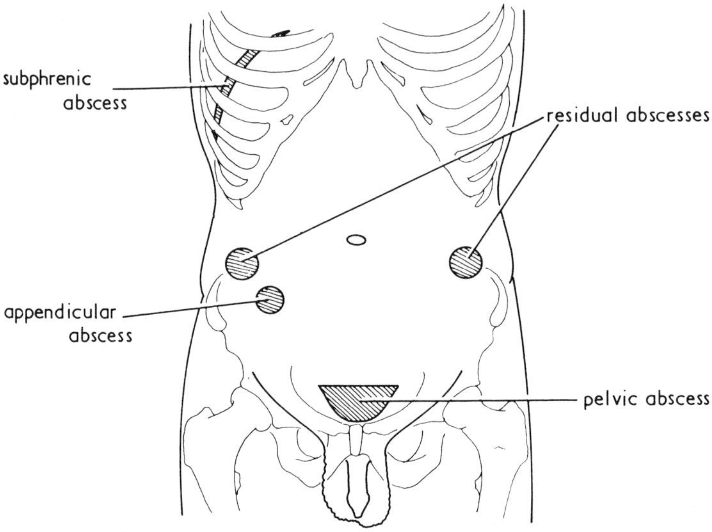

Fig. 17.3 *Common sites of abscesses arising after appendicectomy.*

Paralytic ileus

This is a condition in which there is a paralysis of the small intestine, so causing an intestinal obstruction. There is always some degree of this after an abdominal operation in which the intestines have been handled, but it may become more severe if the operation was long and complicated or if peritonitis is present. The bowel sounds are completely absent and there is no passage of faeces or flatus. As a result, the abdomen becomes distended with gas and fluid and the patient vomits repeatedly without effort. If a nasogastric tube is in position, the amount of aspirate will increase. X-ray films taken with the patient in the upright position will show fluid levels and gas in the small intestine.

A nasogastric tube must be passed to relieve the distension and the contents carefully recorded on a fluid balance chart. If severe distension is present, a Miller–Abbott tube is used (this is described in Chapter 11). An intravenous infusion will be commenced to restore the large amounts of fluid and electrolytes lost in vomiting and into the abdominal cavity. Sodium and potassium are the most important of these electrolytes, and frequent blood tests will be taken to monitor their levels so that they can be accurately replaced. Low levels of potassium increase a paralytic ileus and may lead to a cardiac arrest. Once bowel sounds are present, and the aspirate minimal, the patient may start graduated oral fluids. When he is taking adequate amounts of fluid, his electrolytes are in balance and he is no longer dehydrated, the intravenous infusion can be discontinued. The underlying cause of the paralytic ileus must be treated. If this is peritonitis, surgery will be necessary. If it arises following surgery, a drain may have to be inserted. Broad-spectrum antibiotics will also be necessary.

Faecal fistula

This may arise if the appendix stump breaks down allowing leakage from the caecum. If it does not heal spontaneously, an operation may be necessary to close it. Until this is done the abdominal skin will need to be protected from the discharge by applications of aluminium paste or other barrier creams, and a special collecting bag can be applied.

Portal pyaemia and pylephlebitis (liver abscess)

This is due to septic emboli passing up the portal vein to the liver. The patient will have a pyrexia, rigors, a rapid pulse, pain over the liver area and slight jaundice. It can be a rapidly fatal condition, with vomiting and diarrhoea in the final stages. Antibiotics and operative measures to drain the abscess will be taken.

A persistent sinus

Due to a foreign body (faecal concretions) or an unremoved portion of the appendix, this will require surgical treatment.

Deep vein thrombosis and pulmonary complications may also arise and these are dealt with elsewhere (see Chapter 7).

From these complications it will be seen that a wide range of observations will be required, including the regular monitoring of the temperature and pulse, and the recognition of any abnormal abdominal symptoms such as vomiting or a distended abdomen.

PERITONITIS

Although peritonitis may arise following an operation in the abdominal cavity, it can also occur without an operation having been performed. However, in the majority of cases it develops as a result of disease or injury to one of the abdominal organs (Fig. 17.4). The following causes are some examples.

1. Perforation of one of the abdominal organs or an extension of inflammation from one of them. The most common causes are: a perforated appendix, duodenal ulcer, or an acutely inflamed gall bladder. However, regional ileitis, ulcerative colitis, diverticulitis, ulcerating cancer of the stomach or large intestines, acute intestinal obstruction and various pelvic conditions can all lead to peritonitis.

2. Penetrating wounds of the abdominal wall and trauma due to abdominal surgery.

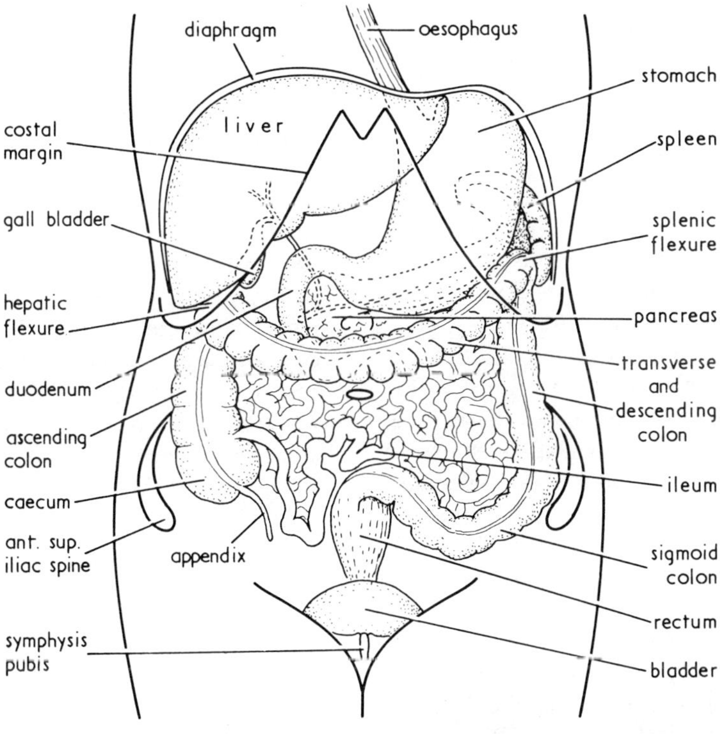

Fig. 17.4 *Diagram showing those organs which may rupture and cause peritonitis.*

3. Infection via the bloodstream (septicaemia). Although the inflammation usually arises from infection by *Esch. coli* or *Streptococcus faecalis*, it is occasionally caused by pancreatic juice or blood in the peritoneal cavity, both of which are irritating substances. Small amounts of blood are frequently found in the abdominal cavity in women without effect, but if larger amounts are released, as with a tubal pregnancy or, rarely, a ruptured aortic aneurysm, then peritonitis will follow. Acute pancreatitis allows the release of the pancreatic juice with its digestive enzymes into the peritoneal cavity.

As a result of the inflammation an excess amount of serous fluid is produced, and if bacterial infection is present, this may be purulent. The peritoneum, and in particular the greater omentum, seeks to seal off the inflamed area, so that initially the peritonitis is localised. If this localisation is successful, it will remain as an abscess. However, if the inflammation is such that it cannot be contained, an acute diffuse peritonitis will be present. This will lead to adjacent peritoneal surfaces becoming adherent, so forming adhesions in which coils of bowel are bound together and peristaltic activity of the intestines is reduced.

Clinical picture

The patient may give some indication of previous abdominal disease which has led to the peritonitis. The most important symptom is the severe abdominal pain and tenderness (Fig. 17.5). The patient tries to avoid any movement, as this increases the pain, in fact he will often lie with his knees drawn up and has an anxious look on his face.

The abdomen is rigid and boardlike due to a spasm of the muscles, but later it becomes distended, as the paralysis of the small intestine occurs. Nausea and vomiting are early signs. Initially the vomit is of gastric contents, then bile, and later copious, slightly faeculent fluid. Diminishing bowel sounds lead to constipation and lack of flatus. Eventually there will be no bowel sounds at all. The pulse rate rises steadily, becoming more and more difficult to feel as the blood pressure falls. The temperature is raised up to 39°C and respirations are shallow as the patient tries to minimise the pain. The tongue is thickly furred, becoming dry and brown, and the breath has an unpleasant smell. Blood taken for examination shows a marked increase in white cells of 20 000 per litre or more. In the final stages the patient has a pinched appearance with sunken eyes, the temperature falls to subnormal, the abdomen is distended with gas and intestinal contents, the breathing becomes even more shallow and the pain disappears.

Management

Unless the peritonitis is due to pancreatitis, an operation will be necessary to remove the cause. The patient should have nothing by mouth, and a nasogastric tube is passed to aspirate the contents of the stomach. In order to replace the large amounts of fluid and electrolytes lost, an intravenous infusion is commenced. To combat the infection, large amounts of antibiotics are given which will continue after surgery. Once the patient has been diagnosed, analgesics such as morphia will be necessary to relieve the pain and therefore reduce shock. The patient is best in a sitting position or with the head of the bed raised to encourage drainage into the pelvic region rather than under the diaphragm. Because the mouth is dry and unpleasant (due to many factors), it will need careful attention. The patient will need frequent washes to keep him cool and fresh, but care should be taken when moving him as he will find it very painful. If the patient becomes very restless and disorientated, he may require cot sides. An x-ray will be taken with the patient in the upright position to see if there is any gas or fluid in the peritoneal cavity.

Observations while awaiting operation

The nurse should note any change from the boardlike rigidity to a softer more distended abdomen as this will indicate a deterioration in the patient's condition. Measuring the girth will give an objective measurement. At the same time she should notice whether there is any change in the intensity of the pain, or if it changes position. She will be monitoring the temperature, pulse and respiration for relevant changes. A fluid balance chart will record vomit and aspirate and any increase will be reported. This care will be continued postoperatively.

CHRONIC PERITONITIS

This condition is less common and is usually a result of infection by the tubercle bacillus. The inflammatory changes mainly affect the parietal peritoneum and the surface of the intestines. It may go on to cause adhesions and intestinal obstruction, ascites or a number of cold abscesses and fistulae.

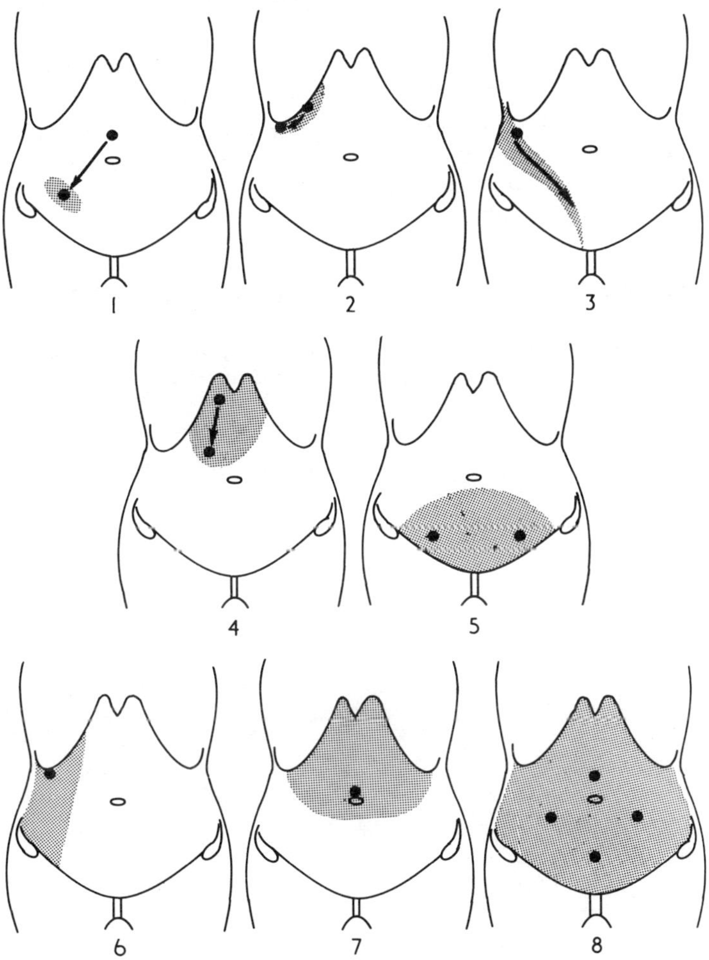

Fig. 17.5 *Sites of rigidity and pain in acute abdominal lesions.* **1.** *Appendicitis.* **2.** *Biliary colic and acute cholecystitis.* **3.** *Renal colic and pyelitis.* **4.** *Peptic ulceration.* **5.** *Acute gynaecological lesions.* **6.** *Pneumonia (right).* **7.** *Acute pancreatitis.* **8.** *Acute diffuse peritonitis.*

The treatment is that for tuberculosis unless an obstruction is present, in which case surgery will be required.

Intestinal Obstruction

This may arise within a few days following peritonitis due to adhesions, but because the adhesions are soft and fibrinous it may subside if treated by gastrointestinal aspiration. The obstruction which can arise at a later date is described elsewhere (see Chapter 19).

Residual abscesses

These may also occur following peritonitis and are indicated by vomiting and fever. They are found in the pelvis, the right and left iliac fossa, and near the liver, and will require drainage and antibiotics.

MECKEL'S DIVERTICULUM

This is a congenital abnormality in which there is a blind-ended tube 6–7 cm long and about 1 m above the ileocaecal valve. In the first few weeks of fetal life this tube was a duct connecting the intestinal tract to the yolk sac, which normally disappears early in fetal life. Like the appendix, inflammation, perforation or twisting leading to gangrene may occur. It presents in a similar manner to appendicitis and is treated by removal of the diverticulum.

SUGGESTED WORK

1. Note the incidence of the various complications arising following an appendicectomy in your hospital. Why did they occur? Could they have been prevented?

SUGGESTED READING

Silver E., Silver A. J. (1984). Acute abdomen. *Medicine in Practice*; **2**: 1.

18

Gastric Conditions

Any operation breaching the gastrointestinal tract within the abdominal cavity presents certain problems. The first of these is the spillage of the contents containing gastric juice which is acid and irritating to the organs it comes in contact with. If the operation involves the tract below the stomach, there will also be a large number of potential pathogens. Without adequate preoperative preparation these factors will lead to peritonitis.

The tract is necessary for the introduction of food and for its absorption into the body. However, where an incision has been made it must be given the opportunity to heal. It will therefore be necessary to find some other means of supplying nutrients to the patient, which will require much more accurate monitoring.

The higher the operation is in the abdominal cavity, the more likely it is that the surgeon will have retracted the diaphragm during surgery. This leads to the patient suffering pain if he breathes deeply, so causing shallow breathing and the possibility of respiratory disorders. Operations including the tract below the stomach may require extensive handling of the intestines, resulting in a paralytic ileus. This disruption to the activity of the tract may cause an electrolyte imbalance, with nausea and vomiting.

It can therefore be seen that apart from the general considerations that are required to nurse any surgical patient, there will also be some which need to be emphasised more fully when nursing the patient who has had gastric surgery.

Specific emphasis in the nursing history

Social. Note any factors contributing to the condition, such as divorce, bereavement or other family problems.

Occupation. Note not only the type of work but the patient's attitude to it and to his colleagues at work.

Nutrition. Note the type of food eaten and its nutritive value, regularity of meals, appetite and the presence of nausea or vomiting.

General appearance. Note any loss of weight.

Attitude. Note the presence of anxiety or tenseness and find the cause.

Respiratory function. Note the evidence of heavy smoking and the presence of a cough.

Pain. Note the relationship of the pain to meals and the effect on it of eating.

Previous medication. Find out what prescribed drugs the patient has been taking, particularly any antirheumatic or steroid drugs. Also find out from the patient if he has been taking any non-prescribed drugs such as aspirin.

CARCINOMA OF THE STOMACH

Carcinoma of the stomach is more common in males over the age of 45 in the lower social groups. It is the fourth most common cancer in Great Britain and there appears to be a familial tendency, those with group A blood having a higher incidence. The cause is unknown; however, chronic conditions of the stomach such as gastritis, gastric ulcers and polyps appear to be predisposing factors. There is also a high association of gastric cancer with pernicious anaemia in which there is achlorhydria and gastric atrophy.

Because there are not usually any symptoms in the early stages of the disease, it tends to be diagnosed late, after it has spread to neighbouring organs and via the lymphatics to the liver, lungs, brain and bones. Symptoms which may arise are anorexia associated with weight loss, dysphagia, fullness or bloating after meals, boring epigastric pain, nausea and vomiting. There may also be anaemia due to chronic blood loss.

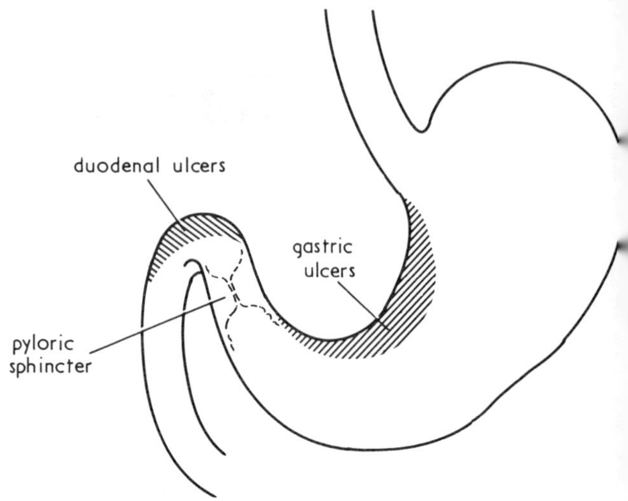

Fig. 18.1 *Positions of peptic ulcers.*

PEPTIC ULCERS

Peptic ulcers may occur in the lower end of the oesophagus, the lower curvature of the stomach, the duodenum or jejenum, the most common being those in the duodenum. The ulcer may be superficial, affecting the mucosa only, or it may penetrate the submucosa and even through the muscle layer perforating into the abdominal cavity. Haemorrhage will only occur if the ulcer erodes a blood vessel. The cause of peptic ulcers is unknown, and although gastric and duodenal ulcers have some factors in common, it is thought that there are sufficient differences to suggest that they are two distinct conditions (Fig. 18.1). Severe physical stress, such as multiple fractures and severe burns, and emotional stress are associated with both types of ulcer.

The gastric ulcer

There is a greater incidence of this condition in the lower social classes, particularly after the age of 50. It occurs equally in men and women but there does not appear to be any family history. Drugs containing salicylates, such as aspirin, and those drugs used in the treatment of rheumatic conditions predispose to gastric ulcers. When aspirin is ingested it may enter the gastric epithelial cells, particularly if the stomach is empty. The change in the pH causes the drug to remain localised, so allowing it to damage the mucosa. Analysis of the gastric contents shows no increase of acid.

The individual will complain of a dull, gnawing, epigastric pain, usually within 30 minutes of a meal. Anorexia and weight loss may be present and vomiting often relieves the pain. In a small percentage of patients the condition may become malignant.

The duodenal ulcer

Although this condition appears to affect most social classes, there is a strong family history. Men are much more likely to acquire the condition than women, and it is often first apparent in the younger adult. Patients with chronic bronchitis and coronary artery disease have a higher incidence than the general population. The ulcer usually appears in the duodenal cap and is associated with an increased level of acidity in the stomach.

The epigastric pain, which is also dull and gnawing, usually occurs at night when there is a long gap between meals and is relieved by antacids or food. This condition is characterised by remissions and relapses and does not become malignant.

Diagnosis

Fibreoptic endoscopy with biopsy and barium meal studies are the most useful diagnostic aids for both carcinoma of the stomach and peptic ulcers. Faecal occult blood will indicate any bleeding. Blood tests for iron deficiency anaemia and pernicious anaemia, particularly in gastric cancer, are necessary. Analysis of gastric secretions will show hyperacidity in a duodenal ulcer or achlorhydria in carcinoma of the stomach. A laparoscopy may be done if secondaries are suspected in the liver or peritoneum.

Surgery

Truncal vagotomy

This is only done for a duodenal ulcer if medical treatment has failed (Fig. 18.2). The gastric glands which secrete hydrochloric acid are stimulated by the vagus nerve (Fig. 18.3) which secretes acetylcholine at its terminal ends. Therefore cutting the vagus nerve, as is done in this operation, causes the stimulation of the gastric glands, and thus the amount of hydrochloric acid produced, to be reduced. However, this also reduces the muscular activity of the stomach and therefore delays its emptying. In order to help the stomach to empty, a pyloroplasty is performed (Fig. 18.4). The pyloric opening is enlarged and the sphincter put out of action by a longitudinal incision which is sutured transversely. Alternatively, a gastroenterostomy or antrectomy may be carried out to aid gastric drainage. Although it is possible to carry out a more highly selective vagotomy which avoids the necessity of a drainage operation, this is a much more complicated operation which takes longer to perform.

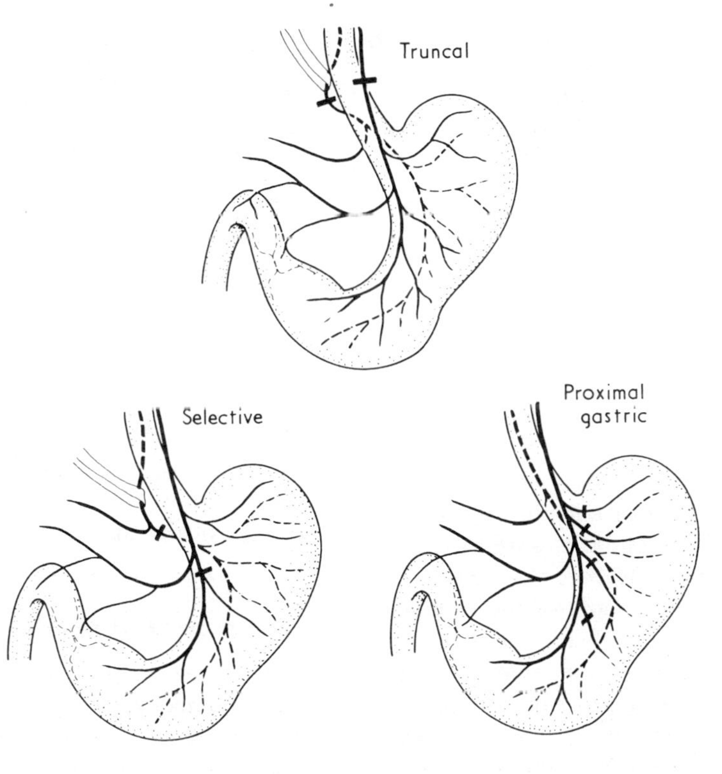

Fig. 18.2 *Various types of vagotomy.*

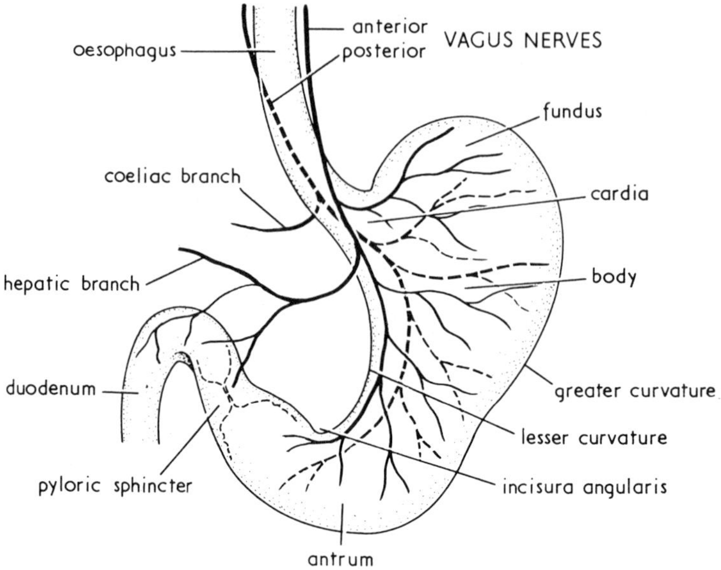

Fig. 18.3 *Position of vagus nerve.*

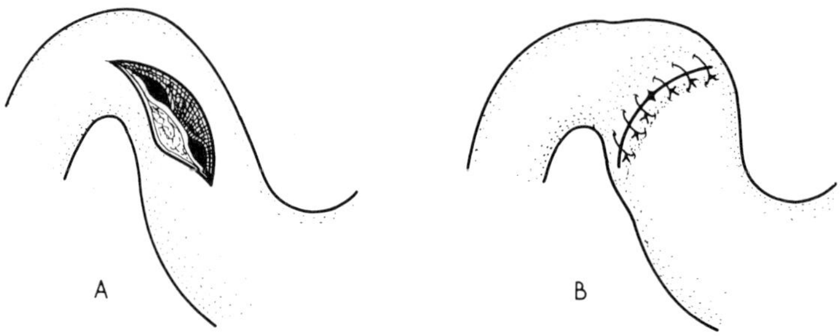

Fig. 18.4 *Pyloroplasty.*

Gastrectomy

This is occasionally done for a duodenal ulcer but much more commonly for a gastric ulcer where the possibility of malignancy requires surgery to be carried out earlier. Various degrees of gastrectomy may be performed for carcinoma of the stomach (Fig. 18.5), although the prognosis is poor. In the polya type of partial gastrectomy, two-thirds to three-quarters of the lower part of the stomach is removed and the remaining portion is anastomosed to the jejenum. In the Bilroth I, the stomach is joined to the duodenum.

In the elderly or those with ulcers high on the lesser curvature, a vagotomy and drainage operation are more likely to be undertaken, with local excision of the ulcer.

Management of peptic ulcers

Medical treatment consists of cimetidine to relieve pain and encourage healing. Histamine and gastrin are substances circulating in the bloodstream which stimulate gastric secretion. Cimetidine acts as an antagonist to histamine and suppresses the

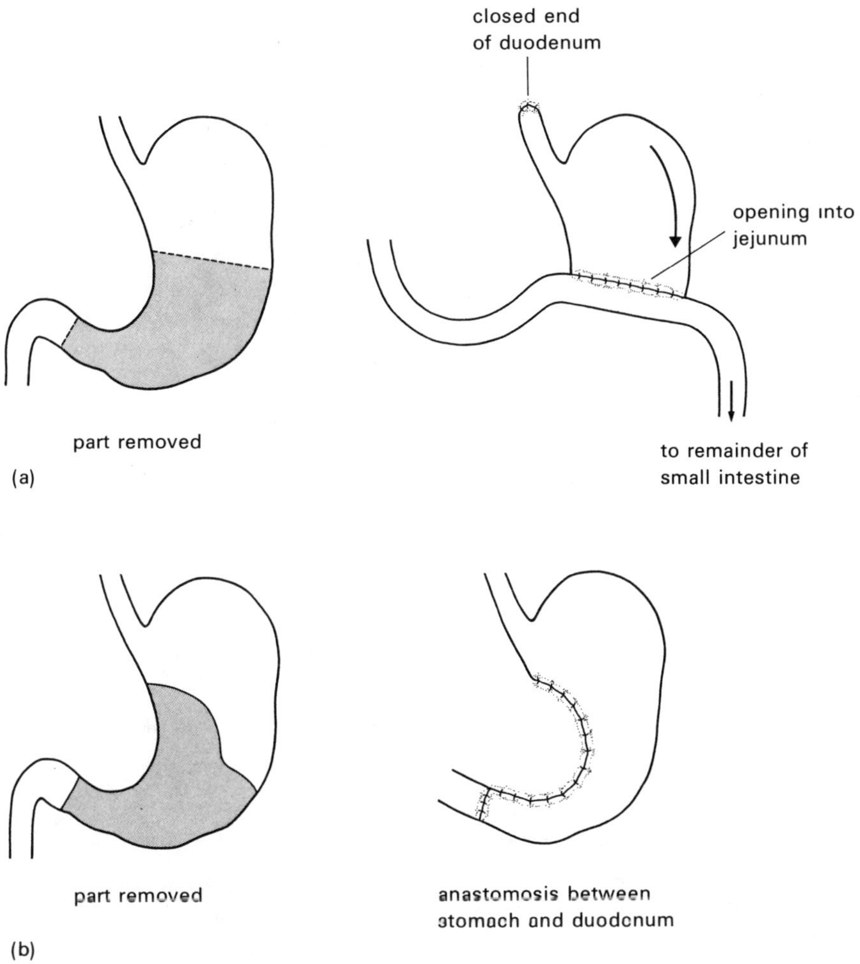

Fig. 18.5 *Types of partial gastrectomy. (a) Polya type. (b) Bilroth I.*

effects of gastrin, thus reducing gastric secretion. Carbenoxolone may also be given to increase the rate of healing, although it frequently causes retention of sodium and water resulting in oedema, altered electrolyte balance and occasional hypertension. Bedrest is advocated for 1 to 2 days during an acute exacerbation of the condition, and small frequent meals are preferable, avoiding highly spiced food, alcohol and strong tea or coffee. Salicylates and other ulcer-producing drugs are not given and the patient is advised to stop smoking.

Unfortunately, when treatment is discontinued the ulcer may recur and therefore the patient is kept on a maintenance dose of cimetidine. Particular care must be taken if the patient is also put on anticoagulants, sedatives or beta-blockers as the action of these drugs may be prolonged because of the effect of cimetidine on the enzymes in the liver.

Another treatment being introduced for a bleeding ulcer involves the insertion by the radiologist of a long catheter up the femoral artery through a small incision made in the groin. The catheter is then moved around until it is sited in the bleeding vessel at the base of the ulcer. The position is then checked by introducing a radio-opaque substance and x-raying. Gel-foam is then injected into the catheter which blocks the vessel.

Complications

Haemorrhage

Haemorrhage may take place from a peptic ulcer due to erosion into a vessel at the base of the ulcer. When a large artery is involved the bleeding is profuse and may be rapidly fatal. Blood transfusions are given to restore the blood volume and the patient is nursed flat. Once the haemorrhage is under control and the patient's condition improved, an elective partial gastrectomy is frequently done to prevent further haemorrhage. Sealing of the blood vessel may be effected by surgery or laser beam.

Perforation

This may occur if the ulcer erodes through the wall of the stomach or duodenum. It is a surgical emergency. The patient initially complains of a vague discomfort which eventually develops into a sharp, severe, localised pain, and the abdomen will be hard and boardlike. Nausea and vomiting will probably be present. Peritonitis is present and the sooner that the patient is taken to theatre the better the prognosis. An intravenous infusion and a nasogastric tube will be passed. The perforation may be closed or a partial gastrectomy carried out. If the patient is not operated on immediately, after 3 to 4 hours the pain diminishes, the rigidity lessens and the patient feels a little better. However, this improvement is transitory and the evidence of an acute, diffuse bacterial peritonitis will rapidly return and the patient will die if not operated on.

Obstruction

Obstruction occasionally occurs due to pyloric stenosis or hour-glass stomach, which is the result of fibrosis from a chronic peptic ulcer. The patient complains of distension and nausea which will progress to vomiting large amounts of stale food. The obstruction will be removed by performing a gastroenterostomy and possibly a vagotomy.

Malignancy

Malignancy is very uncommon in a duodenal ulcer but it is always a possibility when a gastric ulcer is present. Therefore diagnostic procedures are always very carefully carried out in the latter condition to exclude malignancy.

Specific preoperative preparation

The aim is to have the patient in the best possible condition for surgery, to ensure that the upper gastrointestinal tract is empty, and to prevent postoperative complications. Therefore, where possible an elective operation will be carried out following medical treatment and the correction of any anaemia, dehydration and electrolyte disturbance. If the patient has lost weight, his diet will need to be supplemented. However, a patient with a perforated peptic ulcer will require urgent surgical intervention or he will die from peritonitis.

The patient with gastric problems tends to be anxious and must therefore have an adequate explanation and an opportunity to discuss his fears. A tranquilliser such as diazepam may be prescribed by the doctor, as well as a night sedation.

In order to empty the stomach, a nasogastric tube will be passed and aspirated prior to surgery. If there is any obstruction, stomach washouts will be required.

In any upper abdominal operation, chest complications are liable to arise. It is therefore important that the patient has stopped smoking prior to admission and that physiotherapy in the form of deep breathing, coughing and leg exercises is commenced.

Specific postoperative care

The patient will return from theatre having had some form of anastomosis. This suture line needs the opportunity to heal without undue pressure. There will also have been handling of the abdominal contents which causes some delay in gastric emptying and sluggishness in the activity of the small intestine.

To minimise pressure on this internal suture line, a nasogastric tube will be kept in the stomach. Usually this is on open drainage to allow air to escape, but may be attached to a drainage bag or low-pressure pump. Aspiration will be carried out hourly initially and reduced as the amount of secretion becomes less. The nature of the aspirate must be observed carefully and any fresh blood reported as this may indicate the onset of haemorrhage. If the tube enters the afferent loop of the jejenum, bile will appear in the aspirate, and the doctor will need to alter the position of the tube. An increase in the amount of aspirate will occur if a paralytic ileus develops. The tube will be kept in position and aspirated until the aspirate is minimal and bowel sounds have returned, which is usually in about 48 hours.

The patient will also not be given anything by mouth for the first 8 to 12 hours. As the aspirate lessens and bowel sounds return, so 15–30 ml of clear fluid will be introduced hourly. If this is tolerated well, the amount will gradually be increased until the patient is able to take a light easily digested meal.

Because of the limited fluids being taken by mouth and the removal of gastric contents by aspiration, the patient will become dehydrated and develop an electrolyte imbalance unless intravenous fluids are given immediately postoperatively. While these are being given, a fluid balance chart should be maintained and the doctor will take blood regularly to check the electrolytes. Iced water mouthwashes will help to keep the patient's mouth moist until he is able to drink adequate amounts by mouth.

The high abdominal wound will mean that retractors will have been used near the diaphragm during the operation and it will therefore be painful for the patient to breathe deeply. Pain and distension in the abdomen may also cause him to lie very still. The patient should be encouraged to move, breathe deeply and to cough, and the physiotherapist will help him to do this. Adequate analgesia should be given to enable the patient to perform the actions without too much discomfort. The wound should be supported firmly when the patient coughs. Early mobilisation will help to disperse distension and prevent deep vein thrombosis, but when the patient is in bed he is better sitting well up to encourage drainage.

Sutures or clips are removed about the eighth to tenth day, and the haemoglobin is checked on the fourth day postoperatively. The patient is usually discharged on the tenth to twelfth day.

Advice on discharge

The patient is advised to have small frequent meals which are rich in protein and contain a limited amount of carbohydrate. It is important that he has an adequate amount of food for his body requirements and he should keep a check on his weight to see that this is remaining steady. Fluids should not be taken at mealtimes and iced water also avoided. These precautions will help to prevent the dumping syndrome occurring.

The dumping syndrome may arise soon after a meal due to the rapid emptying of the stomach, particularly if that meal had a high carbohydrate content. It may also occur about 2 hours after a meal due to oversecretion of insulin in response to the rapid absorption of carbohydrates. This latter condition is usually relieved by having a meal.

In the dumping syndrome the patient complains of feeling giddy and may feel faint, with a low blood pressure and a fast weak pulse. He may also complain of abdominal cramplike pain and nausea.

Diarrhoea is another after-effect which occurs in some patients and this can be treated by regulating the diet, and by taking drugs such as codeine phosphate or diphenoxylate hydrochloride (Lomotil). The patient should go to his general practitioner regularly for checks on his weight, and for blood tests for iron deficiency or pernicious anaemia and any evidence of calcium deficiency. Occasionally the patient may develop dysphagia and oesophagitis, but these usually do not last. If they do persist, surgery may be necessary. If the stomach remnant is very small, vomiting may be a problem, and meals will need to be small and frequent.

CONGENITAL HYPERTROPHIC PYLORIC STENOSIS

This is a congenital condition in which there is thickening (hypertrophy) of the circular muscle fibres at the pyloric end of the stomach. It most commonly affects the male child who is often the first born; it appears to run in families. Although it is congenital, it does not manifest itself until somewhere between the second and fourth weeks after birth.

The hypertrophied pyloric sphincter acts as an obstruction, so causing food to remain in the stomach. The stomach contracts more forcibly in an effort to overcome the obstruction but instead the contents are ejected forcibly out of the mouth (projectile vomiting). The vomit consists of the recent feed plus stagnant curds. However, a small amount of the feed is left in the stomach causing gastritis. Because the baby has vomited his feed he remains hungry and therefore cries lustily, taking any feeds offered greedily. The obstruction causes a complete constipation, although occasionally the baby may pass loose, green motions. If not treated, the baby will rapidly become dehydrated and show evidence of electrolyte imbalance. The baby also has a characteristically worried expression.

Diagnosis is by giving the baby a test feed when the doctor is able to feel a small 'tumour' the size of a cherry in the abdomen. Peristaltic waves may sometimes be seen crossing the abdomen. If there is any doubt, barium x-rays will be taken.

Treatment

Although the condition can be treated with atropine methonitrate (Eumydrin), it is usually dealt with by a Ramstedt's operation, in which the circular muscle is cut down to the mucous membrane, which is allowed to bulge through it (Fig. 18.6). Before the operation the stomach must be washed out until the saline used returns clear, to prevent gastritis postoperatively. An intravenous infusion will be set up to correct any dehydration or electrolyte imbalance. The operation may be carried out under a local or general anaesthetic.

Specific postoperative care

The baby may be fed after 4 hours with clear fluids (dextrose 5 %). In many hospitals the baby returns to his normal feeds very quickly. However, it is still the practice in many others to adhere to a stricter regime for 4 to 6 days, in which the strength of the feed is gradually increased from clear fluid to the full-strength feed. The amount given at each feed is also increased from 30 ml to the baby's normal requirement and the length of time between the feeds is increased from 2 to 4 hours.

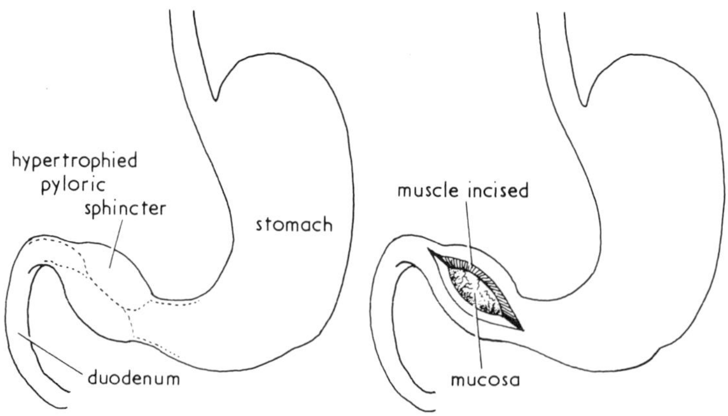

Fig. 18.6 *Ramstedt's operation for congenital hypertrophic pyloric stenosis.*

SUGGESTED WORK

1. Look at the nursing and medical histories of patient's in your ward with gastric conditions and find out how closely they fit to those of the type of patient expected to develop this condition.

2. Find out what are the most common surgical gastric conditions admitted to your ward.

3. Compare and contrast the methods of specific pre- and postoperative care given to patients having gastric surgery in your hospital with those described in this chapter. Find out why they differ.

4. Evaluate the effectiveness of the preoperative preparation of patients for gastric surgery in preventing complications.

5. Find out from the patient if there was any way he would have liked to alter the care given to him.

SUGGESTED READING

Gribble H. (1977). *Gastro-enterological Nursing.* Nursing Aids Series. Special Interest Text. London: Baillière Tindall.

19

Herniae and Intestinal Obstruction

Specific emphasis in the nursing history

General appearance. Note any distension of the abdomen. Does the patient look pale and shocked or grey due to pain?

Pain. Find out the character of the pain, where it is and how strong it is.

Elimination. Find out when the patient last had his bowels open and observe any motions or the passage of blood or mucus per rectum.

Nutrition. What has the patient's appetite been like?

Vomiting. Note the presence of nausea or vomiting, its character, the amount, and how long it has been present.

Vital signs. Note any increase in the pulse rate or temperature or reduction of blood pressure.

HERNIAE

A hernia is the protrusion of an organ or part of an organ through an opening in the cavity in which it is normally contained (Fig. 19.1). The main problem is the possibility of the hernia eventually causing an obstruction in the intestinal tract. This means that although the patient will normally be put on the waiting list for hospital admission, it is always possible that he may be admitted as a

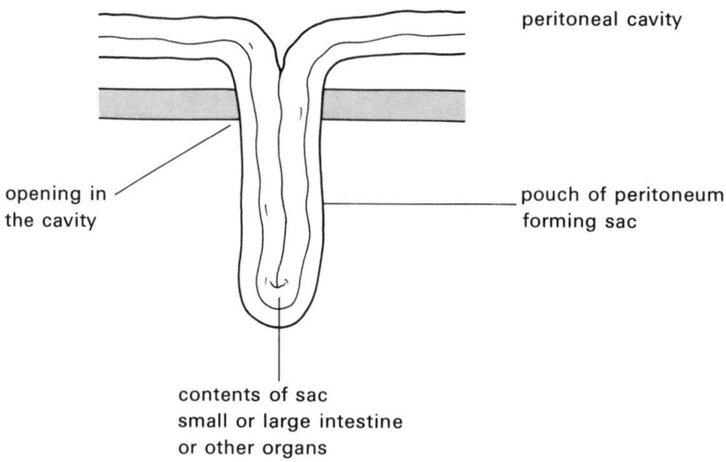

Fig. 19.1 *Typical hernia.*

surgical emergency with an obstruction in the meantime. If this does happen, the emphasis will be on getting him to theatre as quickly as possible. In which case the nurse will have to identify the priorities in preparing him for theatre.

Inguinal hernia

The spermatic cord in the male passes down through the inguinal canal in its journey from the abdominal cavity to the scrotum. There is therefore a natural gap in the muscles of the abdomen. During the development of the male fetus the testes descend, taking with them a pouch of peritoneum, part of which forms the tunica vaginalis (Fig. 19.2). The remaining part of the pouch of peritoneum normally disappears. If this pouch persists, it forms what is called an *indirect* inguinal hernia, which usually presents in infancy but which may not be evident until adulthood. The extent of the

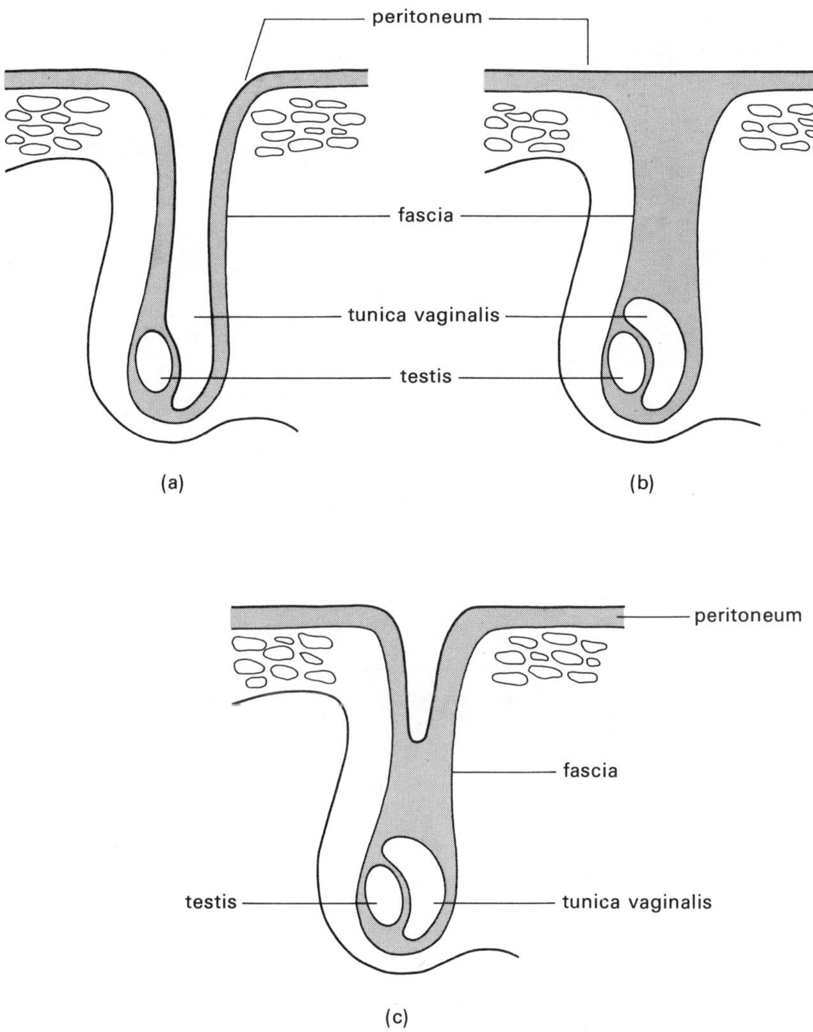

Fig. 19.2 *(a) and (b) Normal development of the tunica vaginalis. (c) Indirect inguinal hernia.*

protrusion varies from just a swelling in the groin to a *scrotal hernia* in which it has descended into the scrotal sac. In obese and elderly people the posterior wall of the inguinal canal can become weakened and so stretch or rupture, allowing abdominal organs to herniate. Both types are much more common in men than in females.

Repair of an inguinal hernia by herniorrhaphy

Care has to be taken to preserve the spermatic cord. With the indirect type the sac is removed, and if it is in a young adult, the opening in the fascia made smaller. In a direct hernia the fascia is reinforced with tantalum metal gauze, a synthetic material, or tissue from the patient. If a patient is unable to have an operation, then a truss can be applied once the hernia has been reduced, to keep it in position. If the hernia cannot be put back, it is said to be *irreducible* and will require an operation.

Femoral hernia (Fig. 19.3)

The femoral ring is formed by the inguinal ligament which allows the femoral artery and vein to pass between it and the pelvis. It is immediately underneath the inguinal canal. In the elderly this ring becomes enlarged, allowing the sac of peritoneum to prolapse causing a small lump to appear in the groin. Occasionally a small piece of the wall of the small intestine or pelvic colon becomes caught in the opening and its blood supply becomes cut off. As this does not involve the lumen there is not an intestinal obstruction, but the wall of

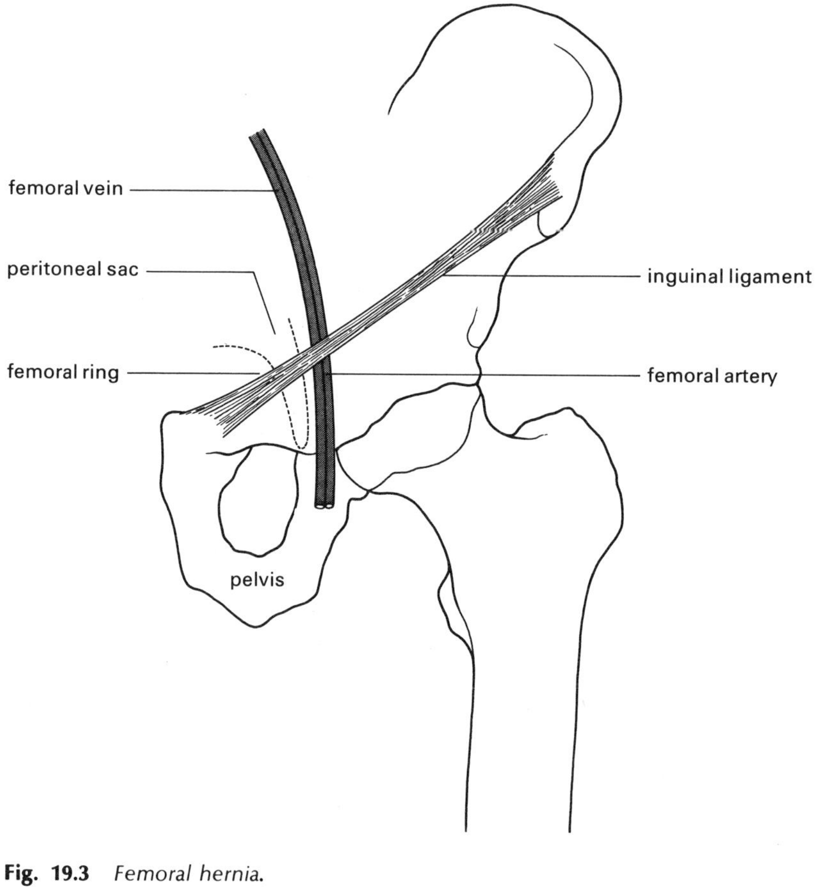

Fig. 19.3 *Femoral hernia.*

the intestine which has lost its blood supply may become gangrenous and break down, so allowing the contents of the bowel to escape into the peritoneal cavity. A femoral hernia must be treated by surgery because it may not be possible to reduce it and even if it is, the pad of a truss cannot be kept in a suitable position because of the movement of the leg.

Umbilical hernia

This may occur in infants due to a failure of the opening through which the umbilical blood vessels pass to close after birth. If it is small, it may close spontaneously in the first 2 years, but larger ones will need surgical repair. Umbilical herniae may also occur in the adult, most commonly in obese, elderly females. The hernia prolapses above or below the umbilicus and is usually large and irreducible. A common complication of this type of hernia is strangulation, therefore surgery is considered at an early stage, with removal of the hernial sac and closure of the defect in the abdominal wall.

Exomphalos

This is an abnormality of development which is uncommon. There is a defect of the abdominal wall, present at birth, through which the intestines escape. It requires immediate surgery.

Incisional hernia

If an abdominal wound is put under more strain than it is able to bear due to heavy lifting or coughing, the scar becomes stretched and allows the abdominal contents to prolapse through it. This is more likely to happen if the wound has had a drain in it. It is normally treated by herniorrhaphy, although a truss may be worn.

Strangulated hernia

This complication most commonly occurs in femoral and umbilical herniae. The neck of the hernial sac may become constricted so that the soft-walled veins in the mesentery are unable to drain that part of the bowel. This causes engorgement and therefore further constriction, cutting off the arterial supply. As a result, there is an acute intestinal obstruction and gangrene of the part affected. The bowel will eventually rupture, causing peritonitis. The clinical picture and the management are those of an acute intestinal obstruction.

Specific preoperative care for a herniorrhaphy

The preparation is as for any abdominal operation, with particular emphasis on preventing chest complications. The patient will have been told to stop smoking and will be given deep-breathing exercises. This is because excessive coughing postoperatively will put a strain on the wound.

Postoperative care

Again the patient must be encouraged to deep breathe even though the pain makes him disinclined to do so. Although he is usually got up on the first day postoperatively; he may be kept in bed another day if the repair was large. He must be encouraged to hold the wound when he coughs. A careful watch should be kept on the urinary output because retention may occur as a result of an enlarged prostate. It is possible for the bladder to be damaged during operation for an inguinal or femoral hernia, therefore any haematuria should be reported. On discharge the patient should be advised not to lift for at least 6 weeks.

INTESTINAL OBSTRUCTION

An obstruction may arise at any point along the length of the small or large intestine from a variety of reasons. If the obstruction occurs suddenly, it is termed an *acute* obstruction and the symptoms will be severe. However, if the symptoms build up slowly over a period of time, it is called a *chronic* obstruction. Frequently the acute form is superimposed on the chronic and this is called *acute-on-chronic* obstruction.

Causes of acute intestinal obstruction

These can be divided into two main groups: those due to a mechanical obstruction, and those due to paralysis of the intestines.

Mechanical obstruction

This may be caused by the following: strangulated herniae (as mentioned in the previous section); adhesions or bands resulting from previous inflammatory conditions or operations, causing strangulation; a volvulus, which is a twist in the bowel (Fig. 19.4), and may be in the small intestine, the caecum or the pelvic colon; intussusception (Fig. 19.5), a condition which occurs in children under 1 year of age, and in which the bowel becomes telescoped into itself (early reduction is essential); foreign bodies in the lumen, such as a large gall-stone; mesenteric thrombosis; and an imperforate anus.

Paralysis of the intestine (neurogenic)

This is called paralytic ileus and may happen as a result of an abdominal operation, particularly if the bowel has had much handling. It may also arise as a result of peritonitis, chemical disorders such as reduced potassium, uraemia, or diabetic coma, and some drugs such as Pro-Banthine given in large doses. (See Chapter 17.)

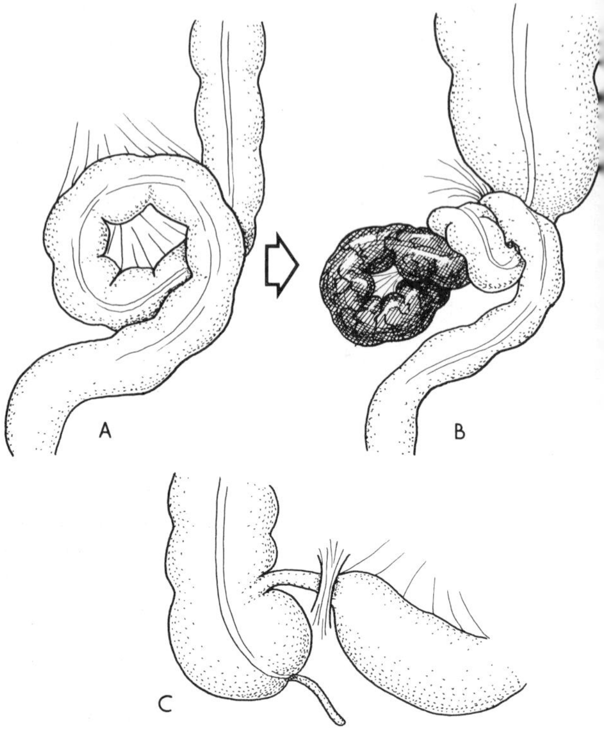

Fig. 19.4 *Volvulus.*

Clinical picture

In an acute intestinal obstruction there will be a severe colicky pain due to spasmodic contractions of the bowel above the obstacle in an attempt to overcome the obstruction. In the later stages there

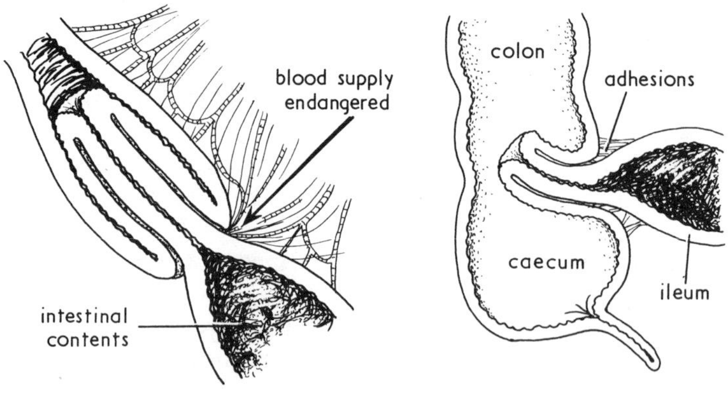

Fig. 19.5 *Intussusception.*

may be visible peristalsis. The intestines above the obstruction become distended with fluid and air, the former from the digestive juices which are normally absorbed. These fluid levels can be seen on an x-ray if the patient is in an upright position. Beyond the obstruction the bowel is collapsed. The higher the obstruction, the less opportunity there is for fluid to be absorbed and therefore the more vomiting will occur. If the obstruction is in the beginning of the small intestine, the vomiting can be copious, leading to rapid dehydration and electrolyte imbalance. To start with it is clear, it then becomes bile stained and eventually faeculent. If the obstruction is at the further end of the small intestine, there will be little vomiting or dehydration, and in a large-bowel obstruction the main problem is abdominal distension. Nothing can pass the obstruction so there will be complete constipation and no flatus. However, contents already in the lower bowel may be passed. If the blood supply to the bowel is affected, as in intussusception and a mesenteric thrombosis, the patient may pass blood and mucus *per rectum*. Shock is present, the patient looking pale, drawn and anxious, and the blood pressure is low. The temperature usually remains normal at first but the pulse is variable.

Management

Emergency surgery is required to relieve the obstruction and minimise the damage to the bowel from gangrene. If strangulation is present, the operation is done as quickly as possible. However, in other cases if there is much dehydration, shock or electrolyte imbalance, these are dealt with first. Blood is taken to check the electrolytes, blood urea, and haemoglobin, and the blood is also grouped and cross-matched.

Specific preoperative care

When taking the nursing history, only that information which is essential or which the relatives can provide is gathered, the remainder being left until a more suitable time. Essential preoperative preparation only is carried out.

A nasogastric tube is passed and aspirated frequently to remove the fluid accumulating in the stomach. Aspiration will be continued until the patient goes to theatre. An intravenous infusion is commenced to replace fluids and electrolytes and, if necessary, may be given fairly quickly.

The aim is to remove the cause of the obstruction. If this is due to a volvulus or band of adhesions, it may be possible to untwist the bowel, or divide the adhesions. However, if the blood supply has been cut off, gangrene may be present and this will have to be resected. Sometimes the obstruction cannot be removed immediately and a temporary colostomy, caecostomy or ileostomy may have to be done to relieve the obstruction before the operation can be carried out. In malignant conditions the growth may have advanced to such a stage that it is inoperable and a permanent colostomy to bypass it is necessary.

Postoperative care

This is the same as for any abdominal surgery. Nasogastric suction is continued until aspiration is minimal. The intravenous infusion is continued until the patient is able to take adequate amounts by mouth and the fluid and electrolyte balance have been restored to normal.

Chronic intestinal obstruction

This is most commonly caused by malignancy of the large bowel, but may also arise as a result of chronic inflammation such as diverticulitis or regional ileitis leading to fibrosis, peritoneal bands or adhesions. Impaction and accumulation of faeces, pressure from abdominal tumours or cysts outside the bowel, and Hirschsprung's disease may also lead to chronic obstruction.

Clinical picture

The patient appears anaemic with a yellow, muddy complexion and wasting. He may have had a history of dyspepsia followed by intermittent attacks of colicky pain which is often associated with eating. There is usually some degree of constipation, although early morning or spurious diarrhoea may be present.

Management

The patient will be investigated by means of a sigmoidoscopy or colonoscopy and barium enema. If possible a resection of the affected bowel will be done with an anastomosis. This is usually carried out in two stages with a temporary colostomy or caecostomy in the first stage, the anastomosis being done when the patient's condition has improved. In some cases a permanent colostomy is all that can be done.

SUGGESTED WORK

1. Find out from theatre which items of pre-operative care may be omitted in an emergency operation and which are essential.
2. Find out which is the most common cause for a patient to be admitted to your hospital with an intestinal obstruction.
3. Which is the most common type of hernia operated on in your hospital?
4. Compare the methods of surgery used in your hospital with those quoted in this chapter.
5. Compare and contrast the specific pre- and postoperative nursing described in this chapter with that you have seen. If there was any difference, why was this?

* * *

Mr PETER JONES (aged 52) is married. He is a driving instructor who manages his own business. He is slightly overweight, a heavy smoker and allergic to penicillin. He has been admitted as an emergency with a strangulated inguinal hernia.

Medical plan
Emergency surgery to relieve the obstruction. Restoration of electrolyte balance.

Identification of the patient's needs and problems prior to surgery and action arising from these

Pain
Find out from the doctor whether analgesics may be administered. If not, explain to the patient why not, and when he will be given some relief. Ensure that as soon as he is allowed an analgesic this is given promptly. Find the position he is most comfortable in, for example with his knees drawn up.

Psychological
Explain briefly what is to be done and what to expect after the operation in the way of drainage tubes etc. Be ready to answer any questions or to let him rest quietly.

Relatives
Ensure that the wife has seen the doctor and understands the situation. Give her some idea of how long her husband is likely to be in hospital and how she can best help him. Advise her when to ring.

Worry about the driving school
Find out from Mr Jones the immediate problems and who would be the best person to deal with them. If this is not his wife, arrange for the appropriate person to be contacted. Explain that the social worker will see his wife initially, and himself when he is fit enough.

Prevention of respiratory complications
Explain the importance of deep breathing on his return from operation. Ensure that the physiotherapist will see him on the first postoperative morning. Ensure that his cigarettes have been removed and he realises he must not smoke.

Allergy
Check that this has been clearly entered on the drug sheet and notes, and that he has not been prescribed any medicines in the penicillin group. He will probably be prescribed antibiotics because of the risk of chest or abdominal infection, and must therefore be carefully observed for any allergic reaction.

Prevention of peritonitis, paralytic ileus
After explanation to the patient, pass nasogastric tube and aspirate frequently. Note amount and nature of aspirate on fluid balance chart and inform the doctor of any marked change. Note and report

any change in the nature of the pain or any undue distension.

Electrolyte imbalance and dehydration
Inform the doctor of any blood electrolyte results when received. Monitor the rate of the intravenous infusion carefully, particularly if it is being run rapidly. Observe for any lethargy or confusion and monitor the pulse rate to detect overloading of the circulation.

Slight overweight
Arrange for the dietitian to see him and his wife when he is fit enough.

Immediate preparation for operation
Ensure that he has been seen by the doctor and that he has signed the consent form. Go through the operation checklist. If it has not been possible to shave him, alert theatre.

SUGGESTED READING

Gribble H. (1977). *Gastro-enterological Nursing Aids Series.* Special Interest Text. London: Baillière Tindall.

20

Conditions of the Lower Gastrointestinal Tract

Surgery of the lower gastrointestinal tract will alter the way in which faeces are excreted from the body. This may only be on a temporary basis, such as the constipation which normally occurs in the first few postoperative days. However, many of these patients will have undergone a colostomy or ileostomy and will require particular nursing care and psychological support for some time after the operation. The higher the surgical intervention, the more fluid the faeces will be, so giving rise to more potential problems.

Specific emphasis in the nursing history

Elimination. Note the frequency of defaecation, the presence of diarrhoea or constipation, and any bleeding.

Nutrition. Note the type of food the patient eats, including the amount of roughage and any food avoided.

General appearance. Note any loss of weight.

Attitude. Is the patient anxious and did this anxiety precede his present complaint or is it a result of it?

Skin. Note any soreness around the anal region.

Vital signs. Is there any evidence of infection or toxaemia such as a raised temperature and pulse?

Previous medication. Note particularly if the patient is on any steroids as these will have to be increased over the period of surgery.

CARCINOMA

Adenocarcinoma arising from gland cells is a common condition resulting in as many as 10 000 deaths a year in the UK, although there are probably many more cases which are undiagnosed. It most commonly occurs after the age of 50 and although it may arise anywhere in the colon, nearly 50% of cases concern the sigmoid colon (Fig. 20.1); the ascending colon and the rectum being the next most common sites. Carcinoma of the colon may be proliferative, with a cauliflower appearance, or ulcerative. Although the cause of carcinoma of the colon is not usually known, patients with benign polyps, and in particular familial polyposis, have a high incidence. It is also known that those people who have had ulcerative colitis recurring for 10 years or more are likely to develop it.

Spread

This may be directly to other parts of the intestine and may lead to fistulae; via the lymphatics to the nodes around the aorta; via the portal vein to the liver and eventually to the lungs or as seedling deposits in the peritoneum which may cause ascites (Fig. 20.2).

Clinical picture

There is usually some alteration in bowel habit, with either diarrhoea or constipation, and the stools may be streaked with blood and mucus. The

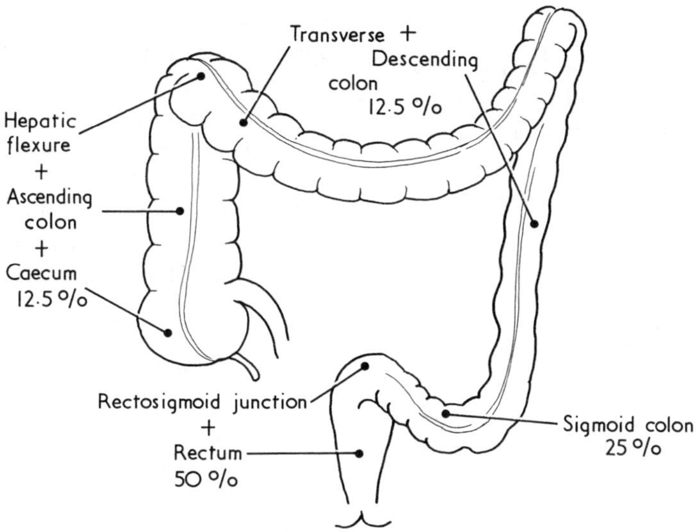

Fig. 20.1 *Diagram showing where carcinoma is most commonly found.*

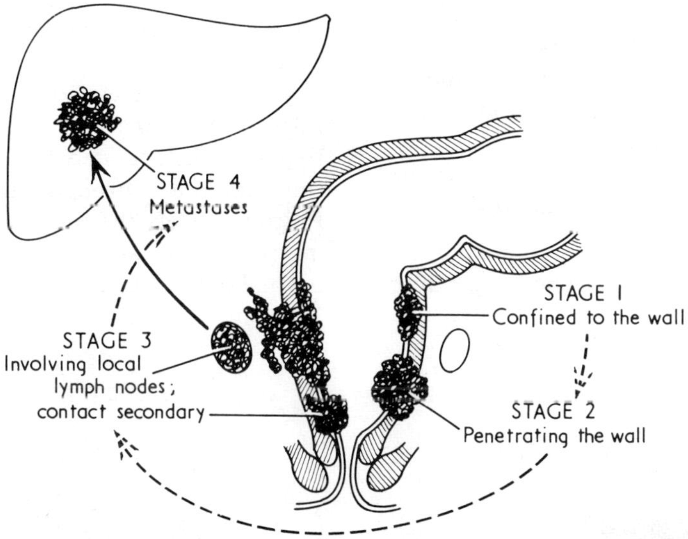

Fig. 20.2 *The spread of carcinoma of the rectum.*

loss of blood leads to an iron deficiency anaemia and the individual feels generally unwell with a loss of weight. There may also be a constant feeling of fulness in the rectum. The individual may not seek advice until the growth is far advanced and may present with an acute obstruction, perforation leading to fistulae or generalised peritonitis, and liver involvement causing jaundice or ascites.

Diagnosis

A careful rectal examination will be carried out by the doctor, followed by a sigmoidoscopy or colonoscopy and biopsy. A barium enema is usually done as well, and a liver scan or intravenous pyelogram may be used if secondaries are suspected.

Management

A resection and anastomosis will be done where this is possible, with the removal of the lymph nodes draining the area (Fig. 20.3). In carcinoma of the rectum the growth is usually too near to the rectum for an anastomosis, and it is necessary to remove the anal canal, rectum and pelvic colon. In order to remove sufficient lymph nodes, an abdominal operation is necessary. Both the abdominal and pelvic operations are usually carried out at the same time and the operation is therefore called an *abdominoperineal excision of the rectum.* There is thus not only an abdominal wound but also a perineal wound and a colostomy. However, if an anastomosis is done using a stapling gun to staple the ano-rectal stump to the colon, a colostomy is avoided (Fig. 20.4).

There are various other operations which will be carried out according to where the growth is.

1. *Right hemicolectomy* involves removal of the last few inches of the ileum, caecum, ascending colon and first part of the transverse colon. The ileum and transverse colon are then joined together.

2. *Left hemicolectomy* involves removal of the last part of the transverse colon, descending colon and beginning of the pelvic colon. The transverse colon is then joined to the pelvic colon.

3. *Transverse colostomy* removes a section of the transverse colon, and the hepatic and splenic ends are anastomosed.

4. *Resection of the pelvic colon* involves removal of a segment of pelvic colon, the two ends then being joined together.

If there is an intestinal obstruction, the bowel cannot be adequately prepared and therefore a *transverse colostomy* (Fig. 20.5) may be done. A loop of the transverse colon is brought to the surface of the abdomen through an incision separate to that of the main operation and is held by a glass rod. Once the main incision has been sutured the colostomy is opened. The glass rod is usually left in situ for a week. When the anastomosis has healed, after 3 or 4 weeks, the colostomy may be closed, following a check barium enema.

5. *Caecostomy* is carried out by some surgeons instead of a transverse colostomy as a temporary bypass to the operated area. A tube is inserted into the caecum through the abdominal wall. Postoperatively the tube has to be kept patent by means of normal saline washouts. After 8 days, normal bowel function may have been restored, in

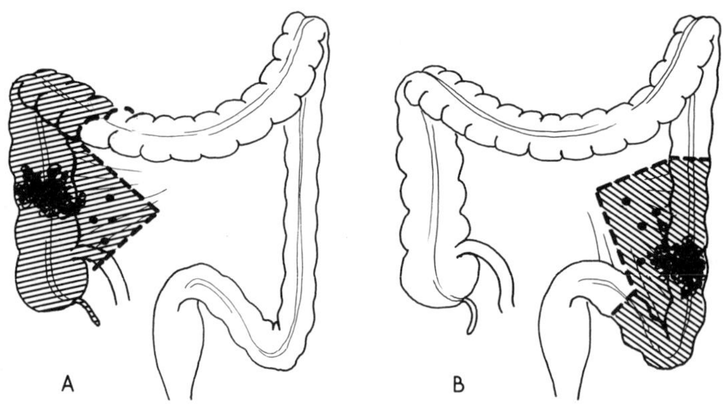

Fig. 20.3 *Diagram demonstrating the extent of surgical excision in carcinoma of the colon. (a) In the ascending, and (b) in the sigmoid colon.*

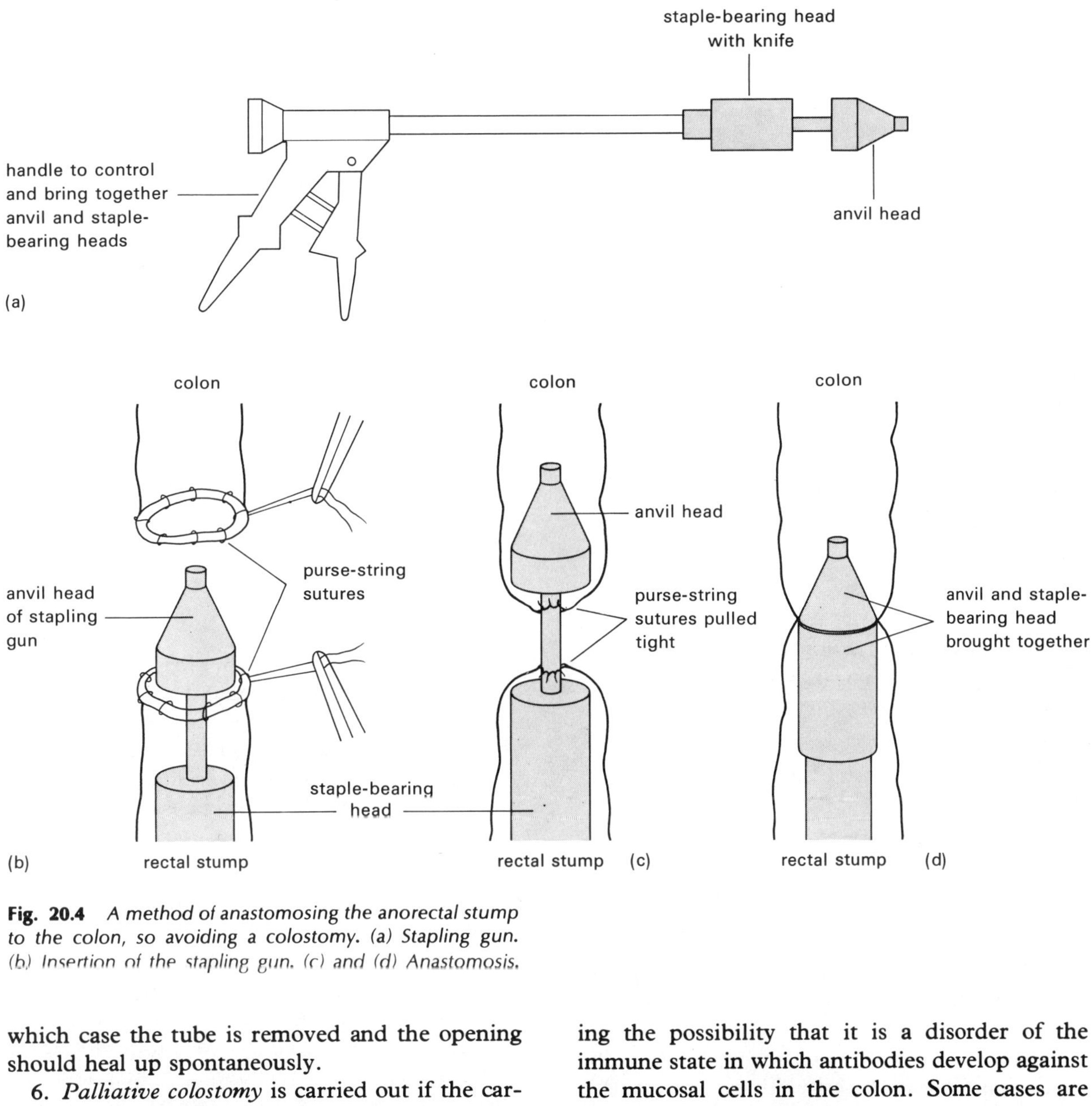

Fig. 20.4 *A method of anastomosing the anorectal stump to the colon, so avoiding a colostomy. (a) Stapling gun. (b) Insertion of the stapling gun. (c) and (d) Anastomosis.*

which case the tube is removed and the opening should heal up spontaneously.

6. *Palliative colostomy* is carried out if the carcinoma is inoperable to relieve or prevent the effects of complete obstruction.

ULCERATIVE COLITIS

Ulcerative colitis is an inflammatory disease of the colon, the cause of which is unknown. Many suggestions as to its cause have been made, including the possibility that it is a disorder of the immune state in which antibodies develop against the mucosal cells in the colon. Some cases are known to be due to an allergy to certain foods such as milk. Viral infections and a high anxiety state may also be factors.

Patches of the intestinal mucosa become detached, leaving ulcers. This superficial ulceration of the mucosa may affect part or the whole of the colon and sometimes may even spread into the small intestine and rectum. It usually affects young adults in the 20–40 year age range but can attack

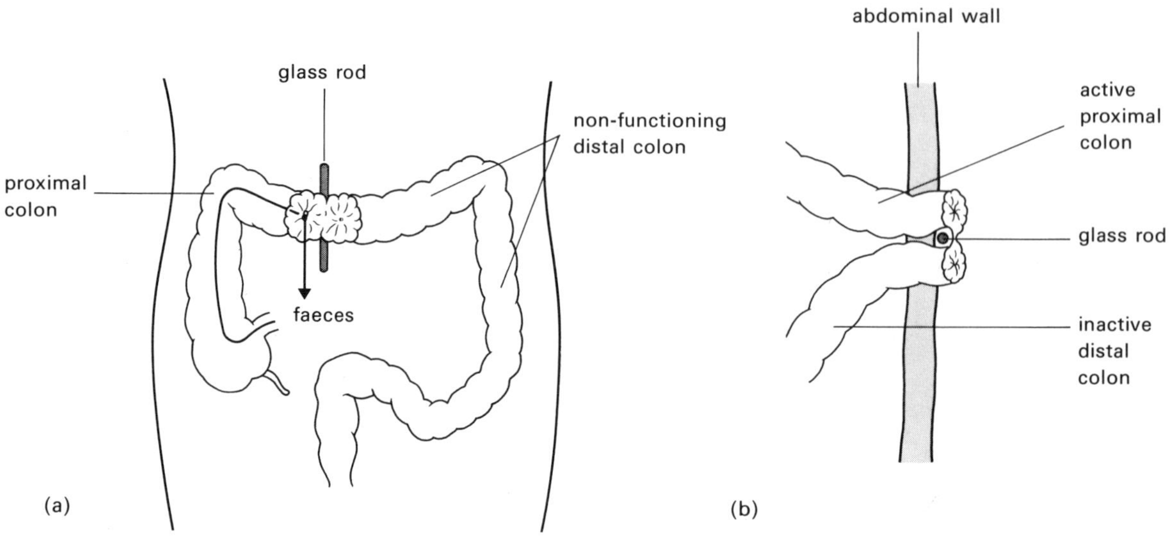

Fig. 20.5 *(a) Transverse colostomy. (b) Side view.*

children and the elderly. As the ulceration heals, scarring may occur leading to a narrowing and thickening of the colon. There may be a superimposed secondary infection.

Clinical picture

The individual suffers from episodes of acute diarrhoea, passing as many as 20 or more stools a day. The stools are loose, with blood and mucus intimately mixed with the faeces. As a result of the loss of blood, fluid and electrolytes, the individual is dehydrated, anaemic and has an electrolyte imbalance. He may develop toxaemia, with a raised temperature and a rapid weak pulse. If the condition is not adequately controlled, fissures, abscesses, perforation or peritonitis may result. If it persists for longer than 10 years, there is a high incidence of cancer of the colon. Ulcerative colitis may be associated with other conditions in the body such as iritis, arthritis, jaundice and skin rashes. Most patients with ulcerative colitis have a series of relapses and remissions, although with some the condition may be continuous, or there may be long breaks between episodes.

Diagnosis

Specimens of the stools are sent to the pathological laboratory to exclude the possibility of infection. A record is kept of each time the patient has his bowels emptied, and what is passed. A sigmoidoscopy and biopsy will be done to examine the mucosa, and a barium enema will also be distinctive.

Management

If the patient is not responding to medical treatment, or if the condition has persisted for more than 10 years, an elective operation of colectomy and ileostomy will be done. Occasionally the patient's condition is such that an emergency operation will have to be carried out, in which case an ileostomy may be undertaken first and the colectomy done at a later date. If an elective operation is being done, steps are taken to reduce colonic inflammation and diarrhoea and to replace substances lost from the body.

Reduction of inflammation

Enteric-coated sulphasalazine (Salazopyrin) 1 g is given four to six times daily. It may cause stomach upsets, and sometimes haemolytic anaemia, therefore regular blood tests will be done. Prednisolone (Predsol) enemas and, where necessary, oral steroids are very effective. It must be remembered, however, that when the patient is having surgery he will need an increased dose.

Reduction of diarrhoea

Methylcellulose adds bulk to loose stools and can be given as diphenoxylate with atropine (Lomotil). Codeine phosphate and morphine derivatives slow down the activity of the intestines.

Replacement of substances lost from the body

Fluids and electrolytes are the most important substances to be replaced and may necessitate intravenous infusions. Blood transfusions and iron preparations may be necessary to correct anaemia. The patient's diet may have become very restricted and he may therefore need a diet high in protein, calories and vitamins B and C. If necessary, parenteral nutrition may be given.

The patient may also require general rest and sedation. A bedside commode, good ventilation and a deodorising wick will help the patient not to feel quite so embarrassed. Prevention of pressure sores is necessary in these often very thin patients. Particular care should be taken to protect the anal area as this may become very sore; a barrier cream may be used.

Specific preoperative care of a patient undergoing an abdominoperineal excision of rectum or colectomy

The patient is admitted 3 to 4 days prior to operation to ensure he is suitably prepared. The bowel must be cleared and each surgeon has his own particular method. It may be by a series of rectal washouts and aperients or suppositories and enemas, or Hartmann's or mannitol solution may be introduced via a nasogastric tube or orally in large quantities to wash through the gut. Another method used is to give magnesium sulphate until diarrhoea is established. Whichever method is used, the nurse must be able to recognise when the patient cannot tolerate any further treatment. If there is any danger of the patient vomiting with a procedure such as the introduction of large amounts of Hartmann's solution, then he should not be left alone. Usually this preparation is associated with a low-residue diet for several days prior to the operation and fluids only the day before.

Medicine will be given to reduce the bacterial population in the bowel, usually in the form of antibacterial substances which are not absorbed by the bowel and therefore have a local action. Colistin sulphate 1.5 mega units 12-hourly for 2 days, and neomycin 1 g 6-hourly for 2 days are two such substances. Patients on these medicines may require nystatin as destruction of the normal bacteria allows *Monilia albicans* the opportunity to enter.

The position of the stoma is decided by the stoma therapist or appliance officer and the surgeon (Fig. 20.6). There should be a diameter of at least 5 cm around it without any skin folds to allow the appliance to fit snugly. Therefore previous scars or folds of fat are avoided. Unfortunately some patients have lost a lot of weight prior to their operation, and when they regain this postoperatively it will have an effect on the positioning of the stoma. If they can wear an ileostomy bag prior to the operation, this is also helpful.

Any patients on steroids must have a booster dose over the operation period, and a careful watch must be kept on their blood pressure. Psychologically, the patient will need to be prepared for a colostomy or ileostomy if he is going to have one. Patients with ulcerative colitis are usually only too happy to be relieved of their present condition; they are also often in the younger age range and therefore find it easier to adapt. The patient having a colostomy is older and may not see the immediate need for it, he may therefore find it much harder to accept. The attitude of the relatives will be crucial in helping the patient to accept this fundamental change to his body image. The social background of the patient will be investigated as this can also affect his attitude.

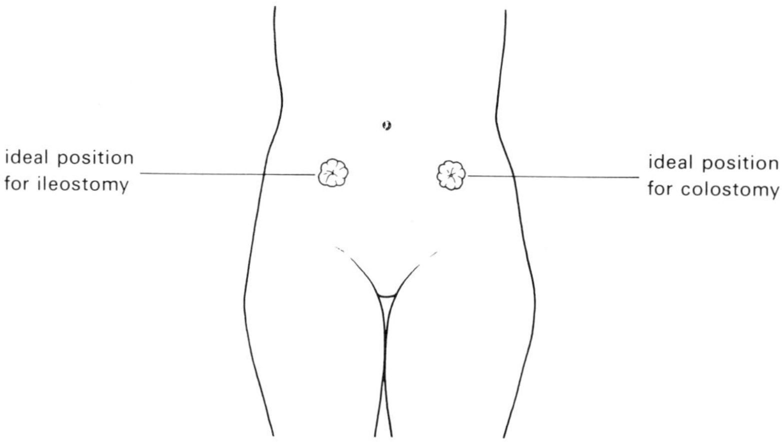

Fig. 20.6 *Stoma sites.*

The specific postoperative nursing care plan

On return to the ward the patient is made comfortable, in a semi-recumbent position if he is conscious. The possibility of haemorrhage is the immediate problem so the blood pressure, pulse, colour and respirations must be observed carefully every half-hour. Any abnormality should be reported immediately to the doctor. The wounds should be checked. A straightforward anastomosis will only have an abdominal wound, but sometimes there is a temporary transverse colostomy and the colour of this should be observed. If a colostomy or ileostomy has been formed, it should be a healthy pink colour; blueness or blackness suggests interference with the blood supply and should be reported at once. The stoma always protrudes a little from the abdominal wall; if this is not apparent or, conversely, it has prolapsed, the surgeon will need to be informed. Following an abdominoperineal operation there will also be a perineal wound which usually has a Redivac drain in position. This wound should be kept as dry as possible with spirit-based lotions.

The patient may return with a Foley catheter in position and the output should be watched very carefully in case damage has been done to the urinary tract. This may remain in for 5 days, and its removal should take place in the morning and a careful note made when the patient first passes urine.

Intravenous therapy is usually continued for 48 hours, depending on the condition of the patient prior to operation, and how soon he is able to take fluids after it. A nasogastric tube will be in position and this will be aspirated half-hourly and then 4-hourly, according to the amount of aspirate. Any increase will suggest a paralytic ileus or peritonitis. Nothing will be given by mouth until bowel sounds are heard, although the patient may appreciate some ice to suck. Usually fluids are withheld up to the fourth postoperative day, when they are gradually increased until the patient is able to take a normal diet. Oral care will obviously be important, as will a fluid balance chart. The patient will also require physiotherapy to encourage movement and deep breathing.

Care of an ileostomy

The stoma is usually fashioned into a spout 3.5 cm long to make it easier to manage (Fig. 20.7). The faeces are in a fluid state, being excreted every hour or two. The stoma still has small intestinal contents and therefore digestive enzymes are present, which can be very destructive to the overlying skin. It usually takes 3 to 4 days before it begins to work, but then the output is copious and the patient may suffer an electrolyte imbalance. Plenty of fluids are therefore very important. The patient also needs to be reassured that eventually some of the fluid will be reabsorbed.

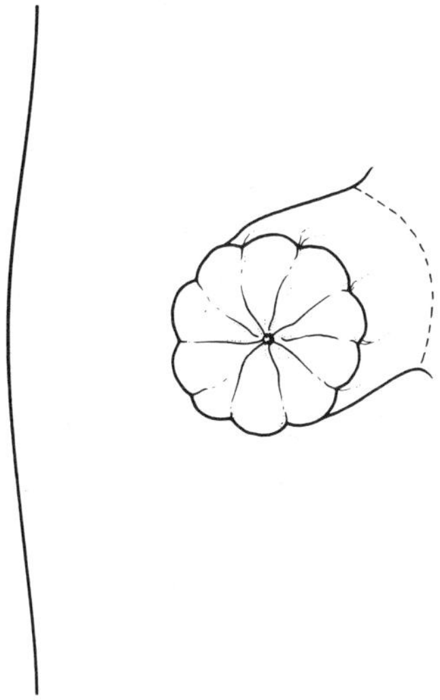

Fig. 20.7 *Ileostomy stoma, 3.5 cm in length.*

It is important that there is no pressure on the ileostomy, so causing it to recede. About the fifth or seventh day, the stitches attaching the mucosa to the skin are removed. Sometimes the stoma will prolapse if it is not fixed adequately and the pressure on the surrounding tissue is increased by something tight such as a corset. The stoma is insensitive and if the appliance is fitted carelessly, it may cause pressure necrosis. Therefore, when placing the phlange there should be a thin margin of skin between the phlange and the stoma. Necrosis can lead to a fistula which can be a very difficult situation to manage.

Because there is an increase in the fluid excreted via the ileostomy, the urinary output is reduced, this means it is more concentrated and more acid, so increasing the possibility of stones forming. The patient must therefore be encouraged to drink plenty, and may be advised to take regular doses of soda bicarbonate to make the urine alkaline. Occasionally a large amount of the ileum has been resected and as this is responsible for reabsorbing bile salts, they are lost from the body. As a result there are fewer bile salts in the bile, and gall-stones may develop. This is much more likely to happen in Crohn's disease.

The appliance used in an ileostomy is not disposable. It is opaque and is emptied from below. The substance from which it is made has had a deodorising agent added to it. The patient will have exemption from prescription charges.

If the patient has a high-residue diet in the first few months following operation, he may develop an obstruction which will need urgent attention or there will be a rapid loss of electrolytes.

The patient with an ileostomy has poor tolerance of gastrointestinal upsets, and a mild attack of food poisoning could have very serious effects on his electrolyte balance. For mild disturbances methylcellulose or codeine phosphate may be effective. Salt supplements may be necessary for patients in a hot climate as they are unable to control salt loss.

Care of the surrounding skin is of great importance as it is much more difficult to restore excoriated skin than to prevent it from breaking down in the beginning. A good projecting stoma, well positioned so that there are no creases in the skin, is of first importance. Protective Karaya gum rings and protective barrier creams are essential.

The patient will require much support in the early days following discharge; he may also benefit from joining the Ileostomy Association whose members have already overcome many of the problems he will have to face. Before he is discharged he will have been given advice on where to obtain fresh appliances, creams etc. He will have discussed with the dietitian those foods best avoided, and how to maintain an adequately balanced diet. He will also have been given advice on how to dispose of tissue used to clean his stoma. Extended bathroom facilities may be required as he will spend a fair amount of time there.

Care of a colostomy

The patient returns from theatre with a Chiron-type plastic colostomy bag applied. If he has a permanent colostomy, there is one opening onto the surface of the abdomen, the distal bowel having been removed. If the colostomy is temporary, such as the transverse colon, to allow an anastomosis or fistula to heal there will be a proximal and a distal opening (see Fig. 20.5). The proximal opening is the active orifice through which the faeces coming from the upper gastrointestinal tract leave the body. The distal opening is not active and only discharges some mucus. It links with the descending colon and rectum. Quite often there is very little drainage from a colostomy in the first 48 hours. To minimise the removal of the adhesive Chiron bag, a Schacht colostomy bag may be used in the early stages (Fig. 20.8). This is a ring of light plastic which can be attached to the abdominal wall. The plastic bags can then be fitted on to the ring instead of the skin itself.

The patient is taught how to clean the colostomy with soap and water, and how to attach the bags. By careful control of diet and fluids it is possible to regulate the colostomy, although some patients prefer to do a daily washout to ensure that the colostomy does not work when they do not want it to. The dietitian will discuss a suitable diet and the problems which may arise from drinking beer, and from eating onions and sometimes green vegetables. Hot drinks act as a stimulant on the gut.

Before going home the patient will have been linked to the Colostomy Welfare Group and may have met and discussed his problems with a person already having a colostomy. He should know how to use the appliance he is going home with and where to obtain further supplies. If the patient is unable to manage, then a relative will need to be shown and the district nurse should visit. If the patient has not got an incinerator, the bags will have to be emptied into the lavatory and rinsed before putting into a plastic bag and the dustbin.

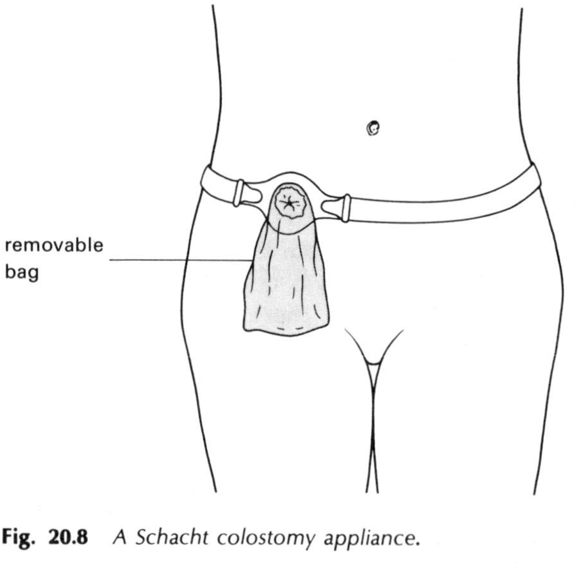

Fig. 20.8 *A Schacht colostomy appliance.*

These patients need even more psychological support once they get home than do patients with an ileostomy because they tend to be in the older age group. Disgust at the colostomy or ileostomy may interfere with the desire for sexual activity, particularly as pressure on the bag may cause leakage. Some patients with a colostomy become impotent.

DIVERTICULITIS

Diverticulitis is a condition in which small pouches form in the walls of the colon as a result of the mucosa herniating through the circular muscle close to a blood vessel. The herniated pouches of mucosa are called diverticula (Fig. 20.9) and are the result of abnormal pressure in the bowel thought to be due to a diet low in roughage and high in refined sugar. These diverticula may become infected causing diverticulitis, or they may rupture, leading to abscesses or peritonitis. If fibrotic adhesions develop, they may cause an obstruction. Fistulae can also form between the colon and the bladder.

The main line of treatment is to give a diet high in residue, that is bran, wholemeal bread, appropriate cereals, fruit and vegetables. A bulk-forming aperient may also be given. If surgery is required, the diseased area is resected and an anastomosis of the remaining bowel carried out. Fistulae usually require surgery and abscesses drainage.

Regional enteritis (Crohn's disease)

This is an inflammatory disorder mainly affecting the ileum and colon but it can affect any part of the gastrointestinal tract. The inflammation jumps from one part of the tract to another, with normal tissue spared between. The submucosa is the layer which is inflamed, with ulceration in the mucosa which has a 'cobblestone' appearance. The bowel wall is thickened and the lumen narrowed. The ulcers may perforate causing fistulae which connect with the adjacent organs, bowel or skin. Strictures may develop as a result of the fibrosis.

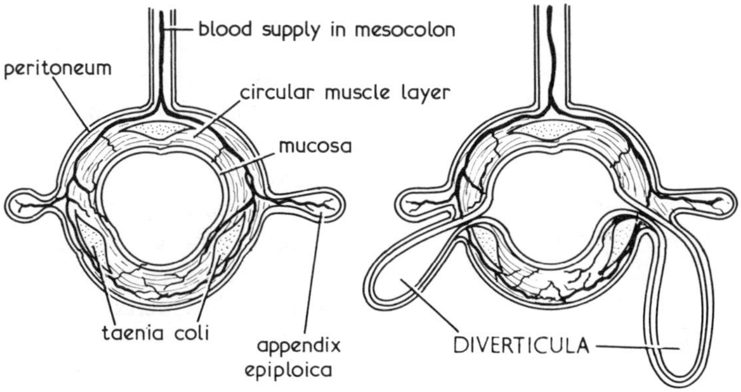

Fig. 20.9 *Diverticula.*

The cause of regional enteritis is unknown, although there have been many theories about it, suggesting that it is an allergic or autoimmune response.

Clinical picture

This condition is found in young adults between the ages of 20 and 35 years. They present with episodes of abdominal cramplike pain and diarrhoea. There may be blood in the faeces, anorexia and a low fever. It tends to be a chronic condition with relapses and remissions, the patient losing weight and showing evidence of malnutrition, anaemia and electrolyte imbalance. It is frequently mistaken for appendicitis. The patient may present with fistulae or an anal fissure, or even an intestinal obstruction.

Management

A rectal examination, barium enema and sigmoidoscopy with biopsy will be done. The barium enema may show the 'string sign' in which normal segments of bowel are seen to be separated by a very narrowed portion like string. A barium meal and follow-through may be given to discover if there are any lesions higher up.

Surgery is avoided if possible because there is a high incidence of recurrence within a few years. The aim of the medical treatment is to treat the pain, diarrhoea and any secondary infection which may arise (in a similar way to ulcerative colitis). Exclusion of milk and its products is also tried as a small group of patients appears to be allergic to it. The diet will be high in protein and calories, and extra iron, hydroxocobalamin (vitamin B12) and folic acid may be necessary.

However, invariably the patient will require surgery at some point, either to remove the diseased part with a resection and anastomosis or to deal with fistulae, abscesses, adhesions or intestinal obstruction. In order to ensure that the patient is in the optimal condition for this operation, parenteral nutrition may be commenced. Otherwise the preparation and aftercare of this patient is the same as for an abdominoperineal excision of rectum or colectomy. Some patients have so much small intestine resected that they are unable to absorb sufficient nutrients to sustain life and therefore have to be maintained on parenteral feeding for the rest of their lives.

Hirschsprung's disease (megacolon) (Fig. 20.10)

In this condition there is an absence of the nerve ganglion in the rectum which is therefore unable to contract and acts as an obstruction. As a result the bowel above it becomes greatly distended and its muscle hypertrophies. It is an inherited abnormality more commonly found in boys.

The baby presents with chronic constipation (the bowels acting less frequently than once a

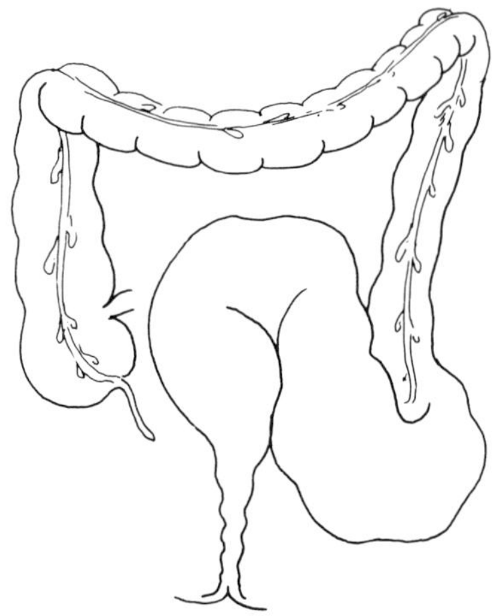

Fig. 20.10 *Hirschsprung's disease.*

week), wasted limbs and a distended abdomen. Marked signs of toxaemia and malnutrition soon arise and without treatment death occurs due to acute obstruction, perforation or malnutrition. In the later stages vomiting may occur and the abdomen becomes barrel shaped and very prominent.

Management

Surgical excision of the aganglionic segment of bowel with an anastomosis of the two ends may be carried out. A temporary colostomy is frequently performed at the same time to allow the anastomosis to heal. Another method used is Duhamel's operation in which the bowel is divided at the upper end of the rectum and the ends closed. The colon is then drawn down into the space behind the rectum. The adjoining walls of the rectum and colon are destroyed by crushing, thus providing a channel in which the front half is without ganglia but the back half is normal and able to produce the necessary contraction to empty the bowel (Fig. 20.11).

The child is not operated on until his general condition has been improved, unless it is considered that emergency surgery to relieve the obstruction is necessary. If this is so, a temporary colostomy will be done, with further surgery at a later stage. Otherwise the obstruction is relieved by rectal washouts and fluids are replaced intravenously.

Congenital atresia of the bowel

Atresia may occur at any point along the bowel and may affect several places. Atresia of the duodenum will cause vomiting soon after birth and this

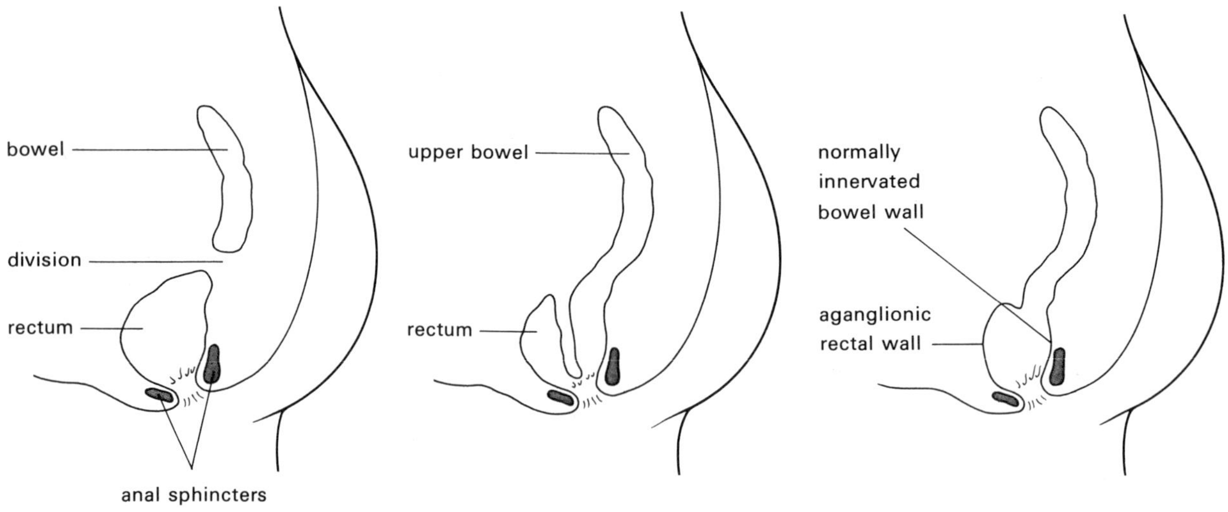

Fig. 20.11 *Duhamel's operation.*

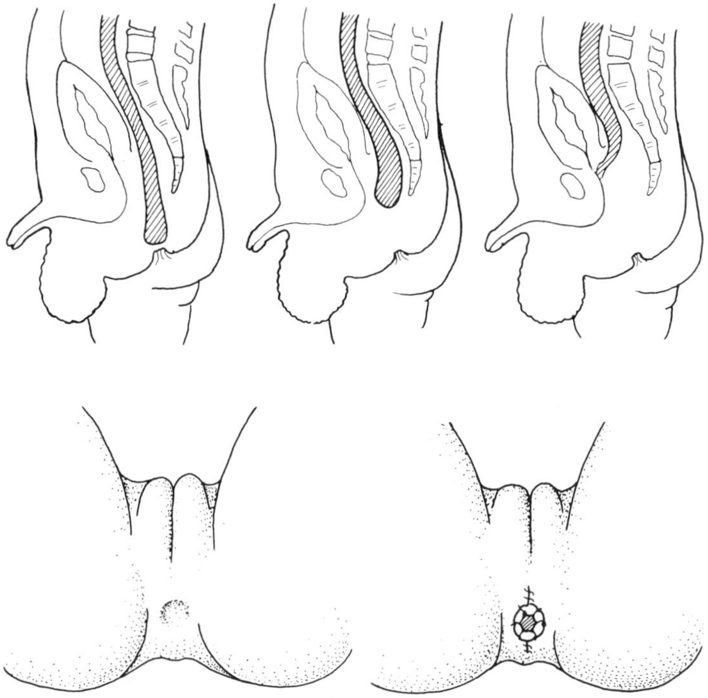

Fig. 20.12 *Types of imperforate anus, and its repair.*

requires urgent operation. An imperforate or deflected anus may also arise due to faulty development. During fetal development the skin in the anal region invaginates to unite with the descending bowel; failure to unite results in an imperforate anus (Fig. 20.12). This may merely consist of a thin layer of skin obstructing the outlet or there may be a considerable distance between the two ends. Sometimes there is only a slight deflection which interferes with the normal process of defaecation. It is diagnosed at birth at the first examination when a thermometer or the finger cannot be introduced into the rectum. A colostomy will be done in the first place to relieve the obstruction and later a plastic operation to correct the defect.

SUGGESTED WORK

1. Find out how different surgeons in your hospital prepare patients for surgery on the colon. Why do they choose their particular methods? What are the advantages and disadvantages?

2. Find out from the stoma care nurse what after-care patients receive on discharge from your hospital if they have had a colostomy or ileostomy. Do all patients receive the same follow-up care on discharge? If not, why not?

3. Find out from a patient who has had either a colostomy or ileostomy what problems worry him most.

SUGGESTED READING

Alexander N. B. (1982). Stomas. Self help groups Parts 1 and 2. *Clinics in Gastroenterology*; **11** (2): 405–419.

Brady V. A. (1980). Community care of the stoma patient. *Nursing*; **17**: 741–3.

Life with an ileostomy (editorial) (1982). *Lancet*; **2**: 1079–80.

Tiffany R. (1978). Oncology for Nurses and Health Care Professionals. Volume 2: *Care and Support*. London: George Allen & Unwin.

* * *

Mr DAVID CROSS (aged 56) a businessman, married with three children in their teens, has been admitted with carcinoma of the rectum.

Medical plan
Abdominoperineal excision of the rectum.

Identification of the patient's needs and problems in the continuing postoperative period and action arising from these

Pain
Administer prescribed analgesics as required. Monitor their effectiveness.

Fluid and electrolyte balance
Regulate and monitor the intravenous infusion carefully. Report any blood electrolyte results to the doctor promptly. Maintain a fluid balance chart. When Mr Cross is taking adequate fluids by mouth, check with the doctor if the intravenous infusion can be discontinued. Encourage him to drink freely.

Wounds
Check that the abdominal wound is clean and dry. If necessary, cover with a waterproof dressing. Remove the sutures after 10–14 days. Check the colour of the colostomy; report any discoloration. Observe if the colostomy is protruding adequately and report if not. Remove the Redivac drains from the perineal wound when drainage minimal and keep this wound clean with a spirit-based lotion.

General observations
Once the patient's condition is stable the blood pressure can be taken less frequently. Four-hourly temperature and pulse will continue for the first few days after operation to monitor for infection.

Nutrition
Nothing will be given by mouth until the fourth postoperative day, but Mr Cross may have ice to suck and frequent mouthwashes. The nasogastric tube will be removed once the aspirate has become minimal. Gradually introduce fluids, then light solids, until the patient returns to a normal diet. Arrange for the dietitian to come and discuss his diet and those foods which are best avoided.

Excretion
Ensure the catheter is comfortably secured and draining satisfactorily. Maintain catheter toilet and empty the drainage bag as required. It should not require changing. Remove the catheter on the fifth day postoperatively in the morning and check when the patient first passes urine, and the amount.

Colostomy
Note the first colostomy action and change the bag as necessary, washing the skin with soap and water. Note the condition of the skin around the stoma. Report any soreness and if necessary apply protective barrier cream. Help Mr Cross to look at his colostomy and gradually take over the management of it himself.

Prevention of respiratory complications
Arrange for the physiotherapist to continue breathing and leg exercises and supplement these. Mobilise the patient as soon as his condition allows.

Hygiene
Bedbath, giving as much assistance as is needed. When Mr Cross is fit enough he may have a general bath, keeping the colostomy covered with a Chiron or other bag. Pressure areas should be inspected and appropriate preventative measures taken. He will be able to attend to his own mouth care.

Psychological
Discuss with Mr Cross his feelings regarding the stoma. If he is agreeable, arrange for a former patient who has adapted well to having a colostomy to come and talk to him. Discuss his needs with his wife and encourage them to talk together. Discuss what the children should be told and who is the best person to tell them. He may be worried about the smell and how he can continue at work. He may decide that he would like to do a daily washout and will therefore need to be taught how to do this. Arrange for the stoma nurse or appliance officer to continue their visits after his discharge home. They will be able to give him advice on the appliances available and how they may be disposed of.

21

Haemorrhoids, Fistulae, Fissures and Abscesses

Most of the conditions affecting the region of the anus are extremely painful, as is the resulting surgery. The individual is therefore very reluctant to defaecate, and can be very demoralised by the pain. Thus the nurse's main role in caring for these patients is to ensure that they receive adequate relief from pain and to give any support required. Infection is another hazard the nurse will need actively to prevent and, if it does occur, she must recognise it at an early stage.

Specific emphasis in the nursing history

Elimination. Note bowel habits and in particular the degree of constipation present. Is blood or mucus present? Is pain associated with defaecation?

Nutrition. Note the amount of roughage the patient has in his diet and his fluid intake.

General appearance. Is there any indication of anaemia such as pallor, tiredness or lethargy?

Skin. Note any skin irritation or soreness of the anus.

Mobility. Note the amount of exercise the patient has each day.

Previous medication. Note what aperients the patient is taking. Is he on any drugs which have a tendency to constipate?

HAEMORRHOIDS

The blood supply to the rectum is mainly from the superior rectal arteries, and the venous drainage is via the superior haemorrhoid veins. These veins become engorged and varicosed as a result of increased pressure in them. The pressure is usually as a result of straining to pass a constipated motion. (This constipation is thought to arise due to a lack of roughage in the diet.) Anything which adds to the abdominal pressure, such as pregnancy, pelvic tumours, cirrhosis of the liver and carcinoma of the rectum, increases the possibility of haemorrhoids. Heredity and occupations requiring much standing also predispose to the condition.

Internal haemorrhoids develop above the internal sphincter and are covered in mucous membrane. If they remain within the canal, they are said to be first degree. Sometimes they descend on defaecation and are visible; these are second degree and can be manually returned to the canal. If the haemorrhoids become prolapsed, they will eventually descend on walking or coughing and are termed third degree (Fig. 21.1).

Clinical picture

Haemorrhoids may bleed slightly over a long period of time before the patient does anything about them. He may therefore present with anaemia, and on further questioning and examination, be found to have haemorrhoids. There is usually a small amount of bright red blood on the surface of the stool when passed, and a mucous discharge may also be present which causes anal irritation. The patient usually complains of pain during and after defaecation. A proctoscopy is necessary to establish the diagnosis.

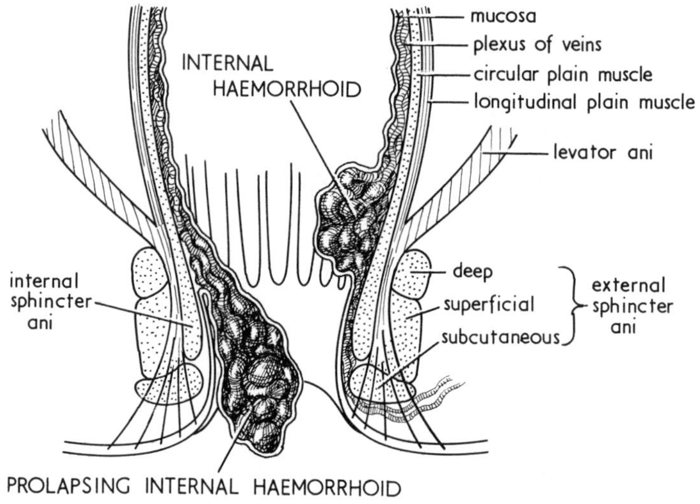

Fig. 21.1 *Internal haemorrhoids.*

Management

The patient is examined to exclude carcinoma of the rectum and this will include a sigmoidoscopy. Any anaemia is treated with iron preparations.

Conservative

The fibre content of the diet is increased with bran, wholemeal bread, fruit and vegetables. At the same time the quantity of food containing a large amount of refined sugar is reduced. Bulk-producing aperients such as methylcellulose are taken until the diet has been adjusted to form a soft bulky stool. Rectal suppositories containing bismuth subgallate, such as Anusol, may ease the local discomfort, but they can cause an allergic skin reaction.

Injection

A submucous injection of phenol 5% may be introduced into the base of each haemorrhoid. This fibroses the tissue around the vein, so constricting it. It may be necessary for several injections to be given before this method is effective which takes 2 to 3 weeks (Fig. 21.2).

Anal dilatation

This involves stretching the anus under an anaesthetic and is useful with small haemorrhoids.

Prolapsed haemorrhoids are treated by raising the foot of the bed, and returning the haemorrhoids to the anal canal if possible. If they are strangulated, a Eusol pack may be applied, and antibiotics given to control the infection. In this case analgesia will be required.

Ligation

This can be carried out with a rubber band and causes necrosis and sloughing of the tissue after a week. To prevent the rubber band being removed, the patient is given an enema prior to the procedure and a low-residue diet immediately after it.

Haemorrhoidectomy

Prior to admission the patient is given a bulk laxative to control the constipation. He may already be apprehensive about the pain to be experienced postoperatively; to add to this, his operation will probably be late in the day, as being a 'dirty case' he will be last on the list. He should

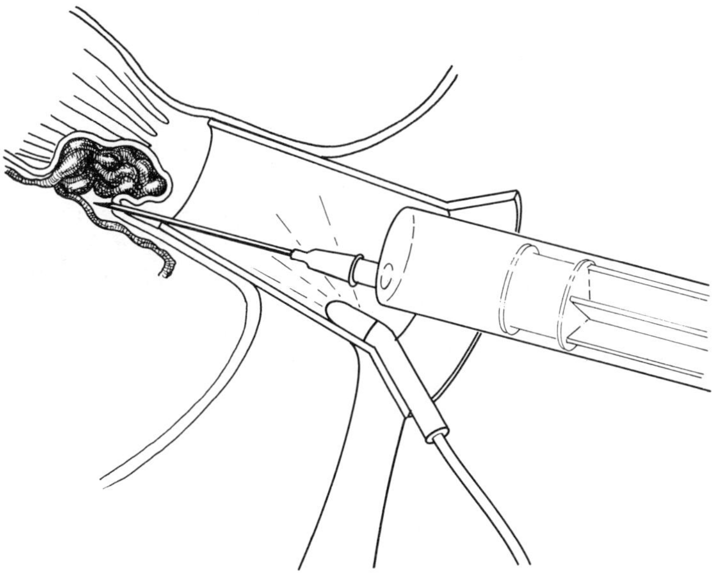

Fig. 21.2 *Injection of haemorrhoids.*

therefore be given a night sedation. His diet is usually normal up to the time of fasting, although some surgeons prescribe a low-residue diet to avoid an early bowel action postoperatively. Suppositories or an enema are usually sufficient to empty the lower bowel. A perineal shave is necessary.

Postoperative care

The patient is usually more comfortable in a lateral position. The wound must be carefully observed for haemorrhage, but as this may drain into the rectum, general observations such as pulse and colour or restlessness may be more significant. Management of the wound varies. There may be no dressing at all, gauze dressings tucked into the anus, or a drainage tube. The last-mentioned are usually left in position until the patient has the first bowel action. The urinary output should be carefully observed, particularly in male patients as retention due to an enlarged prostate may develop. This is a very painful operation and therefore analgesia is essential. The patient is able to get up the first day, and if the bowels have not been opened, a bulk aperient is given on the second day. The passage of the first stool is acutely painful and can cause the patient to faint. He should therefore be given something to ease the pain, Entonox is particularly useful as it is effective at the time required only. Once the pack or tube is out, the patient has saline baths twice a day and after any bowel action. Dilatation with a well-lubricated finger may be necessary to prevent stricture. The bowels are regulated by increasing the fibre content of the diet and with bulk aperients. Once the haemoglobin has been checked the patient is discharged on the fourth to seventh day.

Advice

The patient is advised to increase the amount of fibre in the diet by taking regular amounts of bran and wholemeal bread. He should keep the stools soft, with the addition of aperients as necessary. The saline baths and anal toilet should be continued until completely healed. He should drink plenty and establish a regular bowel habit. He must be told that small amounts of blood may be passed on defaecation for a short while and this is quite normal, but if larger amounts are passed about the seventh to tenth day, he must contact his doctor immediately as this may be a secondary haemorrhage. He may also feel a ridge in the anal passage due to fibrous tissue, and should ignore this and not strain. After 3 to 4 weeks the patient will return to out-patients and the doctor will decide if he is fit to return to work.

External haemorrhoids are caused by haemorrhage and thrombosis at the end of a branch of the inferior rectal vein, causing bleeding into the loose anal skin which presents as a small red cherrylike swelling. If compresses do not relieve the pain, the clot is evacuated by an incision under a local anaesthetic.

FISTULA-IN-ANO

This is a tract in the region of the anal sphincter. It may be complete, one end opening onto the skin and the other onto the mucous surface of the bowel, or incomplete, opening either into the bowel only or onto the skin surface only. There is a continual purulent discharge which irritates the skin. If the fistula becomes blocked, an abscess forms. In a complete fistula there will be leakage of faeces.

Inflammation spreading from the rectum and anal canal to the surrounding tissues, such as an ischiorectal abscess, may cause a fistula. Fistulae are occasionally due to tuberculosis or syphilis.

Management

The patient is examined to exclude any other disease of the colon which may have led to the fistula. A *fistulectomy* will be done in which the surgeon cuts down into the fistula and lays it open. Healing is allowed to take place from the bottom of the wound by granulation. Paraffin gauze or warm wet dressings may be used to cover the exposed area, and any excess granulation removed with a silver nitrate stick. Aperients are given to soften the stool. Twice-daily saline baths are also given. If there is any danger of damaging the anorectal ring, the operation will be performed in stages. The anorectal ring is formed by the deep part of the external sphincter, a part of the levator ani, and the internal sphincter muscles. Division of the ring causes permanent faecal incontinence.

ANAL FISSURE

This is a tear in the anal mucosa, usually caused by the passage of a constipated stool. It becomes infected, sloughs and will not heal. There is a small triangular ulcer with a tag of oedematous skin (which is called a sentinel pile) below it (Fig. 21.3). Because of acute pain there is spasm of the anal sphincter. It is so painful that the patient avoids having a bowel action, so becoming very constipated. The pain which occurs on defaecation and for some time after is burning and stabbing. There is also an associated pruritus ani and there may be slight bleeding and a purulent discharge. As the patient finds a rectal examination extremely painful, it is usually done under an anaesthetic.

Management

The aim is to relax the external sphincter and so allow the fissure to heal. If the fissure is recent, the muscle and surrounding tissue will be infiltrated with lignocaine. Digital dilatation may be done under anaesthetic. Regular aperients are given and dressings applied to the fissure.

The only satisfactory treatment for more long-standing cases is to excise the fissure, the fibrous tissue surrounding it and the sentinel pile, and divide the underlying sphincter. The wound must be allowed to granulate from the base, as with a fistula. Saline baths, analgesic ointments and aperients to keep the stool soft will also be used. A dilator will be necessary after the fifth or sixth day (Fig. 21.4).

PILONIDAL CYST OR SINUS

This condition is thought to be congenital and consists of a cyst filled with epithelium and hair over the sacrococcygeal area. From the cyst to the skin there are one or more small channels lined with epithelium and hair. These hairs may show on

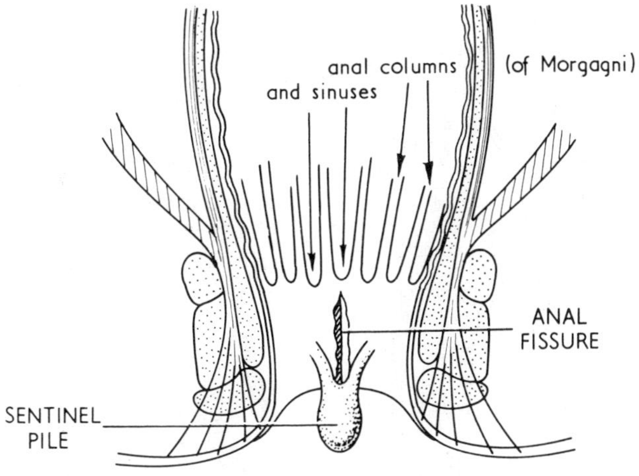

Fig. 21.3 *Anal fissure with sentinel pile.*

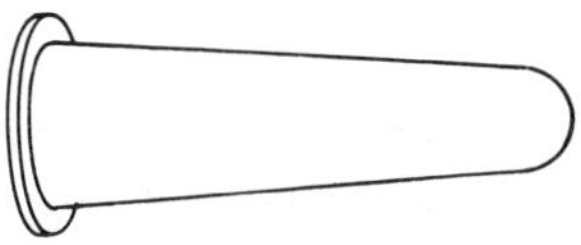

Fig. 21.4 *Anal dilator.*

the surface of the skin. Normally it causes no problems, but if it becomes infected, an abscess forms which has to be incised and drained. A chronic infection is treated by surgery.

The cyst may be removed and the resulting wound closed with stitches, or it may be left open to granulate. With the first approach the aim is to avoid tension on the suture line. The patient is therefore nursed prone and, when allowed up, discouraged from sitting for long periods. A bowel action is inhibited for the first few days. The second approach is cared for in the same manner as a fistula or fissure which has been laid open.

ISCHIORECTAL AND PERIANAL ABSCESS

Abscesses may arise in the ischiorectal fossa (a fatty mass) from conditions of the rectum and anal canal or from skin infections such as boils, or they may be due to infection elsewhere. If an abscess occurs near the anal margin, it is called a perianal abscess. Either of these may lead to fistulae (Fig. 21.5).

The patient complains of persistent pain which becomes severe on defaecation. Redness will be evident near the anus and the patient will have a temperature. Treatment is by incision and opening up of the abscess. It must be allowed to heal by granulation from the base of the wound or further abscesses may form. Twice-daily saline baths and frequent changes of dressing are necessary. The doctor usually prescribes antibiotics and a mild analgesic.

PROLAPSE OF THE RECTUM

Most commonly, the prolapse is incomplete, with only the mucous membrane prolapsing, and is associated with haemorrhoids. Complete prolapse with protrusion of the whole rectal wall most commonly occurs in children, but it can arise in adults, particularly elderly women. Prolapse is the result of weak muscles and straining due to chronic constipation. It is therefore associated with the elderly and those who have had an operation in that region.

The red mucous membrane of the prolapsed

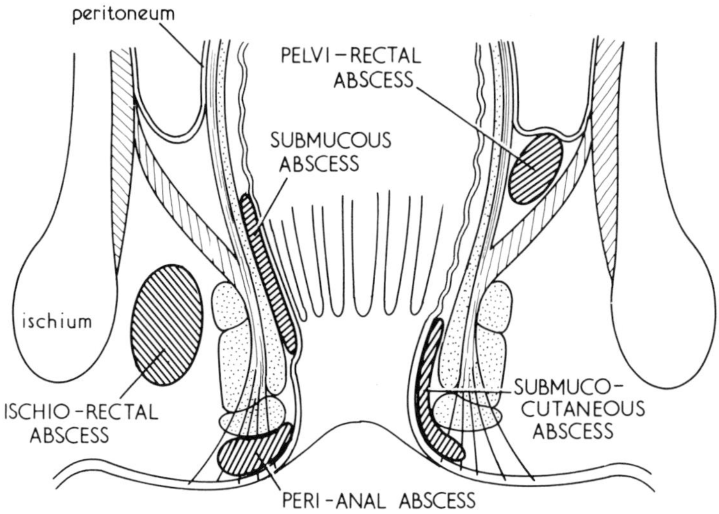

Fig. 21.5 *Rectal abscesses.*

rectum is visible on examination, and there is an associated discharge and bleeding. There may even be incontinence of faeces in the chronic case. An incomplete prolapse can be treated by phenol injections which cause adhesions, or by removal of the prolapsed mucous membrane. A reparative operation is necessary for a complete prolapse.

PROCTITIS

This is an inflammation of the rectum which may arise in association with inflammatory conditions of the colon, infection, threadworms and following treatment locally with radium. The patient passes frequent stools, which are mixed with blood or pus. Pain and pruritus ani may also be present. The causative condition is treated.

PRURITUS ANI

This is the term used to describe intense itching around the anus. Haemorrhoids, fissures, fistulae and proctitis may be the cause. Diabetes mellitus and dermatitis may also give rise to it, but often no cause can be found and it is then thought to be due to tension. Possible causes have to be looked for, and if found, treated. Personal hygiene must be maintained but excessive washing with soap may be an aggravating factor. Soothing lotions and steroid preparations may reduce the irritation. Mild sedation may be given to help reduce the tension.

SUGGESTED WORK

1. Find out the most common form of treatment for haemorrhoids in your hospital. Are any patients treated as day cases?
2. Discuss with a patient who has had a haemorrhoidectomy or surgery for a fistula or fissure how his postoperative care compared with what he expected.

SUGGESTED READING

Silver E., Silver A. J. (1984). Acute abdomen. *Medicine in Practice*; **2**: 1.

* * *

Mrs SARAH CHURCH (aged 40) is married with four children. She has been admitted with internal haemorrhoids for a haemorrhoidectomy. She tends to eat easily prepared food with little roughage and is not interested in active sport, being slightly overweight. She has a tendency to constipation, despite taking various aperients, frequently seeing bright red blood on the stool passed. Associated with the haemorrhoids she has pruritus. She also complains of pain during and after defaecation. Prior to admission she commenced ferrous sulphate, methylcellulose and Anusol suppositories.

Medical plan
Continue medication as on admission. Sigmoidoscopy. Haemorrhoidectomy.

Identification of the patient's needs and problems in the immediate post operative period and action arising from these

Possibility of haemorrhage
Observe for any soaking of the perineal dressing. Take particular note of restlessness, raised pulse or pallor, as haemorrhage may be hidden.

Pain
Administer prescribed analgesics as required, do not withhold. Note their effectiveness and ask the doctor for something stronger if not sufficient. Make sure the patient is not inhibited from asking for analgesia if required.

Dressing
Change as required, noting how frequently this is necessary. The drainage tube will be left in until the first bowel action.

Pruritus
Keep the anal area clean and dry and apply soothing ointment as prescribed. Make sure the patient is not allergic to the ointment.

Anaemia
If there was a heavy blood loss in theatre, she may require injections of iron or even a blood transfusion. The haemoglobin will be checked.

Hygiene
Once she has fully recovered from the anaesthetic she will be given a wash and her nightdress put on. A mouthwash will freshen her mouth. She may also have sips of water.

Worry about pain on defaecation
Explain that her bowels will probably not act until the following day, at the earliest, and that if they have not acted then, a special type of aperient will be given. Reassure her that on passing her first motion Entonox will be used, which she will have already handled.

22

Conditions of the Biliary Tract, Liver and Pancreas

The patient suffering from a disease of these organs may, as a result, have jaundice. He presents the nurse with a number of what may appear to her as minor problems, but which to the patient can be very important. In some forms of jaundice, skin irritation can be quite distressing for the patient and nursing measures added to the medical preparations may afford him considerable relief. Encouraging the patient to drink large quantities of fluids may take all the nurse's ingenuity, as will the need to make a low-fat diet appear as palatable as possible. The nurse will also need to encourage the patient in deep breathing exercises before and after the operation on the gall bladder and to ensure that he has adequate analgesia to control pain, so making his co-operation easier.

Specific emphasis in the nursing history

Elimination. Note the colour of the stools and the urine.

Nutrition. Does the patient have to avoid fats because of association with pain or vomiting?

Skin. Note the presence of jaundice, skin irritation or petechial haemorrhages.

General appearance. Is there any obesity or wasting?

Pain. Note the presence of pain, where and when it occurs and its duration. What type of pain is it and is it related to nausea or vomiting?

Vital signs. Raised temperature.

The reticuloendothelial system breaks down damaged red blood cells releasing the pigment bilirubin, a fat-soluble substance. This is carried to the liver where it is converted into a water-soluble compound which is suitable for excretion in the urine and faeces. From the liver the bilirubin is secreted in the bile, passing down the biliary tract to the gall bladder, where the bile is concentrated. The gall bladder stores about 30 ml and releases the bile under the stimulus of the hormone cholecystokinin when fat enters the duodenum. The bilirubin is converted to stercobilinogen by bacteria in the bowel. Some of the bilirubin is reabsorbed into the bloodstream and is excreted by the kidneys as urobilinogen.

JAUNDICE (ICTERUS)

Jaundice is the yellow staining of the tissues occurring as a result of an increase in the amount of bilirubin in the blood; the normal range is 3.4–13.6 μmol/l. The sclera of the eyes, skin, mucosa and some body fluids become stained yellow.

Pre-hepatic jaundice

Before the red blood cells reach the liver they are broken down in large numbers, so releasing excessive amounts of bilirubin into the blood plasma. The liver is unable to deal with this increased amount of bilirubin and so it remains at a high level in the bloodstream. Breakdown of red blood cells in this way is called *haemolytic jaundice* or *anaemia*. Although this may be due to a number of causes, the only one requiring surgical intervention is *acholuric jaundice* (absence of bile pigment in urine). This arises as a result of a congenital abnormality in the shape of the red blood cells. The spleen and the reticuloendothelial system destroy the abnormal cells more quickly than normal. The excess bilirubin has not passed through the liver and therefore normal amounts of stercobilinogen and urobilinogen are excreted in the bowel and bladder, and as nothing is obstructing their excretion, the stools and urine are a normal colour. There is an indirect Van den Bergh reaction because the bilirubin is still in its fat-soluble state.

Hepatic jaundice

This is due to disease in the liver itself, such as hepatitis or, less commonly, cirrhosis. In this case too little bilirubin is removed from the blood in its passage through the liver. There is therefore less passed on to the bowel to form stercobilinogen, and less to the kidneys to form urobilinogen. The stools are therefore clay coloured and the urine dark. The plasma albumin falls and the plasma globulin, transaminases and alkaline phosphatase rise.

Post-hepatic jaundice

This arises as a result of some form of obstruction of the common bile duct preventing the bile from entering the duodenum (Fig. 22.1). The most usual causes are gall-stones in the duct, and carcinoma of the head of the pancreas obstructing the duct from outside. The excess bilirubin is reabsorbed back into the bloodstream, so giving a direct Van den Bergh reaction and raised serum alkaline phosphatase. Bile pigment is excreted in the urine which becomes dark, but as the bilirubin does not reach the duodenum, no stercobilinogen is formed and the stools are clay coloured. Its absence from the bowel also interferes with the absorption of fat

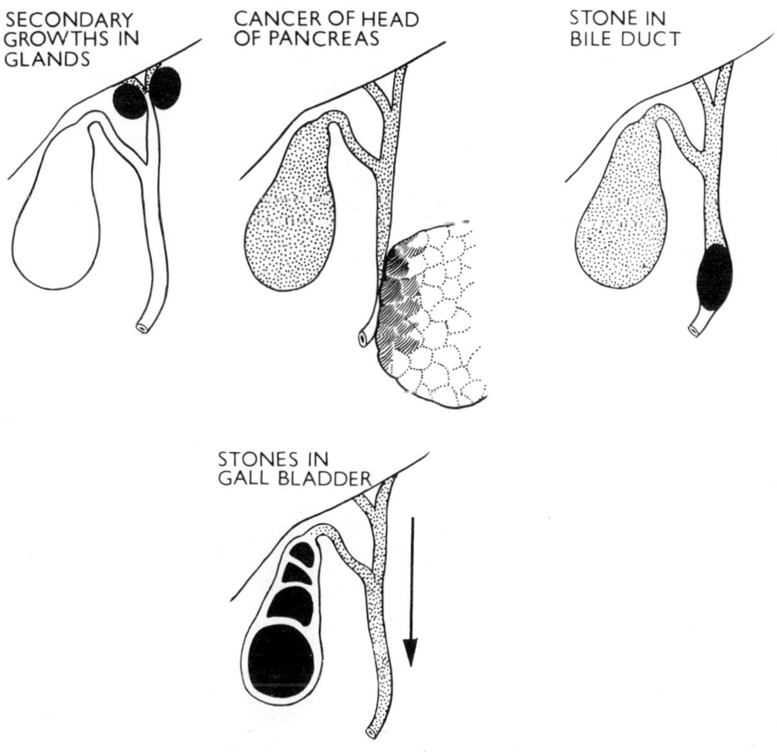

Fig. 22.1 *Obstruction of the biliary tract.*

and fat-soluble vitamins. Skin irritation may be severe due to the excess bile salts.

GALL-STONES

Gall-stones are very common but only cause problems when infection is present or the stones cause an obstruction. They are most common in middle-aged, obese women, but their incidence increases in older men. They are associated with a less active gall bladder which is present in pregnancy, and infection which may be the result rather than the cause. An increase in the ratio of cholesterol to bile salts is thought to be the main cause. Increased viscosity of the bile due to greater amounts of mucus being secreted by the gall bladder may precipitate the salts. These changes may be due to familial factors, certain diseases or diet.

There are three types of stone, consisting of cholesterol, bile pigments, or a mixture of cholesterol, calcium and bile pigments. Those consisting of cholesterol are usually large and single, the pigments being arranged in a radiating fashion. Bile pigment stones are black and usually numerous; they occur in haemolytic conditions. Mixed stones are the most common, and vary in size from as small as a grain of sand to those rather larger. If cut, alternating dark and pale rings can be seen, the former being the bile pigments and the latter cholesterol. The calcium is combined with both. At the centre there may be a nucleus of organic matter such as pus cells or mucous debris.

The stones may occur anywhere in the gall bladder or biliary tract, but only those in the common bile duct cause jaundice. They will also cause biliary colic. A stone obstructing the outlet from the gall bladder will cause biliary colic and cholecystitis. If one becomes impacted in the outlet of the common bile duct at its junction with the duodenum, there will be severe pain, jaundice, and pancreatitis. If the stone ulcerates through the gall bladder wall, it may enter the gastrointestinal tract and be excreted with the faeces. Large stones can cause an acute intestinal obstruction (gall-stone ileus).

BILIARY COLIC

Sudden, severe pain in the hypochondrium radiating round to the back which increases in intensity and lasts 2 to 3 hours or more is characteristic. The pain is such that the patient may roll about in the bed in an effort to gain relief from it. He is pale and sweaty.

ACUTE CHOLECYSTITIS

Inflammation of the gall bladder most commonly occurs as a result of obstruction to its outlet by a gall-stone. However, in a very small proportion of cases the obstruction is caused by inflammation and oedema resulting from an infection in a neighbouring organ spreading via the bloodstream, lymphatics, duodenum and biliary tract or directly. The organisms most commonly isolated are: *Esch. coli*, *Streptococcus faecalis*, *Streptococcus viridans*, *Salmonella typhi* and the staphylococci.

Clinical features

The patient has usually had a history of flatulent dyspepsia, and tends to be the type of person who develops gall-stones, possibly having episodes of biliary colic brought on by eating fat. The pain may be a dull ache due to the inflammation. There is nausea and vomiting and a raised temperature and pulse. On examination of the abdomen, the patient complains of extreme tenderness and will find taking deep breaths painful. Jaundice will be present if there is an obstruction of the common bile duct.

Management

If biliary colic is present, the patient will rest in bed and be given an analgesic such as intramuscular pethidine. Occasionally an anticholinergic drug which reduces secretions, such as propantheline, is given. Local application of heat helps reduce the pain. If the temperature is raised, a suitable antibiotic will be prescribed. Initially the patient may only be given fluids and a nasogastric tube may be passed for aspiration, but once the attack subsides he will be given a low-fat diet and, if necessary, a reducing diet. Straight x-rays of the upper abdomen may reveal some stones. In the absence of jaundice, an oral cholecystogram will be done to demonstrate the efficiency of the gall bladder. If required, an intravenous cholangiogram will also be carried out to show the bile ducts. Ultrasonography may also be used where this is available.

Chenodeoxycholic acid (CDA) 12–15 mg/kg/day, orally alone or combined with other drugs to dissolve the gall-stones and reduce the saturation of bile with cholestrol (alternative—ursodeoxycholate acid). This treatment is only effective for those stones composed of cholestrol in a functioning gall bladder, the stones reforming when the treatment is discontinued.

Cholecystectomy—removal of the gall bladder

Cholecystostomy—removal of stones and drainage of the gall bladder.

A self-retaining drainage catheter is left in situ.

Choledochostomy—drainage of the common bile duct.

Choledocholithotomy—removal of stone from common bile duct.

If the common bile duct is obstructed by a growth the following operations may be done.

Cholecystogastrostomy—anastomosis of the body of the gall bladder with the stomach.

Cholecystojejunostomy—anatomosis of the body of the gall bladder with the jejenum.

Specific preoperative care

The importance of deep breathing after the operation will be explained to the patient. He will be told that analgesics will be given to lessen the pain and so enable him to co-operate in this way. The presence of the two drainage tubes will also be explained to him. The physiotherapist will teach the patient diaphragmatic breathing, because the diaphragm is retracted during the operation, causing pain on deep breathing postoperatively and therefore a tendency to shallow breathing and chest infection. Blood tests will be taken for liver function and prothrombin as well as for grouping and cross-matching. Vitamin K is administered to prevent haemorrhage if there is any jaundice. Some surgeons request a nasogastric tube to be passed.

At the end of the cholecystectomy an operative cholangiogram is done to make sure that there are no stones in the ducts. The surgeon inserts a drain into the gall bladder bed to drain serous fluid, and if the bile ducts have been explored, he will also insert a 'T' tube into the common bile duct. The latter enables bile to drain while the ducts are inflamed.

Postoperative care

If there was any jaundice, the patient will continue on injections of vitamin K. He will be sat up in bed as soon as his condition enables it, and breathing exercises will be encouraged. Adequate analgesia will be required to enable the patient to breathe deeply without too much distress. Any intravenous therapy is discontinued once the patient is taking adequate fluids. Observations are related to the complications which may arise, the most likely being atelectasis, and bronchopneumonia, therefore the temperature and the patient's breathing will be observed. A subphrenic abscess or a biliary fistula may also arise, the former causing a raised temperature and the latter a discharge. Other more general complications may also arise, in particular a deep vein thrombosis.

The drain to the gall bladder bed is usually removed after 48 hours once significant drainage has ceased. The 'T' tube usually remains in for 8 to 10 days, after which a cholangiogram is done, but it may remain in longer than this and be removed when the stools are a normal colour and there is no pain when the tube is clamped off. While it is in position the drainage is measured and recorded. Before removal the patient may require pethidine. The 'T' tube will require firm traction to pull it out, the retaining suture having been removed first. There is usually some leakage of the bile from the remaining fistula but the latter heals up within a few days. Any jaundice or clay-coloured stools following the removal of the tube suggests that there is still some blockage in the ducts.

CHRONIC CHOLECYSTITIS

This condition may follow repeated minor attacks of acute cholecystitis or develop as an ill-defined condition. The main symptom is chronic dyspepsia with epigastric discomfort which is not related to meals. There is usually a sensation of fullness in the epigastrium which appears worse after large fatty meals, and tenderness in the region of the gall bladder on palpation. The patient may complain of 'bilious attacks' which consist of nausea and vomiting with some pain. Jaundice and pyrexia are not signs of a chronic cholecystitis, although referred pain in the shoulder or back may occur. The patient is treated conservatively unless gall-stones are shown to be present when a cholecystectomy will be done.

CARCINOMA OF THE GALL BLADDER

This is a rare condition and associated with gall-stones. The patient presents with the clinical features of chronic cholecystitis, intractable pain or discomfort in the right hypochondrium, wasting, and jaundice, and the doctor may feel a tumour and enlarged liver on examination. The treatment is a cholecystectomy and excision of the adjacent liver where possible. However, many cases are not diagnosed until they have become inoperable. The prognosis is poor and the operative mortality high. Cytotoxic drugs may be used instead of operation.

CARCINOMA OF THE BILE DUCTS, AMPULLA OF VATER AND HEAD OF PANCREAS

All of these conditions cause an obstruction of the bile duct and will present with similar clinical features. Carcinoma is rare in the bile ducts and only slightly more common in the ampulla of Vater. However, carcinoma of the pancreas is a moderately common tumour, usually affecting the head of the pancreas. They all cause a progressively deepening obstructive jaundice which may be painless or may cause bouts of epigastric pain which extends into the back. The stools are pale and the urine dark. The patient appears depressed, generally unwell and weak, having lost weight. He will have anorexia and vomiting, chronic diarrhoea and an intense irritation of the skin. There may be a raised temperature, mild diabetes, thrombosis in the leg veins or even mild fits. Melaena is sometimes present if the tumour has spread to the duodenum and ulcerated.

Investigations which may be carried out include: a barium meal to show distortion of the duodenum; pancreatic biopsy; scanning with selenomethionine-75; and eventually an exploratory laparotomy.

If an operation is possible, a pancreatoduodenectomy (Whipple's operation) is done, in which the head of the pancreas, the lower and of the stomach, the lower part of the common bile duct, all of the duodenum and the first part of the jejenum are excised. The bile duct, stomach and pancreas are then anastomosed separately to the jejenum. The prognosis is poor. Postoperatively the patient will require phytomenadione, blood transfusion and antibiotics. If the pancreas is completely removed, the pancreatic enzymes are replaced in the form of pancreatin which is usually sprinkled onto a meal. Insulin replacement is also required.

If the condition is inoperable, some relief may be obtained from the symptoms by a bypass operation—a cholecystojejunostomy, in which the gall bladder is anastomosed to the jejenum. The skin irritation may be relieved with oral cholestyramine 12–24 g daily, which reduces the serum cholesterol. It is ineffective if there is complete obstruction, and may add to the anorexia and nausea. If ascites is present, a paracentesis abdominis will provide relief. As the condition progresses, increasingly strong analgesics will be needed.

ACUTE PANCREATITIS

This is not a surgical condition but may be present on a surgical ward because the signs are typical of a ruptured gastric or duodenal ulcer. The cause of pancreatitis is unknown, although it may be associated with gall-stones in obese women, alcoholism or mumps.

The pancreatic juice escapes into the tissue of the gland, initially causing inflammation but progressing to destruction of the gland. There is also bleeding into the gland from damaged blood vessels, and peritonitis develops. The released lipase causes patches of fat necrosis in the pancreas and peritoneum.

Because the patient may present with clinical features similar to those of a ruptured peptic ulcer—that is, severe epigastric pain, vomiting and collapse—he may be operated on. Preferably, an operation is avoided and the symptoms treated by gastric aspiration, intravenous therapy, analgesics and antibiotics. The condition may resolve or develop into chronic pancreatitis.

Chronic pancreatitis

Although this condition may follow acute pancreatitis, it may present in the chronic form from the start. There is a gradual destruction of the pancreas which may lead to an obstructive jaundice or an intestinal obstruction. Replacement enzymes and insulin may be required. Sometimes calculi develop in the pancreatic ducts.

PANCREATIC CYSTS

These cysts cause a swelling in the epigastrium or left upper quadrant of the abdomen and sometimes grow to a large size, but they are not common. They may cause pain, vomiting or jaundice. There are two types.

True pancreatic cysts are usually benign cystic neoplasms (cystadenoma) and most of them can be removed completely. *False pancreatic cysts* result from pancreatitis or injuries to the pancreas. They are collections of fluid lying adjacent to the pancreas, and it is not possible to remove them. They cannot be drained on to the surface of the abdomen because they often communicate freely with the pancreatic ducts and a persistent fistula of highly irritant pancreatic juice would then result. They are usually dealt with by making an anastomosis between the cyst and the stomach, after which the cyst rapidly becomes smaller and the secretion flows harmlessly into the gastrointestinal tract.

ADENOMA OF THE ISLET TISSUE

This tumour arises less frequently than the others. It gives rise to episodes of hypoglycaemia in which the patient becomes confused, restless and pale, and feels weak, the pulse rate being increased. Repeated attacks cause brain damage. The tumour is removed surgically or a partial pancreatectomy is done.

LIVER ABSCESS AND PORTAL PYAEMIA

The circulation of the intestinal tract, gall bladder, pancreas and spleen drains into the liver via the portal vein. Therefore, if any of these organs is affected by disease, emboli may be taken to the liver where they may form an abscess (suppurative pylephlebitis). The most common source of infection is an infected appendix, although abscesses may arise following diverticulitis or infection of the gall bladder. The organisms most commonly found are *Esch. coli* and *Streptococcus faecalis*, although others may be isolated.

Clinical features

The patient looks toxic, with a raised temperature and rigors, increased pulse rate, weight loss and a dull ache over the region of the liver. There may be some jaundice and anaemia present. Vomiting is common and diarrhoea may occur in the terminal stages. On examination the liver is found to be enlarged. Blood taken for analysis shows a raised white cell count and erythrocyte sedimentation rate. The liver function tests show a raised alkaline phosphatase and low serum albumin. There are filling defects shown on the liver scan.

Management

The abscess is drained surgically and an appropriate antibiotic given; any underlying infection will also be treated. Nursing is as for any pyrexial patient, fluids being encouraged and light easily digested meals. An antiemetic may also be required. General nursing care will be of paramount importance. Unfortunately, treatment is not always successful.

HYDATID CYSTS OF THE LIVER

The tapeworm *Echinococcus granulosis*, not normally found in Britain, may be picked up from dogs, the ova being carried by the portal vein to the liver where they give rise to cysts which may contain daughter cysts. Although the majority of these cysts occur in the liver, they may also be found in the lungs, intestines, brain or spleen.

They may not give rise to symptoms, but as the liver enlarges this will cause abdominal distension and discomfort. If the cyst ruptures, the daughter cysts may spread into the neighbouring organs and, because of the release of protein from the cyst, a severe anaphylaxis results.

X-rays may reveal the outlines of the cysts and a liver scan may help to localise them. The eosinophils in the blood are increased. Cassoni's intradermal test, in which sterile hydatid cyst fluid is injected to produce a wheal, can also help diagnosis.

Because of the danger of rupture, the cysts are surgically removed, but prior to their removal they are injected with formalin to kill the daughter cysts. Great care is taken not to rupture the cyst as this will cause an anaphylactic reaction or spread of the daughter cysts.

NEOPLASMS OF THE LIVER

Benign tumours and primary neoplasms (hepatomas) are rare, but secondary ones (carcinomas) from the gastrointestinal tract via the portal vein are common. They may also arise from a primary carcinoma in the breast and lungs, and melanomas may spread to the liver.

Clinical features

The liver becomes enlarged and nodular causing abdominal distension, and there may also be some abdominal pain. Jaundice and ascites may develop as the condition progresses, and the patient's condition will gradually deteriorate. Liver scanning will demonstrate filling defects and arteriography an abnormal arterial system. The blood alkaline phosphatase and transaminase levels are raised.

Management

If the growth is localised, a wedge resection may be done, but it is frequently spread through the liver and palliative procedures such as a paracentesis abdominis will be carried out as required. Cytotoxic drugs will be introduced directly into the hepatic artery with a cannula. Rarely, complete removal and a liver transplant may be attempted.

RUPTURE OF THE LIVER

This may arise as a result of a road traffic accident or a kick by a horse. The patient will be severely shocked with abdominal tenderness and rigidity. The haemorrhage and shock are treated with a blood transfusion and the torn surfaces of the liver sutured together or the injured lobe resected.

PORTAL HYPERTENSION AND OESOPHAGEAL VARICES

Portal hypertension is a rise in the pressure in the portal vein and is most commonly caused by hepatic cirrhosis. This is a chronic inflammatory condition of the liver in which the damaged cells are replaced by scar tissue (fibrosis), causing obstruction to the flow of blood through the liver. Thrombosis in the veins entering or leaving the liver, and in particular the portal vein, may also give rise to portal hypertension.

As a result of the portal hypertension and back pressure, a collateral circulation develops. As the pressure increases in these unsupported veins under the mucosa, they bulge into the oesophagus and stomach forming oesophageal varices. If the pressure increases too much, they will rupture causing a massive haematemesis with melaena stools.

Management of ruptured oesophageal varices

The immediate care is to control the bleeding, reassure the patient and restore blood volume. The patient may be shocked due to loss of blood and will therefore be nursed lying down, the doctor being informed immediately of his condition. Observations of his temperature, pulse, respirations and blood pressure will be taken quarter-hourly at first. The vomit will be measured, recorded and saved for examination by the doctor. Any stools passed will be observed for blood, recorded on a stool chart and kept for the doctor's inspection. Nothing is given by mouth, but when the patient has finished vomiting he may require a mouthwash.

The doctor will commence an intravenous infusion until a blood transfusion is ready. The bowel is kept empty by means of a lavage and neomycin given to reduce the activity of organisms in the bowel which break down protein and produce ammonia. Pitressin may be given to control bleeding. If the bleeding continues, it may be necessary for the doctor to pass a Sengstaken tube for up to 48 hours (Fig. 22.2). This contains three channels. Channel one leads to an elongated balloon which, when inflated, presses against the oesophageal wall; channel two leads to a smaller balloon which lies just inside the stomach so preventing the tube from going further down; and channel three leads to the stomach for aspiration. The tube is passed via the nose with the balloons deflated, a cuff of foam protecting the nose at its entry point, and traction is applied to it. While it is down, the nurse stays with the patient, regularly aspirating the contents. If there is any excess saliva, suction apparatus is used, and if blood is aspirated from the stomach, a gastric lavage is done with a small amount of iced water. Should there be any difficulty in breathing or choking, the tube is deflated. The patient will need to be carefully watched as he may be confused.

To remove the tube, the oesophageal balloon is deflated and 12–24 hours later the gastric balloon is also deflated, the traction being removed and the tube fixed to the face. The patient is observed for further bleeding during the next 24 hours and, if none, a lubricant such as olive oil is given to the patient to drink. The tube is then withdrawn and the patient observed for any further signs of bleeding. During this period the patient must be nursed on complete bedrest and attention paid to his hydration and nutrition. He will need much support because of the fear of a further haemorrhage. Trauma to the area is avoided by cutting out roughage, raw fruit and vegetables, and by chewing the food well. The patient is also encouraged to have small meals.

If the above measures are not effective or the surgeon wishes to prevent further episodes, some means of bypassing the obstruction and so reducing the portal hypertension is carried out. A portacaval shunt is one method which may be considered in which an anastomosis is made between the portal vein and the inferior vena cava (Fig. 22.3). Preferably these bypasses are planned operations carried out when the patient's condition has improved.

Specific preoperative care

These operations are not carried out if the patient has ascites or is in a hepatic coma. Instead the patient will be given phytomenodione, antibiotics and intravenous fluids. A blood transfusion will also be required and a nasogastric tube will be passed.

Specific postoperative care

The approach may be either abdominal or via the chest. Whichever route is used, the appropriate care should be given. Great care is taken with the drugs used as these may precipitate a coma. The patient will be watched carefully for mental confusion or personality change which may indicate the onset of a coma. The renal function is monitored carefully, a fluid balance chart being kept. The nasogastric tube is aspirated 2-hourly and a note made of any blood in the aspirate. Observations for haemorrhage are maintained. The patient is fed intravenously until bowel sounds return and he is taking sufficient by mouth. At this time the nasogastric tube will also be removed. When he is able to

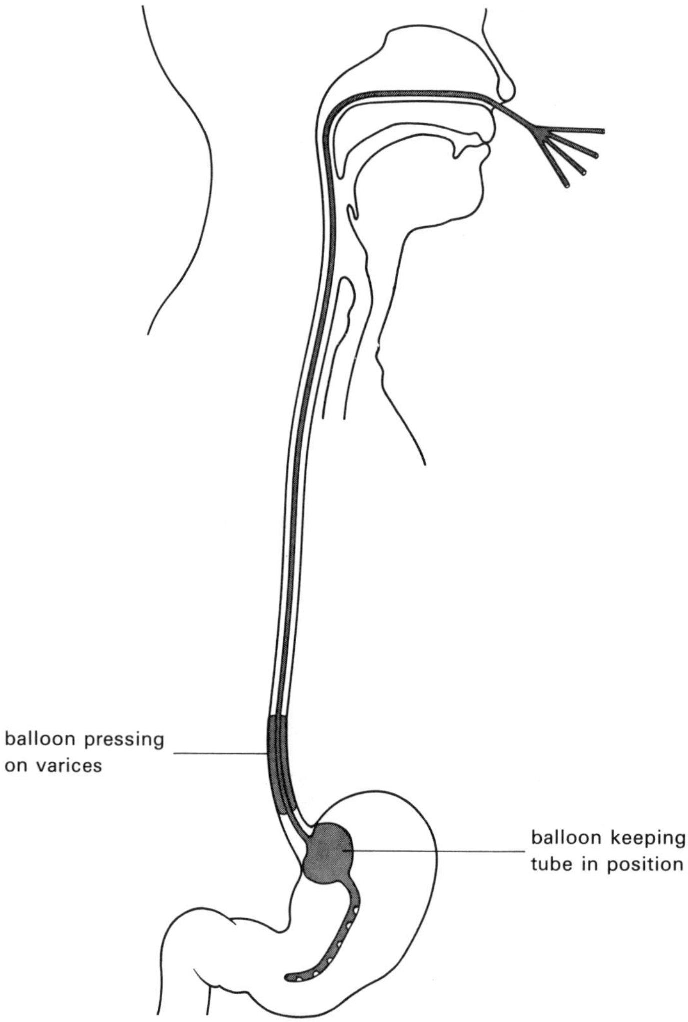

Fig. 22.2 *Sengstaken tube.*

eat he will be given a low-protein diet and commence neomycin. He will also be observed for any evidence of thrombi at the site of the anastomosis which would be indicated by pain, raised temperature, distension and nausea. The nurse will also look out for oedema, ascites and melaena. On discharge the relatives need to recognise the initial symptoms of portosystemic encephalopathy, which arises because the liver no longer deals with toxic substances such as ammonia, and which can be seen to be developing if the patient lacks co-ordination and concentration and becomes confused or even goes into a coma. Reduction of protein in the diet and the use of neomycin to destroy bowel bacteria which break down protein will help.

RUPTURE OF THE SPLEEN

This condition will only arise if there is a severe blow in the region of the lower ribs. It is obviously

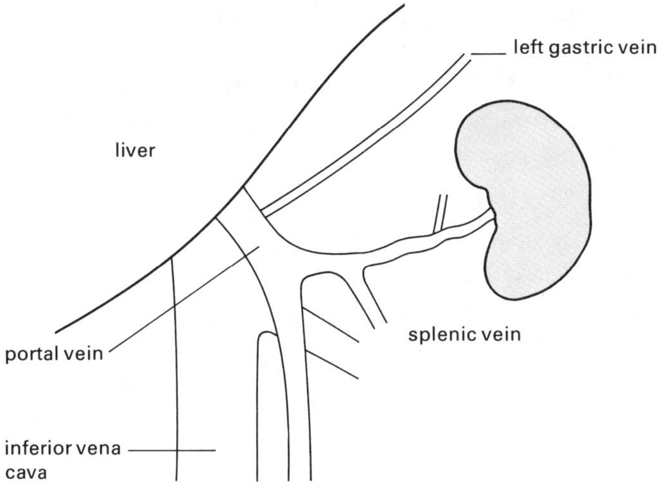

(a)

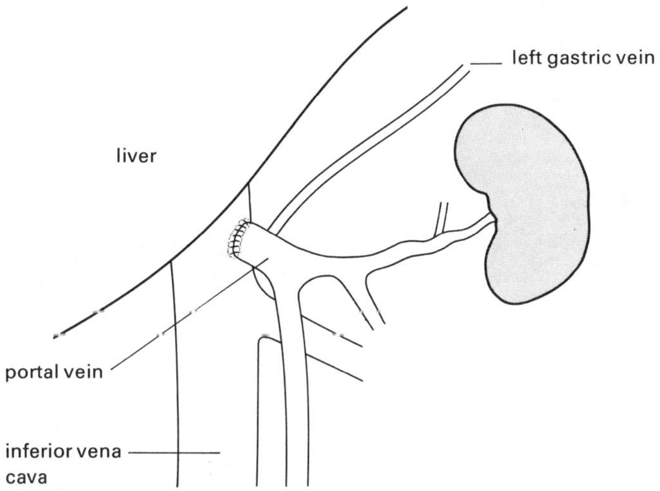

(b)

Fig. 22.3 *(a) Normal circulation to the liver. (b) Portacaval shunt.*

easier for damage to occur if the spleen is enlarged due to disease. Severe haemorrhage occurs which may be contained within the capsule to begin with, but as pressure builds up this eventually ruptures. The patient will present with the signs of an internal haemorrhage and pain in the left shoulder and flank. An emergency splenectomy is carried out. The patient invariably requires a blood transfusion.

SPLENOMEGALY

The spleen may become enlarged in conditions in which the blood cells are abnormal, for example in shape, and it therefore destroys them, causing anaemia. The most effective treatment is by means of a splenectomy.

SUGGESTED WORK

1. Find as many patients with jaundice as you can and compare the degree of jaundice arising from different causes.
2. Find out what preparations are used in your hospital to relieve skin irritation.

SUGGESTED READING

Gotch P. M. (1981). Are you ready for a total pancreatectomy patient? *R. N.;* **44** (11): 55–7.

* * *

Mrs ETHEL BEAN (aged 45) is married with four children in their teens. She is an obese lady with a history of flatulent dyspepsia and some jaundice. She has been diagnosed as having cholecystitis due to gall-stones. Before admission she was commenced on a low-fat reducing diet and antibiotics.

Medical plan
Cholecystectomy and exploration of the common bile duct.

Identification of the patient's needs and problems in the immediate postoperative period and action arising from these

Pain
Administer prescribed analgesics as required. She will particularly need these prior to physiotherapy sessions and for the removal of the 'T' tube.

Recognition of haemorrhage and shock
Monitor the blood pressure and pulse half-hourly until stable. Note any physical signs of shock such as pallor, and the general appearance of the patient. Administer vitamin K if prescribed.

Wound
Check the wound on return from theatre and at frequent intervals after this for haemorrhage. Check the notes for specific instructions. Note any abnormal discharge from drainage tube in gall bladder bed; explain that this will usually remain in position for 48 hours, depending on drainage. Check the drainage from the 'T' tube and record. Explain that this will remain in position for 10 days.

Fluid and electrolytes
May have sips of water as soon as she can tolerate this. Discourage her from drinking large amounts at a time. Monitor the intravenous infusion and explain that this will be discontinued once she is taking adequate fluids.

Prevention of respiratory complications
Observe respirations and report noisy or abnormal breathing. Monitor her temperature 4-hourly. Sit Mrs Bean up as soon as her condition allows. Encourage breathing exercises. Administer the prescribed analgesic before the physiotherapist attends the patient. Continue with the prescribed antibiotics.

Prevention of deep vein thrombosis
Explain to the patient the importance of moving her legs and flexing her calf muscles at half-hourly intervals while in bed. Check the calves for any pain on dorsiflexion or pressure when attending to the patient.

Hygiene
Wash the patient on recovery from the anaesthetic and put her own nightdress on. Give her a mouthwash. Assist her with the bedpan and note when she first passes urine.

Psychological

Encourage her to look her best for her family. Help her with a little make-up.

Relatives
Persuade them to visit her in pairs and not to spend too long the first evening. Arrange for the doctor to see her husband if he so wishes, otherwise the nurse in charge will give an explanation of what Mrs Bean has had done and how she is expected to progress.

23

Vascular Conditions

An intact circulatory system is essential to the life of the individual. If any part of this system is breached, there is danger of death from a haemorrhage and shock. Monitoring of the vital signs and in particular the pulse and blood pressure, must therefore be carried out very accurately by the nurse.

Specific emphasis in the nursing history

Mobility. Is walking limited because of pain?

Vital signs. Check the presence of pulses in the limbs. Note the temperature, and colour of the extremities.

Pain. Where is the pain and what characteristics does it have? Does anything increase or relieve it?

Excretion. Test the urine for the presence of sugar.

Skin. Note any discoloration or ulcers on the fingers or toes.

ARTERIAL CONDITIONS

Arteritis

This is inflammation of an artery. Acute arteritis is due to infection, which may lead to a secondary haemorrhage or at a later date to an aneurysm. Chronic arteritis occurs as the result of many conditions but is most commonly related to *atherosclerosis* (arteriosclerosis), hardening of the arteries with the laying down of yellow plaques of cholesterol, which is most likely to occur at the junction of arteries. Portions of the plaques may separate, leaving ulcers which allow the platelets to settle and narrow the lumen of the artery. This leads to a reduced blood flow to the area—*ischaemia.* Eventually the artery becomes completely blocked by a thrombus and will cease to supply blood. If an adequate collateral circulation has developed, the area will continue to receive a sufficient supply of blood.

The ischaemic limb

If the atherosclerosis occurs in the aorta and common iliac arteries and an adequate collateral circulation does not form, *intermittent claudication* results, mainly affecting the thigh or buttocks. Atherosclerosis in the femoral and popliteal arteries leads to intermittent claudication in the calf. Increased activity of the muscles, such as in walking, requires an adequate blood supply and if this is not present a cramplike pain occurs, which forces the individual to stop walking for a few minutes. After a short rest he is able to recommence walking, only to have to stop again once he has covered a similar distance. If the blood supply becomes completely occluded by a thrombus, and this is more likely to happen in the smaller vessels, gangrene will develop.

In the ischaemic limb the pulses which are normally felt over the femoral, popliteal, posterior tibial and dorsalis pedis arteries are absent. The limb also feels cold to the touch and the skin of the feet and toes looks polished, the toenails being hard and brittle. There is also absence of hair in the skin of the lower leg and foot. Although there is diminished sensation, the patient may complain of a boring or burning pain at rest—'rest pain'. When the patient lies flat and the foot is raised and moved it becomes pale, but if the leg is allowed to hang over the edge of the bed, it becomes red due to the sluggish circulation. Once the skin becomes red and blotchy, gangrene is imminent.

Embolus

The most common form of embolus is a portion of blood clot which has become detached from a thrombus in the heart or blood vessel and travels in the bloodstream until the lumen of the vessel is too small to allow it to pass, and therefore becomes blocked by it. It causes the artery to go into spasm which results in severe pain and whiteness of the limb. If it is not removed within 5–6 hours, the blood in the artery will form a thrombus which will block the artery completely and gangrene will develop. These emboli arise from atrial thrombi which develop in atrial fibrillation, mural thrombosis following a myocardial infarction, subacute bacterial endocarditis, and occasionally from thrombi in the aorta.

The most common place for emboli to become lodged is in the blood vessels supplying the lower limb. This may be at the point where the aorta divides into the common iliac arteries (saddle embolus), where the femoral arteries divide, or at the division of the popliteal artery.

Raynaud's disease

In this condition there is abnormal sensitivity of the peripheral arteries to changes of temperature in the environment, causing a prolonged arterial spasm, mainly in the fingers. It is thought this may be due to overactivity of the sympathetic nervous system. Initially the fingers become white, which may last from a few seconds to an hour, and this is followed by blueness of the digits for a variable length of time during which time the fingers feel dead and useless. As the circulation returns, the fingers become red and begin to burn and tingle. In mild cases control of the environmental temperature, avoidance of undue exposure, and warm gloves are sufficient. But in some people this is not enough and the individual develops ulcers on the tips of the fingers which may become gangrenous.

Buerger's disease (thromboangiitis obliterans)

This is an uncommon condition, almost exclusively affecting young or middle-aged men who smoke. It mainly affects the lower limbs in which the arteries and veins are inflamed, although it can affect the mesenteric or coronary vessels. The patient may present with an ischaemic ulcer on one or more toes, or he may complain of continuous pain in his toes or foot. The pain tends to be worse after resting with the limbs elevated and may be relieved by positioning the legs lower than the body. Sometimes the patient presents with intermittent claudication or phlebitis and will have the signs of an ischaemic limb. The condition may progress to gangrene. The treatment for Raynaud's and Buerger's disease is to **stop smoking**, protection from the cold, vasodilator drugs such as bamethan sulphate (Vasculit) 25 mg four times daily, sympathectomy, and when gangrene presents, amputation.

Gangrene

This involves death of local tissue (necrosis) due to a reduced blood supply with infection and putrefaction. *Dry gangrene* arises due to the obstruction of an artery causing ischaemia to the tissues supplied by it, a lack of oxygen and nutrients and therefore death of cells. If the veins are not affected and no infection occurs, the blood will still be drained from the affected tissues and the area will remain dry. The dying tissue goes through a series of colour changes, becoming green, yellow, brown then black, hard and wrinkled. There is usually a sharp line of demarcation between the dead and viable areas, often with evidence of inflammation at the junction, which is very sensitive (Fig. 23.1). If the infarcted area becomes infected, it putrefies and the lesion is called *wet gangrene*. There is an offensive smell due to the presence of bacteria, and

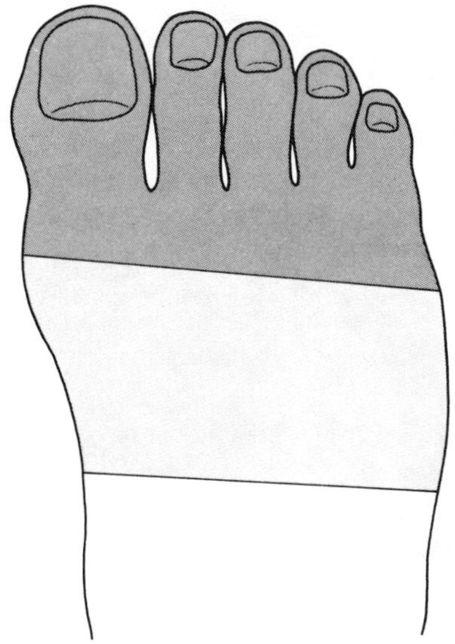

Fig. 23.1 *Diagram showing gangrene and line of demarcation.*

the part appears swollen, soft and cold, the broken areas being moist. This type is more commonly found in diabetics.

Treatment of the ischaemic limb and gangrene

The patient is advised to stop smoking although he may drink alcohol as this is a vasodilator. If the patient is obese, he will be put on a weight-reducing diet. Diabetes should be carefully controlled. Great care is taken to avoid damage to the feet, the chiropodist attending to any corns or ingrowing toenails. The legs are exercised to encourage the flow of blood, and the head of the bed is elevated. Infection of the feet is avoided if possible. If rest pain is present, it may help to keep the feet uncovered, to sleep in a chair with the legs down, or to walk about. The patient will certainly need night sedation. If gangrene is present, the limb must be kept as cool as possible to reduce the requirements of the tissues. In the early stages a lumbar sympathectomy may improve a poor blood supply if this is due to spasm. A thromboendarterectomy can be done to clear short sections of artery, or a bypass operation with a graft. If the thrombus is isolated and short, transluminal angioplasty may also be done, in which a special catheter is guided into an artery in the leg and passed into the narrowed artery. The catheter has a balloon at its end which is blown up, so pushing the fatty deposits against the blood vessel wall. Gangrene usually necessitates an amputation.

Aneurysm

An aneurysm is a weakness in the blood vessel wall which when put under pressure balloons out (Fig. 23.2). Trauma, atherosclerosis and syphilis may all cause this condition in the aorta. Indirect trauma may follow the sudden deceleration of a vehicle causing the aorta to whip forward and tear across at its upper end, usually fatally. Atherosclerosis begins as a plaque in the lining of the blood vessel but the adjacent middle coat may degenerate forming a fusiform aneurysm. Syphilis may damage the minute blood vessels supplying the wall of the aorta, so causing muscle and elastic fibres to die and be replaced with the non-elastic fibrous tissue, which may be stretched by the pressure of the blood and does not return to its normal size. Eventually it will rupture, usually within 2 years of developing. If an aneurysm is diagnosed early as a result of symptoms arising due to the enlarged aorta pressing on other structures, grafting may be contemplated.

Berry aneurysms are those that arise at the junctions of the blood vessels supplying the brain. They are usually clipped, but if they rupture, they will cause a subarachnoid haemorrhage.

Coarctation of the aorta

This is a narrowing of the aorta where it begins to descend (Fig. 23.3). It may present at any age and is frequently without symptoms, being diagnosed on a routine medical examination. Usually a collateral circulation develops ensuring an adequate supply of blood to the lower limbs. The condition is recognised by a difference in the blood pressure of the right arm from that of the left. If not treated, the patient may die in the early thirties from

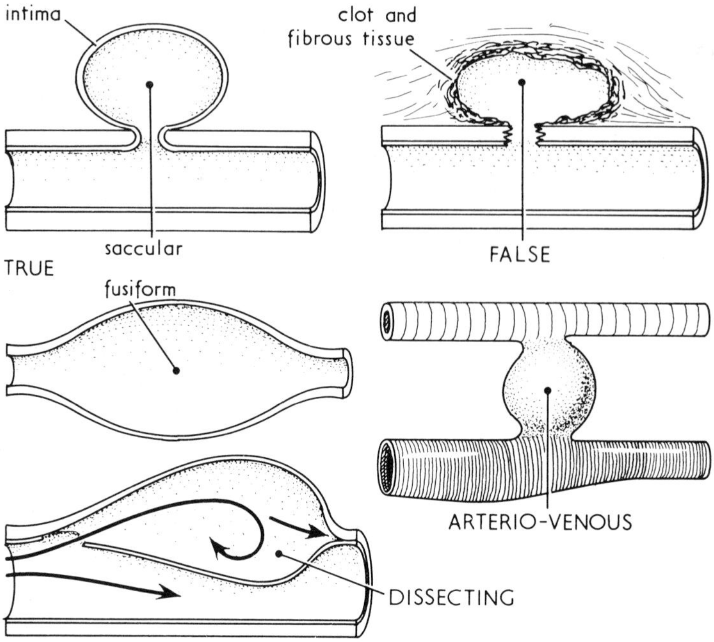

Fig. 23.2 *Aneurysms.*

rupture of the aorta, subacute bacterial endocarditis, left ventricular failure or subarachnoid haemorrhage.

TYPES OF ARTERIAL SURGERY

Grafts

These may be carried out for a severe obstruction of the larger blood vessels due to atherosclerosis, aneurysm or coarctation of the aorta. The blood vessel is bypassed (Fig. 23.4) or the section replaced with a graft which, in the case of aortic or iliac grafts, is usually of a synthetic substance such as Dacron (Fig. 23.5). In smaller vessels the muscular saphenous vein is used. The knitted or woven tubes of Dacron are crimped to prevent kinking. To prevent the graft leaking once in position, Dacron grafts are immersed in some of the patient's blood before he is given heparin and this is allowed to clot. Saphenous veins are removed, dilated, reversed and sutured to the artery.

An operation on the aorta and iliac arteries may be approached via the peritoneal cavity (transperitoneal) or from behind the peritoneum (retroperitoneal). The former involves all the problems of an abdominal operation, and the latter cannot be done in obese patients.

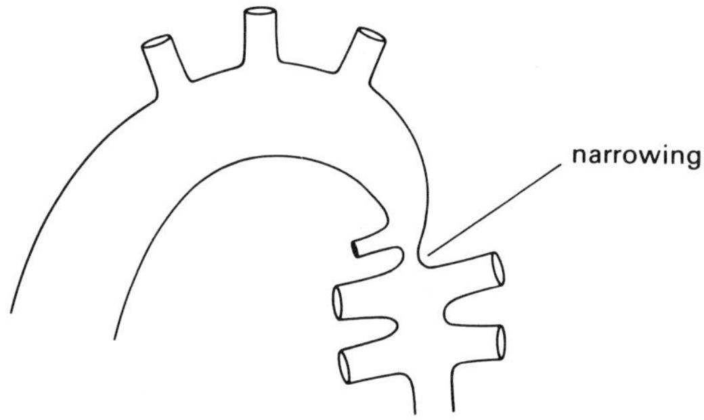

Fig. 23.3 *Coarctation of the aorta.*

Endarterectomy (thromboendarterectomy)

In this operation the artery is opened up, the thrombus plus the intima and the inner part of the

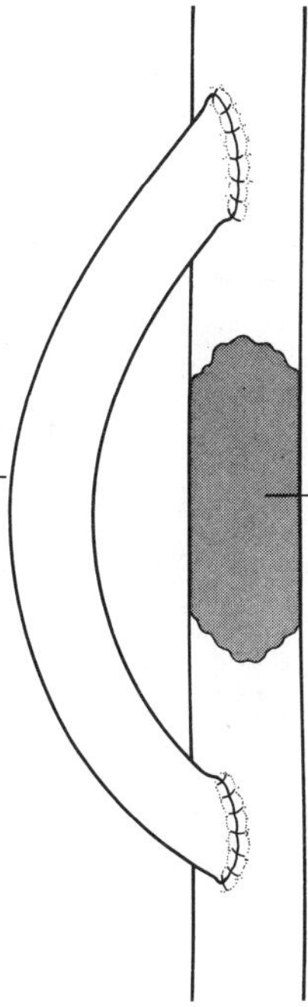

Fig. 23.4 *Bypass graft.*

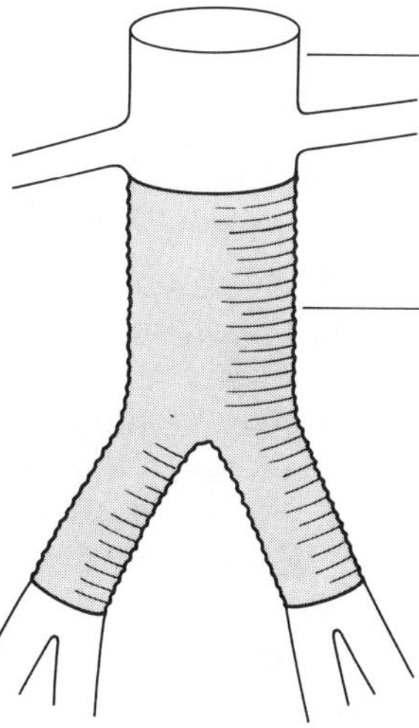

Fig. 23.5 *Aortic graft.*

media removed (Fig. 23.6), and the incision is then closed. Because the inner lining is no longer smooth, anticoagulants have to be given post-operatively and continued for at least a year.

Embolectomy

If an embolus blocks an artery, the latter may be opened and the embolus removed, the artery then being closed with a suture. The most urgent indication for this operation is when an embolus becomes lodged at the division of the aorta, in the common iliac or common femoral arteries. After operation anticoagulant treatment must be continued or further emboli may form.

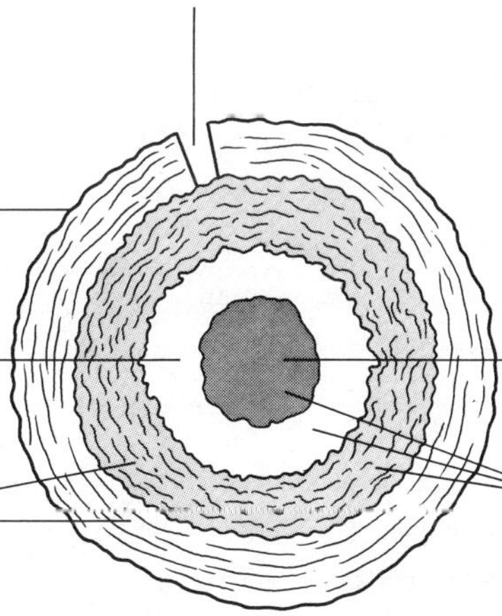

Fig. 23.6 *Thromboendarterectomy.*

Amputation of a limb

The majority of amputations are carried out for gangrene arising as a result of peripheral vascular disease, although a few may have to be done for traumatic conditions or frostbite. The aim of surgery is to remove the dead or unhealthy tissue and leave a healthy stump suitable for a prosthesis. The stump is left smooth, without creases and long enough to fit the prosthesis comfortably and allow movement. The skin flaps are cut in such a way that the scar does not form on the weight-bearing part of the stump. In a lower limb amputation the knee is preserved if possible, as this will make it much easier for the patient to walk.

The surgeon plans and marks out the position of the skin flaps, cuts through the skin, subcutaneous tissue, fat, muscle and nerves, and ligates and clips blood vessels. The bone is then sawn through, unless the amputation is being done through a joint. The surgeon then sutures the various tissues in turn, ensuring that the skin flaps are positioned where he has planned and inserting a drainage tube.

Lumbar sympathectomy

This is most useful in patients with Buerger's disease, although occasionally those suffering from atherosclerosis may benefit. A small section of the sympathetic chain on both sides of the lumbar vertebrae is excised in order to improve the blood supply to the legs. Although the approach to the operation is through the abdominal wall, the peritoneum is not opened up. The main complication is haemorrhage due to damage of the inferior vena cava or the lumbar veins.

Upper dorsal sympathectomy

Raynaud's disease, excessive perspiration, and Buerger's disease of the hands may be relieved by this operation. The approach is in the region of the axilla through the chest wall. The patient may therefore have an underwater seal drain postoperatively.

SPECIAL PREPARATION OF THE PATIENT FOR ARTERIAL SURGERY

The urine will be checked for diabetes and, if present, appropriate care undertaken. Arteriography is carried out to discover the extent of the problem, and x-rays will frequently reveal calcification in the arteries. Because atherosclerosis does not confine itself to one part of the body, an ECG is done to check for any evidence of coronary artery disease. Blood will be taken for estimating the haemoglobin, blood grouping and cross-matching. If there is any evidence of anaemia, this is corrected to ensure that the oxygen-carrying capacity of the blood is at its optimum. If the aorta is to be operated on, and particularly if an aneurysm is present, as many as 10 units of blood may be required.

Measures may be taken to improve the circulation such as exercise and brandy, a vasodilator. For the same reason smoking will be discouraged as this is a vasoconstrictor. The physiotherapist will also encourage breathing exercises and, if an amputation is to be done, strengthening of muscles which will be required later. Any infection must be treated with antibiotics, which may be given anyway as a cover to the patient.

If an abdominal route is required for surgery on the aorta, a nasogastric tube will be passed. In the case of aortic, iliac and femoropopliteal disease, the patient is shaved from the nipple line down to the calves or ankles. Where only one side is being operated on the correct side is marked by the surgeon.

The patient must be prepared for any drainage tubes or apparatus he will have present after the operation. If an amputation is being done, there will have to be adequate psychological preparation of the patient for the loss of a limb. He will need to be given time to talk over the restrictions this may impose in his life and how some of these may be overcome. Depending on his age, he may be troubled about his ability to work, his acceptability to other people, or even whether he will be able to maintain his independence. Talking to another patient who has managed to overcome the difficulties may help him.

SPECIFIC POSTOPERATIVE CARE FOLLOWING ARTERIAL SURGERY

Immediately postoperatively the patient must be observed carefully for any evidence of haemorrhage. The pulse and blood pressure are monitored quarter-hourly until the patient's condition indicates that it may be done less often. His colour is also observed and any restlessness or other signs of haemorrhage noted. If an operation has been done on the aorta or iliac arteries, there may have been a period of profound shock affecting the function of the kidneys, and therefore the urinary output should be watched carefully. Also, if an abdominal operation has been done, the patient will have a nasogastric tube in position and must be observed for signs of a paralytic ileus. The limbs will be checked for an adequate circulation as a clot may form in the graft or stripped artery. The colour and temperature of the limb will be noted and the pulses checked quarter-hourly initially.

SPECIFIC CARE OF A PATIENT FOLLOWING AN AMPUTATION OF THE LOWER LIMB

The patient is usually returned to a divided bed with a cradle in position to make it easier to inspect the stump frequently. He is nursed on a firm bed to prevent a flexure contracture. As already stated, haemorrhage is the main danger initially and if this occurs digital pressure should be applied and medical aid sought immediately. The stump may be kept in position by sandbags and a drawsheet and the patient should be advised not to lift the stump off the bed in order to relieve the pain. Occasionally, if oedema is present, the stump may be elevated on a pillow, but if so this should not be done for longer than 24 hours. If the patient does lie on his side, he is better on the good side with the stump supported on a pillow. Pain from a phantom limb may be a problem and may require analgesics. If the patient exercises as if the limb were still there, it may help, but if the pain is severe and persistent, the nerve endings may require injecting with alcohol. There will be one or two drainage tubes in and these should receive the usual care. A blood transfusion may also be in progress.

The care of the stump is of major importance. A special 15-cm bandage is applied in such a way that it produces a well-shaped stump. It should be firm and even, reaching high into the groin and not causing flexion. If applied properly, it will help to reduce oedema by encouraging the venous return and it will help to mould the tissue and increase its tone. The patient will be assisted to lie on his abdomen for half an hour at least twice a day to prevent flexure contracture. The ischial tuberosities will now have to become weight bearing and therefore have to be hardened up. This is done by getting the patient to sit on an upright chair without a cushion for an increasing amount of time each day. The good leg must not be ignored and should be put through a range of exercises.

The patient is mobilised as quickly as his general condition permits. He is encouraged to stand on the good leg and let the stump hang. This may feel a bit uncomfortable at first but will improve the circulation. The physiotherapist will teach the patient exercises not only for the stump and the good leg, but also to strengthen his arm muscles and improve his balance. He should not sit out in a low soft chair nor should he cross his legs. Usually he is fitted with a light temporary pylon for the first 4 to 6 weeks and then he is fitted with a permanent artificial limb. He will be taught how to dress himself, and to apply the pylon. The physiotherapist will give him the opportunity not only to walk in the ward but also to go out of doors, up and down slopes and stairs, and will show him how to manage getting in and out of a bath. He will be taught how to care for his pylon, to apply his bandages or sock, and how to prevent pressure sores occurring. The stump socks should fit well and have no creases or darns which could cause a pressure sore. Before he goes home an assessment will have been made and ramps or hand bars fitted to his house where appropriate. He will have an appointment to attend the limb-fitting centre for his prosthesis.

A small proportion of patients never progress to using an artificial limb due to age or other disabilities, and these patients will need to be supplied with a wheelchair, which may require doorways to be widened and a hoist to be supplied.

VENOUS CONDITIONS

Varicosed veins

The venous drainage of the legs consists of deep veins running alongside the arteries and superficial veins which are present in the subcutaneous fat and can be seen through the skin. Connecting the deep and superficial veins above the ankle, in the midcalf and below the knee, are the perforating or communicating veins. The two superficial veins in the leg are the long saphenous vein, which runs from the foot up the inside of the leg to the groin where it joins the deep femoral vein, and the short saphenous vein which runs from the foot up the outside of the leg to join the popliteal vein behind the knee (Fig. 23.7).

The pressure of blood arriving from the capillary network, the presence of one-way valves, and the contraction of the powerful calf muscles are all involved in the venous return. As the calf muscles contract they increase the pressure within the deep veins of the leg, so pushing the blood forward. The superficial veins are not buried in muscle and therefore rely on the deep veins for emptying. As the calf muscles relax there is a sudden drop in the pressure in the deep veins and this suctions blood via the communicating arteries from the superficial veins into the deep veins. The valves prevent blood travelling in the opposite direction.

If a valve is incompetent, it allows the blood to flow in the opposite direction causing pooling and congestion, a condition which most commonly occurs in the long saphenous vein at its upper end. The vein becomes dilated, so making the adjacent valves incompetent because they are unable to meet across the vein. Eventually the whole vein and its tributaries become dilated and tortuous (varicosed). Less commonly, the short saphenous vein is affected.

Varicosed veins may develop as a result of a familial tendency to incompetent valves or because of increased pressure in the venous system. The most common contributory factor is pregnancy, although any increased pressure in the pelvic cavity may be a cause. Prolonged standing and obesity may also affect the pressures in the veins, and thrombophlebitis or a deep vein thrombosis will damage the valves and may therefore be contributory factors.

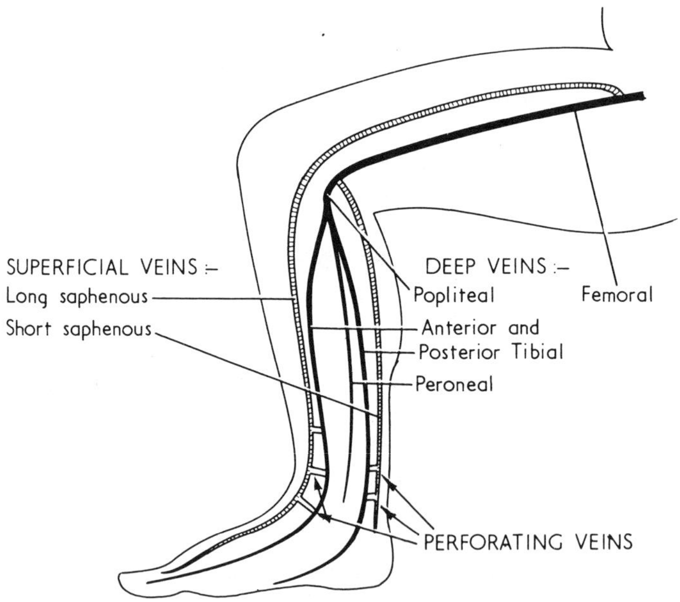

Fig. 23.7 *The veins of the leg.*

Clinical picture

The superficial veins appear swollen and tortuous and have dark blue or purplish swellings. The patient may complain that the legs feel heavy and tired and there may be evidence of mild oedema. There may be a dull ache or cramplike pain in the calf after standing or walking. Pigmentation, eczema or varicose ulcers may be present in the area drained by the vein. Inflammation of the vein and thrombosis, thrombophlebitis, may affect the varicosed veins. The most serious complication is haemorrhage which is treated by elevating the leg and applying firm pressure.

Management

The Trendelenburg's test is carried out to demonstrate the presence of varicosed veins. In this test the patient is asked to lie down flat and his leg is raised to empty the veins of blood. He is then asked to stand up, when the veins should take 30 seconds to refill. In varicosed veins they fill more quickly. By means of applying a tourniquet in the groin, midcalf and knee in turn, it is possible to find out which valves are affected.

Conservative treatment

The patient is advised to avoid anything that will impede the circulation or slow it down, such as standing still, crossing his legs, constrictions such as garters, overweight and excessive cold. He is encouraged to exercise and may wear elastic stockings and elevate the foot of the bed to improve venous return.

Compression sclerotherapy

With the patient lying down, a tourniquet is applied to stop venous drainage. One millilitre of sodium tetradecyl sulphate (STD) is injected and the tourniquet removed. A foam pad is applied to the injection site and kept in position with an elastic bandage or stocking for 24 hours a day for at least 3 to 6 weeks. During this period the patient is encouraged to walk as much as possible, so ensuring a good flow of blood and preventing the extension of a thrombosis. The aim is to cause an inflammation of the lining of the vein so that the walls stick together.

Stripping of the saphenous vein

The long saphenous vein is ligated and cut in the groin and at the ankle, and a wire stripper inserted into the vein at the ankle end, threaded through the vein to the groin where it is attached to a handle. At the lower end there is a bulbous portion called the acorn and the vein in the ankle is securely tied to this. The surgeon then pulls the complete vein out from the ankle to the groin with the stripper. All of the branches of the saphenous vein are torn off and will bleed into the tissue. In order to minimise this a firm bandage is applied to the leg.

Ligation of the saphenous vein

In this operation the long saphenous vein is ligated at the point where it joins the femoral vein. This may be combined with multiple excisions in which short lengths of the vein are removed at various points in the leg. A compression bandage will be necessary to prevent further bleeding.

Specific preoperative preparation

If multiple excisions are to be done, the leg will have been marked by the surgeon and the nurse should take care not to remove these markings. The whole leg will require shaving, and the surgeon will write the correct leg on the consent form. It is important that the nurse checks the notes, operating list and the patients leg to see that they all indicate the same leg. The physiotherapist will teach the patient what he has to do after the operation.

Specific postoperative care

The foot of the bed is elevated and a cradle positioned for ease of observation. The surgeon will have applied an elastic bandage in theatre and therefore the nurse must check the colour, temperature and pulses of the foot so that she will become quickly aware if the bandage is too tight. The wounds must be checked frequently for bleeding (especially the one in the groin) or the bleeding may pass unnoticed. The patient is quickly mobilised to prevent the incidence of deep vein thrombosis and pulmonary embolism. When not walking around, the patient should either lie on the top of his bed or sit with his leg elevated, taking care to avoid pressure on the calf as this will predispose towards a deep vein thrombosis. The patient may be discharged after 48 hours, returning to have his sutures out on the seventh day. His haemoglobin will also be checked for any signs of anaemia.

Advice on discharge

The patient is advised not to stand still but to flex his muscles and move his toes. When sitting down he should continue to elevate his leg. During the first week postoperatively he may be encouraged to have daily saline baths. He will be shown how to apply his leg bandages or stockings, which he will continue to wear until after his out-patient appointment, which may be in 1 month. He may require some advice regarding his work or a reducing diet.

SUGGESTED WORK

1. Find out what exercises the physiotherapist will teach the amputee patient.
2. Visit a limb-fitting centre to discover the different types of prostheses and when these are used.
3. Ask if you can visit an amputee patient's home and see what adaptations to the house have been necessary.
4. Which type of treatment is most commonly used in your hospital for varicose veins?

SUGGESTED READING

Green S., Wickenden A. (1984). Varicose veins. *Nursing*; **2** (26): 779–81.

Horton R. E. (1980). *Vascular Surgery*. London: Hodder & Stoughton.

* * *

Mr ROBERT DALE (aged 54) is a postman who is divorced and lives on his own in a first-floor maisonette. His elderly mother lives 120 miles away. He has been admitted with gangrene of the left foot. He was a fairly well-controlled diabetic but has been rather slack in keeping to his diet since the divorce, and is drinking rather heavily. He has been admitted to the ward from the diabetic clinic. Prior to admission he was on lente insulin 24 units.

Medical plan
Control of his diabetic condition. Below-knee amputation of the left leg.

Identification of the patient's needs and problems in the preoperative period and action arising from these

Pain
Take care in handling the patient and avoid knocking the bed. Give prescribed analgesics as required and monitor their effectiveness.

Management of gangrenous foot
Use a cradle to remove the pressure of the bedclothes. Keep the foot cool with a fan. Do any dressings aseptically. Note any progress of the gangrene.

Diabetic state
Test blood carefully with Dextrostix 4-hourly and chart. Test urine for acetone. Administer soluble insulin as prescribed in relation to blood sugar.

Dehydration and electrolyte imbalance
Find out what he likes to drink and encourage fluids. Monitor and control the intravenous infusion carefully. Report blood tests to the doctor as soon as received.

Anxiety about the effects of the amputation
Allow him to talk about the problems he expects. Arrange for the social worker to come and discuss with him whether he needs to be rehoused or could manage with adaptations to his maisonette. Arrange for his employer to come and discuss the effects of the amputation on his work and the

possibility of other openings. Introduce him to a former patient who has overcome a similar disability. Discuss with him the rehabilitation he will receive to enable him to become independent.

Prevention of respiratory complications
Explain the importance of not smoking because of its effect on the arteries, as well as on the chest. Arrange for the physiotherapist to come and explain about the postoperative exercises and to teach deep breathing.

Hygiene
Assist the patient as much as is required. He will be able to manage his own mouth care. Attention to pressure areas will be required, especially to the sacrum and his right heel. He may find a 'monkey pole' helpful to lift himself.

Prevention of infection
Administer prescribed antibiotics. Aseptic care of gangrenous foot.

Anxiety about the operation itself
Explain to the patient that he will be given an injection which will help him to relax and become sleepy and that before being taken into the operating theatre he will be given another injection which will put him to sleep. Explain to Mr Dale what he should expect on his return to the ward, such as the intravenous infusion and drainage tubes. Reassure him that analgesics will be given for the pain.

Social
He might be amenable to talking to a minister of religion or, perhaps linking with some self-help group.

24

Conditions of the Thorax

Normal breathing is dependent on the fact that there is a negative pressure within the thoracic cavity and only one way through which air can enter it. Any operation which requires entry into the cavity—such as those on the heart, lungs, oesophagus and great blood vessels— will destroy this negative pressure and provide another route through which air may enter. In order to restore the negative pressure and allow the lungs to expand, the surgeon will introduce a drainage tube which must be kept sealed under water. The nurse's role, therefore, is to ensure that the patient's respiratory function is adequate and that no air can enter the drainage tube at any time. It is of vital importance that she understands how to care for the drainage tube and does not attempt to change or remove it before she is considered capable of doing so.

Specific emphasis in the nursing history

Breathing. Degree of breathlessness. Cough. Sputum—type and amount. Is the patient a smoker? Presence of breath that smells.

General appearance. Loss of weight. Flushed face. General malaise or tiredness. Engorged veins in neck.

Vital signs. Raised temperature, pulse and respiration rate.

Pain. Related to breathing.

Social. Social and environmental background.

Nutrition. Any anorexia or vomiting.

Mobility. Is the patient able to walk any distance without becoming breathless?

Skin. Colour of extremities and lips.

CONDITIONS AFFECTING THE LUNGS AND PLEURA

Empyema

Empyema is an abscess in the pleural space, usually arising as a result of infection of the lung as in pneumonia, bronchiectasis and lung abscess. It may also develop following carcinoma of the bronchus or a bronchial fistula. Less commonly, tuberculosis, chest wounds, subphrenic abscess or septicaemia may be causes.

The patient feels generally unwell and has a raised, irregular temperature and a rapid pulse. The respirations are shallow due to the pain experienced on breathing, and there is a dry cough. On examination the doctor will find impaired movement of the chest and dullness to percussion on the affected side, the heart may be displaced towards the opposite side.

The underlying cause is treated and unless the condition is due to tuberculosis, the pus is aspirated. Antibiotics will be given according to the organism isolated, both into the pleural cavity and systemically. If the pus is too thick to be aspirated, streptokinase and streptodornase 20 000 units in 10 ml of sterile water may be injected to liquefy the pus; aspiration is then carried out 12 hours later. An underwater seal drain may be introduced. If re-expansion does not occur, the chest is opened under a general anaesthetic and the thickened membrane of pus adhering to the visceral pleura is peeled off the lung (decortication). The pus and fibrin remaining in the chest are removed by suction and the lung re-expanded. If the empyema is due to tuberculosis, repeated aspiration with the instillation of streptomycin into the pleural cavity is preferred to prevent secondary infection. If secondary infection does develop, open drainage, thoracoplasty or pleurectomy may be necessary.

Tumours of the lung

Benign tumours are rare but lipoma, fibroma, neurofibroma and dermoid cysts are sometimes present. They may cause mechanical pressure in which case they will be removed surgically.

Carcinoma of the lung

About 66% of carcinomas occurring in the lung are found in the main bronchus, a further 25% in the smaller bronchi, and only about 10% in the peripheral bronchi. There are four main types: squamous carcinoma, oat cell carcinoma, anaplastic carcinoma and adenocarcinoma, the last-mentioned being the least common. Anaplastic carcinoma has the fastest growth and the greatest incidence of metastases. Secondary malignant growths may arise in the lung from a primary neoplasm in the breast, gastrointestinal tract, bone, prostate, kidney or chorionepithelioma of the uterus.

The occurrence of lung carcinoma is closely linked with cigarette smoking. The greater the number of years the individual has smoked and the larger the number of cigarettes smoked, the higher the incidence. It is much more common in men than women, particularly between the ages of 40 and 70. People living in industrial areas are more likely to develop the condition than those living in rural areas. Industries dealing with asbestos, chrome ore and nickel are high-risk areas. There is also a higher incidence in patients who already have chronic bronchitis. However, some people do appear to have a greater resistance to the condition, and this may be due to genetic factors or immune response.

There may be no clinical evidence until the disease has become widespread. Otherwise the patient may have a cough, with or without sputum, dyspnoea, haemoptysis and chest pain. Frequently the patient presents with unresolved pneumonia. If the growth obstructs the superior vena cava, the venous system will be engorged, especially in the neck and superficially on the abdomen. Sometimes the patient does not seek medical attention until symptoms arise as a result of secondary deposits, such as the pain arising from deposits in bone or jaundice from involvement of the liver or biliary tract. There may also be loss of weight, anorexia and a general malaise. Carcinoma of the lung also appears to influence the function of some of the endocrine organs, without necessarily spreading to them, so that diabetes mellitus, overactivity of the parathyroids and altered electrolyte balance may arise.

Diagnosis is mainly based on the presence of malignant cells in the sputum and the results of bronchoscopy and biopsy. Chest x-rays and tomograms will also be carried out and sometimes an aspiration biopsy. In cases of doubt or to discover how far the condition has spread locally, a *scalene node biopsy* or *mediastinoscopy* is done. In the former, the fat and its lymph nodes are removed just above the clavicle, and in the latter, lymph nodes alongside the trachea are removed by an incision above the sternal notch.

There is a high rate of metastases because of the good blood supply and lymphatic drainage. Spread occurs via the lymph nodes to the liver and the adrenals, and via the bloodstream to the bones, particularly the vertebrae, the breast and the brain. Often there are many metastases but occasionally there is a solitary one which is therefore more amenable to treatment.

Treatment

Squamous carcinoma is usually treated by surgery, whereas the oat cell and anaplastic forms frequently require radiotherapy; chemotherapy may also be used. Surgery is undertaken where the growth is contained and there are no known metastases. It may require pneumonectomy or lobectomy, or occasionally a segmentectomy, in which the part supplied by one bronchus is removed, is sufficient. A wedge resection in which there is removal of part of a segment is not sufficient if carcinoma is present. In order to enter the chest an incision is made which extends from near the spine to the front of the chest, and part of the fifth rib is removed. After removing the diseased lobe or lung the corresponding branches of the pulmonary artery and vein are ligated and divided. The bronchus is usually clamped in the early stages of the operation and when it has been cut through, the open end is closed with a stainless steel wire suture. The 5-year survival rate is 25–30%.

Specific preoperative preparation

The general health of the patient invariably requires improvement, and any infection or anaemia must be dealt with. Most surgeons do not operate on patients over the age of 65. Breathing exercises are given by a physiotherapist in the days leading up to the operation in order to improve respiratory function. Oral hygiene is important and if the patient has any dental caries, these are attended to. In order to reduce bronchial infection an antibiotic is given, and in some patients postural drainage. Many surgeons prescribe subcutaneous heparin in order to prevent deep vein thrombosis which is a high risk postoperatively. Blood will be taken for grouping and cross-matching. The patient needs to be psychologically prepared for the way he will feel when he returns from theatre and to know what will be expected of him, as his co-operation is essential.

Specific postoperative care

The patient is kept in the recovery room until he has fully regained consciousness. Nevertheless, when he returns to the ward a careful watch will need to be made for signs of shock, haemorrhage and respiratory difficulties. As soon as his blood pressure is stable he will be sat up in bed to encourage drainage and allow the healthy lung to expand fully. At an early stage he will be encouraged to do breathing exercises and to cough every 2 hours. When coughing, the nurse or physiotherapist must support the wound to prevent excess strain on it, as the wounds of these patients may not heal very well. Because deep breathing and coughing are so important to avoid collapse of the lung, the patient will require adequate analgesia to relieve the pain, but not sufficient to depress respirations. Steam inhalations may also loosen secretions and enable them to be coughed up, and fluids must also be encouraged. A high concentration of oxygen will be necessary in the early stages to ensure adequate oxygenation of the blood. The patient will return from theatre with a blood transfusion in progress and this should be monitored carefully to prevent overloading the circulation. There may be one or two drainage tubes in position (Fig. 24.1), an apical

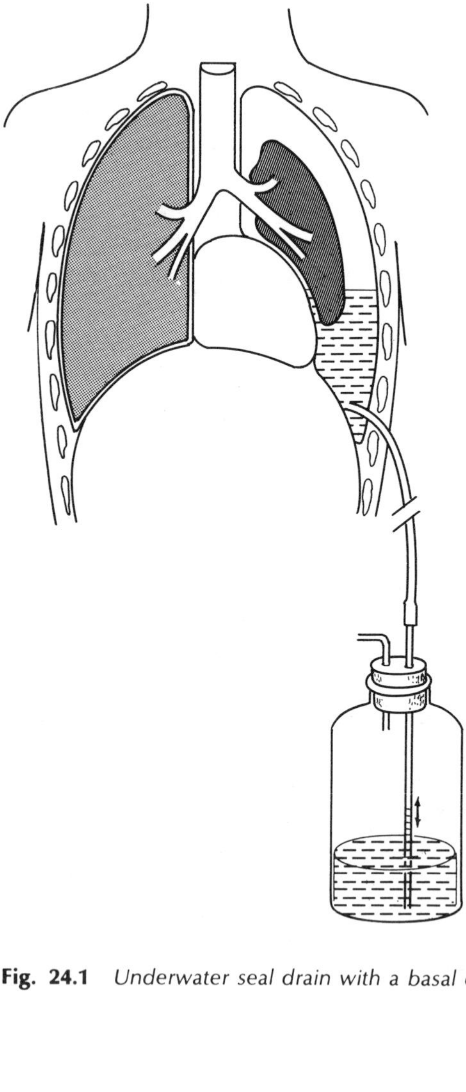

Fig. 24.1 *Underwater seal drain with a basal drain.*

one draining air from the upper part of the pleural cavity, and a basal drain for serous fluid, draining the base of the pleural cavity. For convenience they usually leave the chest alongside one another. This means that the apical drain has a length of tubing threaded through the pleural cavity and will therefore be more difficult to remove. The drains are usually clamped during transit of the patient from the theatre to the ward and therefore these clamps must be removed once the connections have been checked, and the underwater seal bottle is in position. Drainage tubes may not be used in a pneumonectomy, or if they are, they will be removed after 24 hours. If they are not used, the surgeon will measure the pressure in the pneumonectomy space, aiming to keep it at a slightly negative value. If the patient has to be placed on his side to carry out nursing care, this should be on the operated side (particularly in a pneumonectomy) or the breathing will be affected. When the drainage bottle requires changing, the tubes on the patient side must be clamped. Apart from this most surgeons do not like the tubes to be clamped for any other reason than a break in the continuity of the tube because of the danger of tension pneumothorax. During the first 24 or 48 hours following a lobectomy or other operative procedure of the thorax (other than a pneumonectomy) the fluid in the tube of the underwater seal will swing up and down unless there is a blockage or the lung is fully expanded. Before the tubes are removed the lungs are x-rayed to check they are fully expanded. Sometimes a Robert's pump is attached to the underwater seal to speed up expansion. If the pump is turned off, it must be disconnected from the tubing or it will act as a clamp.

Antibiotics are usually continued postoperatively, and possibly also the heparin. The patient must be observed for bronchospasm as this will need bronchodilators to relieve it or, if these fail, steroids. If the patient becomes very dyspnoeic and cyanotic, with a rising pulse and confusion due to cerebral anoxia, this may indicate that atelectasis has developed in the remaining lung which could be fatal and needs urgent treatment by bronchoscopy. If moist sounds develop in the unoperated lung and the patient coughs up sputum with streaks of blood in it, a bronchopleural fistula may have developed. The patient will be x-rayed and the fluid aspirated. If it cannot be dealt with adequately, empyema will develop which will require surgical drainage. Deep vein thrombosis followed by pulmonary embolus is a particular hazard of thoracic surgery. Therefore the patient should have a cradle to allow him to move his legs regularly, and he should be encouraged to do this. Atrial fibrillation may arise in the older patient and is recognised by an irregular pulse. An ECG will be required to identify the problem and the patient may be prescribed digoxin to control the activity of the heart.

Mobilisation is usually started as soon as possible depending on the patient's condition.

Bronchiectasis

This is a condition in which the smaller bronchi of the lung become grossly dilated and retain secretions. Sometimes it is due to a congenital defect of the bronchi but it more commonly follows chronic bronchitis, tuberculosis or other infection. It may be localised to one or more lobes or may be generalised throughout the lungs. It may be symptomless, but eventually there is usually a large amount of foul-smelling sputum coughed up, which may be as much as 0.5 litres a day. Blood may be present in the sputum, or the patient may suffer from recurrent attacks of pneumonia or dyspnoea.

Treatment is by aspirating the bronchi during a bronchoscopy, postural drainage, lobectomy or pneumonectomy if the condition is confined. A bronchogram will be carried out to demonstrate the extent of the condition. Preoperatively a rigid schedule of postural drainage for a large proportion of the day, over a period of 1–3 weeks will be carried out (Fig. 24.2).

Lung abscesses

These are usually due to an inhaled foreign body, blood or mucus, or to a purulent necrosis of a lung carcinoma. An infarction of the lung and influenzal bronchopneumonia are other less common causes.

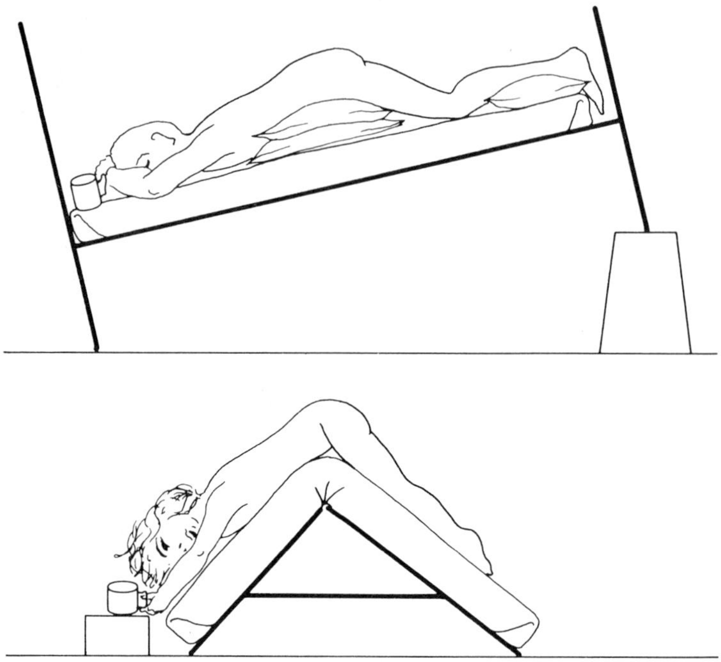

Fig. 24.2 *Postural drainage.*

The patient has a high swinging temperature, marked loss of weight, an unpleasant breath, cough, dyspnoea and pain in the chest, followed by rusty or 'prune-juice' sputum when the abscess bursts into a bronchus. Diagnosis is by x-ray or bronchogram. There may be spread to the brain.

Trauma to the chest

Fractured ribs, contusion of the lung and penetrating wounds of the chest wall are the most common forms of injury. Their importance depends upon the amount of damage caused to the respiratory apparatus. Severe contusion of the lung alone may cause interference with breathing, because the underlying lung has lost the support of the chest wall which then moves inwards on inspiration and outwards on expiration (paradoxical respiration). A penetrating wound of the chest wall may also be fatal, either from haemorrhage or from collapse of the lung due to air passing into the pleural space. Collapse of the lung is particularly liable to occur when the chest wound is valvular.

Treatment

Treatment for shock and oxygen are given, as well as morphia for the pain. Extensive crushing injuries may need a tracheostomy, and possibly assisted respiration by a machine. Rib fractures due to indirect violence are strapped to relieve pain. However, compound and direct rib fractures must never be strapped. If a sucking wound is present, it will be sutured or, as a first-aid measure, covered with a wet or Vaseline gauze dressing. All wounds of the chest wall require excision in the operating theatre, and any foreign bodies are removed from the lungs as soon as the patient's condition allows.

Complications of chest injuries

Surgical emphysema is air in the tissues of the chest wall which has escaped from the wound in the lung. It will be reabsorbed within a few days. If air is present in the pleural cavity, this may need to be withdrawn.

Haemoptysis indicates a damaged lung.

Pneumothorax—air in the pleural cavity. This helps to control haemorrhage by collapsing the injured lung. However, if severe the patient may become very breathless and will die if not treated by an underwater seal drain and a Robert's pump.

Haemothorax—blood in the pleural cavity. Haemorrhage may occur due to a severed vessel or damage to the lung itself. However, the latter normally ceases spontaneously due to the collapse of the lung. The blood is aspirated on the day following the injury.

Empyema—pus in the pleural cavity. This is due to the entrance of pyogenic bacteria through the wound and is prevented by giving antibiotics to all patients with chest injuries. Having developed, it will require closed drainage and appropriate antibiotics.

SURGICAL CONDITIONS OF THE HEART

Mitral stenosis

Rheumatic heart disease if not adequately treated leads on to endocarditis (inflammation of the endocardium), which is usually confined to the valves, the mitral valve being particularly susceptible. Adhesions often develop between the cusps of the valves causing a narrowing of the opening (mitral stenosis). This limits the amount of blood flowing from the left atrium to the ventricle, causing back pressure in the pulmonary system and eventually leading to right-sided heart failure.

In mitral stenosis the patient becomes increasingly breathless on exertion over the years and frequently has a 'malar flush' due to the dilatation of the venules of the cheeks. Because the output of the heart is reduced the patient tires easily. Without treatment the condition progresses to right-sided heart failure, atrial fibrillation with the release of emboli, and attacks of acute pulmonary oedema. Surgical intervention is therefore of great benefit to the patient.

Treatment

A mitral valvotomy is the usual treatment for a straightforward mitral stenosis, otherwise a mitral valve replacement is the treatment of choice. Occasionally a mitral valvuloplasty is carried out for an incompetent valve.

Mitral valvotomy This is a closed-heart operation. The thorax is opened on the left and the pericardial sac is incised. The left atrial appendage is clamped, a purse-string suture inserted, and an opening cut into the appendage just large enough to allow the surgeon's index finger to be introduced through it. The suture is tightened to prevent loss of blood, and the clamp is released. Occasionally the finger will be sufficient to break down the adhesions, but usually a dilator is introduced through a stab incision in the left ventricle, which is used to split the valve. The incisions are then sutured.

Mitral valve replacement In this operation the patient is attached to a heart–lung machine so that the heart may be opened to excise the mitral valve and insert an artificial one. The chest is opened through the sternum, and after attaching the patient to the heart–lung machine the aorta is clamped, the left atrium opened and the diseased valve removed and replaced by an artificial one. The atrium is then closed and the clamps are removed. An underwater seal drain is inserted into the mediastinum and the pericardial cavity.

Coronary thrombosis

This condition may be treated by a coronary artery bypass graft in which the long saphenous vein is taken from the leg and stitched into place to bypass the blockage. The procedure will be carried out as open-heart surgery. If the thrombus is isolated and short, a special catheter can be guided into the artery in the arm and fed up to the blocked coronary artery. The catheter has a balloon at its end which is passed into the narrowed portion of the vessel and then blown up, so pushing the fatty deposits against the blood vessel wall.

Laser angioplasty

A 1.2-metre long fibreoptic tube as thin as a needle is inserted into an artery in the patient's thigh and then fed along the artery towards the heart. Laser energy is then used to burn off fatty deposits on the walls of the artery. This is carried out under local anaesthetic and the patient requires 2 weeks to recover.

Congenital abnormalities

The most common congenital heart diseases requiring surgery are: ventricular septal defect, atrial septal defect, patent ductus arteriosus, and Fallot's tetralogy—ventricular septal defect being twice as common as the others. Pulmonary stenosis, coarctation of the aorta, aortic stenosis and transposition of the great vessels are other important congenital abnormalities.

Ventricular septal defect

In this condition there is an opening of variable size in the septum between the ventricles which allows some of the blood to pass directly from the left to the right ventricle and so to the lungs, bypassing the general circulation—a left-to-right shunt. Surgery is carried out to repair the defect with Dacron, using the heart–lung machine. This is usually delayed until the child is 5.

Patent ductus arteriosus

While the fetus remains in the uterus it does not require a pulmonary circulation and therefore a blood vessel connects the left pulmonary artery to the aorta. At birth this connection disappears, so allowing blood to enter the pulmonary circulation. In patent ductus arteriosus it persists and blood continues to flow through it but in the reverse direction because the pressure in the aorta is now higher than that in the pulmonary artery. Therefore the blood supply in the systemic circulation is reduced and there is increased pressure in the pulmonary circulation—a left-to-right shunt (Fig. 24.3). Surgery is carried out to ligate and divide the connection when the child is aged about 3 years.

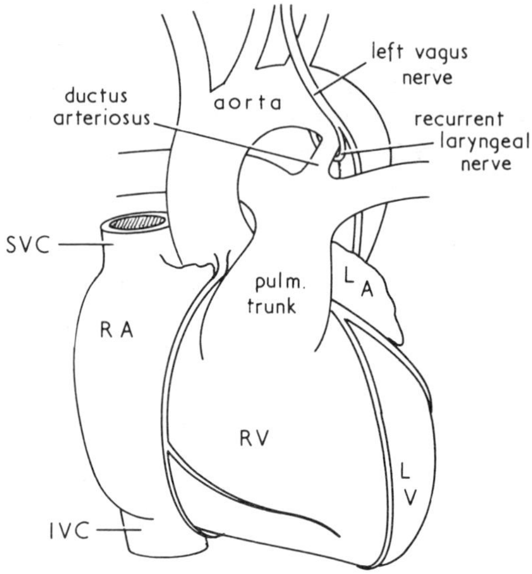

Fig. 24.3 *Ductus arteriosus.*

Atrial septal defect

The defect in this condition is between the two atria, allowing blood to pass from the left side to the right (Fig. 24.4). This results in overloading of the right side of the heart and pulmonary circulation and a poor output to the general circulation—a left-to-right shunt. Surgery when the child is older is undertaken to close the defect with sutures or a Dacron patch using a heart–lung machine.

Fallot's tetralogy

In this condition there are four defects: pulmonary stenosis, ventricular septal defect, hypertrophy of the right ventricle which is displaced to the right of the aorta, the latter being enlarged and communicating with both the right and left ventricle. As a result of these defects the blood flow to the lungs is deficient and the blood is therefore not adequately oxygenated (blue baby). This is a right-to-left shunt (Fig. 24.5).

In addition to severe cyanosis, these children suffer from extreme dyspnoea on exertion which is relieved by squatting, a position which increases abdominal pressure. A large number of children with this condition die in infancy; those surviving suffer from cyanotic attacks. If surgery has to be carried out within the first few years of life, a

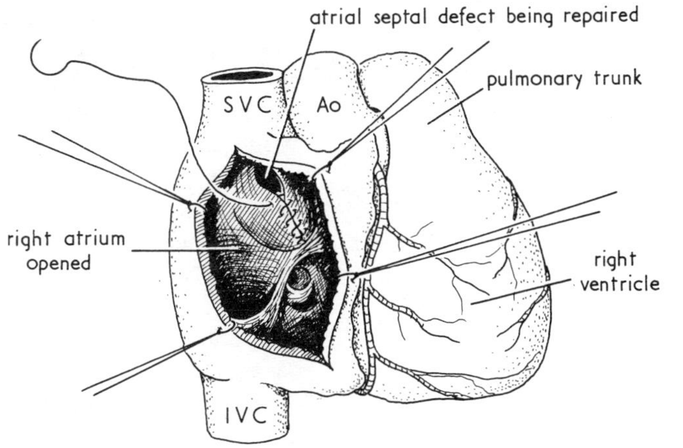

Fig. 24.4 *Atrial septal defect.*

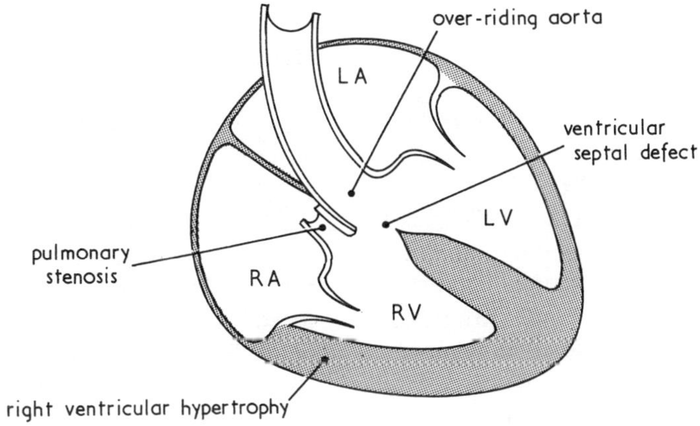

Fig. 24.5 *Fallot's tetralogy.*

Blalock's operation is done as an interim procedure. This consists of an anastomosis between the left subclavian and the left pulmonary arteries to improve the circulation to the lungs, and therefore the oxygenation of the blood. It is possible to correct the defects under hypothermia with a heart–lung machine, although this is usually preferable at a later age.

Pulmonary stenosis

There is either damage to the valves or thickening of the walls of the pulmonary artery as it leaves the ventricle. In either case the stenosis interferes with the flow of blood from the right ventricle which hypertrophies in an effort to overcome the obstruction. It eventually leads to right-sided heart failure. Surgery to cut the obstruction is carried out with the use of the heart–lung machine.

Coarctation of the aorta

This is a rare abnormality in which the aorta has become narrowed just below the origin of the left subclavian artery (Fig. 24.6). The blood supply to the trunk and legs is maintained by an extensive

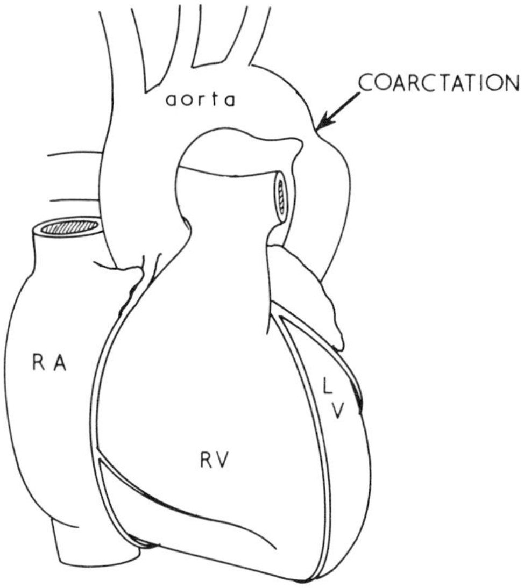

Fig. 24.6 *Coarctation of the aorta.*

collateral circulation, mainly from the intercostal arteries. These vessels become greatly enlarged, resulting in visible pulsation and notching of the ribs which can be seen on x-ray. The blood pressure is raised in an effort to overcome the constriction but beyond the obstruction the pressure is low, and the pulses in the lower limbs are weak or cannot be felt at all. Death may occur before the age of 40 due to the hypertension and its effects or to rupture of the aorta. The constriction is excised and replaced with a graft. Depending on where the constriction is, the heart–lung machine may be used.

Transposition of the great arteries

In babies with this condition the aorta leaves the right ventricle and the pulmonary artery the left, therefore unoxygenated blood is continually passed around the body, and oxygenated blood around the pulmonary circulation. Cyanosis is therefore severe soon after birth. Operation is urgently required to introduce a balloon catheter to make a hole between the left and right atrium. This is carried out during cardiac catheterisation. Further surgery may be possible later.

Heart–lung machine (Fig. 24.7) The heart–lung machine is used to bypass the circulation while open-heart surgery is being carried out. Cannulae are inserted into the venae cavae via the right atrium and the venous outflow led through tubing to an oxygenator. Here the blood absorbs oxygen and is then passed to an arterial pump which returns the blood to a peripheral artery such as the femoral. Some machines have a reservoir to supply additional blood, and a cooling circuit to lower the temperature of the blood before its return to the patient. The patient has to be heparinised prior to the procedure, and the CVP and blood pressure are monitored by means of cannulae. Following the procedure defibrillation is usually necessary. Once the heart is beating satisfactorily the bypass is discontinued. Intravenous protamine sulphate is given to neutralise the effect of the heparin.

Hypothermia If the temperature of the body is reduced, less oxygen is required by the tissues and large blood vessels can be clamped off or the blood diverted into the heart–lung machine for a longer period of time, so allowing the surgeon to operate on the open heart or the large blood vessels. Various techniques, including the heart–lung cooling circuit, are used to reduce the temperature to 30 °C. With a combination of techniques it is possible to reduce the temperature to 15 °C and allow the surgeon as much as 45 minutes operating time.

Cardiac catheterisation Much information can be gained about the functioning of the heart from x-rays and ECGs but if more detailed information is required, cardiac catheterisation will be necessary. This procedure is usually carried out in a special x-ray department under aseptic conditions. An anaesthetic is not usually required. A cardiac catheter, made of polythene tubing, is introduced into the antecubital vein to the vena cava, through the right atrium and ventricle to the pulmonary artery. Its progress is watched under x-ray until it is seen to enter the heart. This procedure is used to record the pressures within the chambers of the heart and the adjoining vessels, to take samples of blood for gas analysis, and to inject a contrast

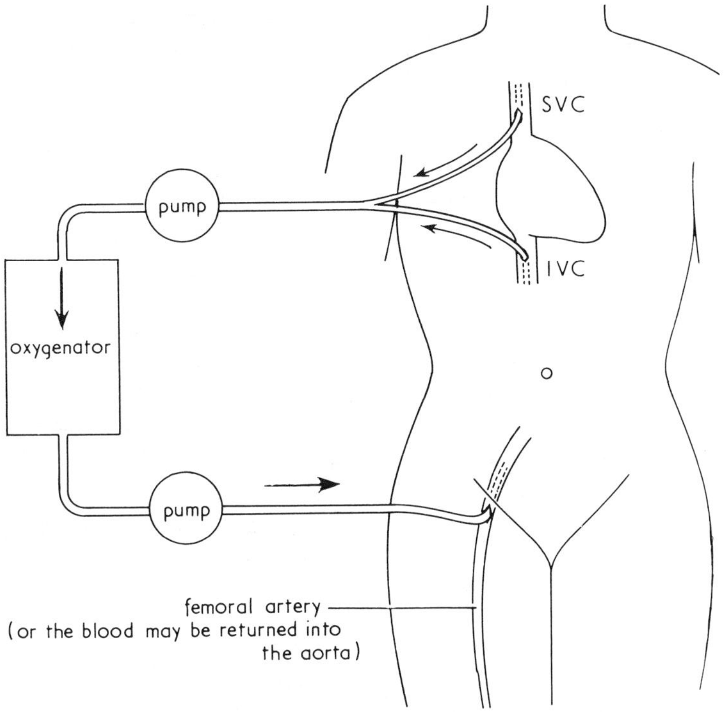

Fig. 24.7 *The heart–lung machine.*

medium to demonstrate abnormalities in the heart or large blood vessels.

Specific preoperative care

Prior to cardiac surgery very thorough tests are carried out to check for anaemia, electrolyte imbalance, disturbance of blood gases, bleeding tendencies, kidney and liver function, and the presence of any infection. Blood is taken for full blood count, haemoglobin, blood grouping and cross-matching, bleeding and coagulation tests, electrolytes, blood urea, liver function tests, and if endocarditis is present, for blood culture as well. Nasal and throat swabs are taken and if sputum is present it is sent to the laboratory. Any infection is treated, and antibiotics and anticoagulants commenced. The temperature, pulse, respirations, blood pressure and apex beat as well as the weight of the patient are monitored carefully. Otherwise the preparation of the patient is similar to that for a lobectomy.

Specific postoperative care

Whether the patient has had open- or closed-heart surgery, the care is similar to that following a lobectomy. The patient will also be connected to a cardiac monitor and a CVP line to monitor any abnormal heart beats and recognise disturbances in the blood pressure at an early stage. A pacemaker may also be used to control the rate of the heart. Great care must be taken in controlling the rate of the intravenous infusion because drugs such as digoxin will have been added to it. In open-heart surgery a nasogastric tube will be in position, as any disturbance of the electrolyte balance may cause a paralytic ileus. Haemorrhage is much more likely to occur in cardiac operations than in those on the lung, and the drainage must therefore be watched for an increased amount. A diminished amount may mean that the bleeding is occurring into the pericardium—pericardial tamponade. Urinary output must be monitored carefully as a low blood pressure will interfere with renal function.

CARDIAC ARREST

Cardiac arrest is the sudden failure of the heart to maintain an adequate circulation, either because it stops beating (asystole) or because the activity of the ventricles becomes unco-ordinated (ventricular fibrillation). In either case there is a lack of oxygen to the tissues and brain, which if continued for more than 3 minutes will cause permanent damage.

The patient collapses, losing consciousness, and on palpation no carotid or femoral pulse can be felt. Respiration ceases and the pupils dilate. The patient should be given a sharp thump on the sternum and then placed flat on a hard surface. The airway is cleared and a Brook airway inserted so that expired air resuscitation may be commenced. To do this the head is extended, the jaw is brought forward with one hand, and the nostrils pinched with the other hand. Either the Brook airway is used or the mouth is placed firmly over the patient's mouth and the lungs inflated by expiration. A deep breath is taken and the whole procedure repeated every 6 to 8 seconds (Fig. 24.8). If an Ambu bag is available, this will be used (Fig. 24.9).

At the same time cardiac resuscitation should

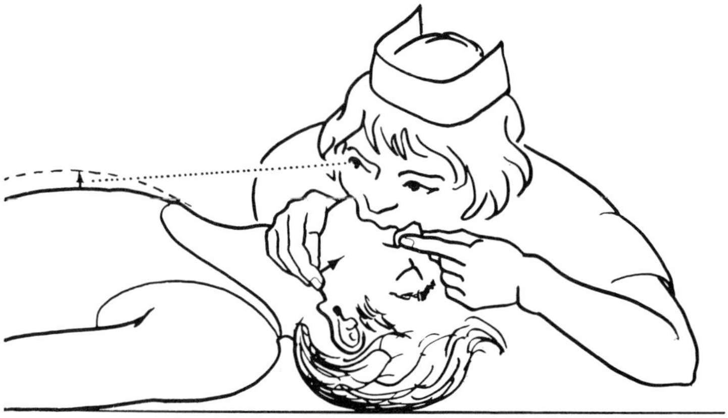

Fig. 24.8 *Mouth-to-mouth resuscitation.*

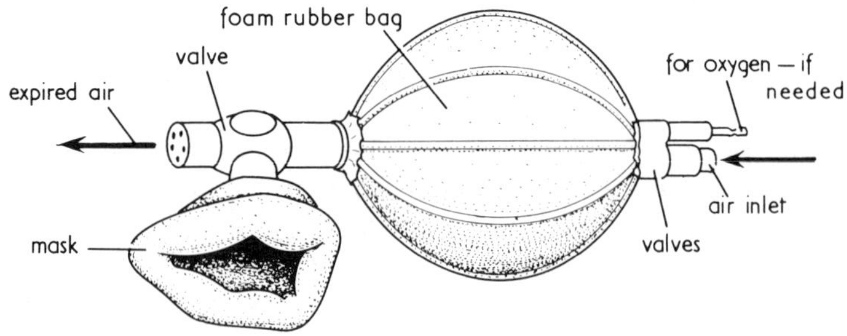

Fig. 24.9 *An Ambu bag.*

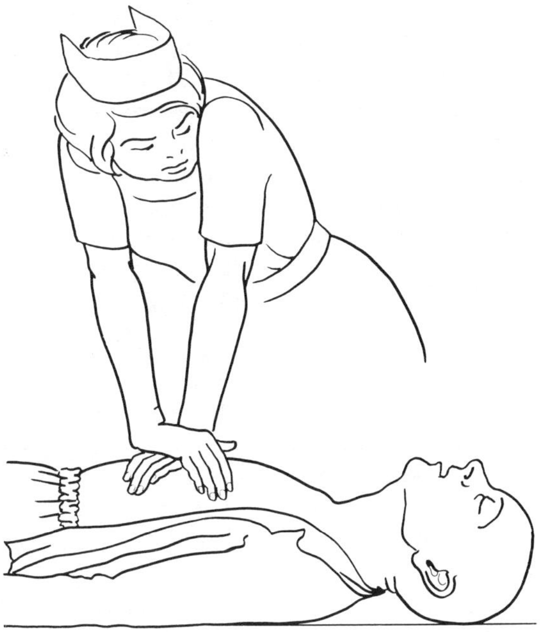

Fig. 24.10 *Cardiac resuscitation.*

take place. The heel of one hand is placed over the lower third of the sternum in the midline with the heel of the other hand on top (Fig. 24.10). The sternum should be depressed 3–4 cm, 60 to 80 times a minute. In the meantime a cardiac call for the cardiac arrest team should have been made by another member of staff.

Cardiac massage and expired air resuscitation are continued until the patient recovers or the medical staff take over. A nurse will make sure that the resuscitation trolley, with all the drugs, ECG machine and defibrillator, is ready. She plugs in the electrical apparatus and assists where required in preparing intravenous drugs or infusions. During this time a nurse will ensure that the patient is curtained off and other patients reassured. Drugs likely to be used during and following cardiac resuscitation are: sodium bicarbonate (to counteract the resultant metabolic acidosis), calcium gluconate, adrenaline, calcium chloride, metaraminol (Aramine), and noradrenaline (to stimulate the heart or raise the blood pressure), mannitol (to reduce cerebral oedema by its diuretic effect), and lignocaine (to act as a cardiac sedative). If ventricular fibrillation is present, a localised shock is applied to the heart with the defibrillator, but care must be taken to follow the instructions.

Following a cardiac arrest the patient will be attached to an oscilloscope, if it is not already in use, to monitor the cardiac rhythm. The pulse and blood pressure and in some cases the venous pressure are recorded every quarter of an hour. Oxygen will be administered and because inhalation of vomit is a common complication after a cardiac arrest, a nasogastric tube may be passed and aspirated regularly. Urinary output is measured carefully to recognise renal failure arising due to the hypotension, and if necessary a catheter is inserted.

Internal cardiac massage

This requires the thoracic cavity to be opened so that the heart can be directly massaged. It is most likely to be done if the patient's heart arrests while he is still in theatre and all the facilities are available to open up the chest under sterile conditions. The patient will require an underwater seal drain, as with any other thoracic surgery, and antibiotics.

CONDITIONS AFFECTING THE OESOPHAGUS

Dysphagia

Dysphagia arises as pain or difficulty in swallowing and may be due to any one of the following conditions.

Diseases of the pharynx such as tonsillitis.
Diseases of the mouth.
Strictures of the oesophagus.
Carcinoma of the oesophagus.
Compression of the oesophagus from outside.
Foreign bodies.
Severe iron deficiency.
Neurological conditions.
Achalasia and hiatus hernia.

Tumours of the oesophagus

Benign tumours of the oesophagus are uncommon; malignant ones occur much more frequently. They are usually squamous epithelioma and are most common in men over the age of 40 years. They may spread rapidly through the wall of the oesophagus into the mediastinum, involving the lungs and major blood vessels. Spread also occurs via the lymphatics. Tumours in the upper part of the oesophagus may involve the pharynx; however, they are more common in the middle and lower third.

These tumours appear to be more common in some families than others but there are also certain factors which predispose the oesophagus to cancer, for example cigarette smoking, excessive consumption of alcohol, long-standing hiatus hernia, coeliac disease, and some forms of iron deficiency. It follows, therefore, that any patient having these conditions should be observed carefully for any evidence of difficulty in swallowing.

Clinical picture

In the early stages of the disease there may be no signs or symptoms. The patient may eventually complain that food is sticking in the oesophagus—dysphagia. Unfortunately the carcinoma may be well advanced by this stage. Initially the dysphagia occurs with solid food, but gradually the patient has difficulty with fluids and may reach the stage where he is unable even to swallow his saliva. He may regurgitate undigested food, and have a foul breath. Because the patient has been unable to eat adequately he may have lost a considerable amount of weight.

Treatment

Surgery is the treatment of choice. Growths in the upper third of the oesophagus may be removed and a graft inserted to restore the continuity of the tube. In the middle and lower third of the oesophagus the tumour may be excised and the end of the oesophagus either anastomosed to the stomach or part of the jejenum used as a graft (Fig. 24.11). The neighbouring lymphatic glands will also be excised.

Although the tumour may be sensitive to deep x-ray therapy, it is difficult to give an accurate dose because the oesophagus is deep in the body and has many important organs around it. This method of treatment may be used if the condition is diagnosed early or palliatively to relieve the symptoms in

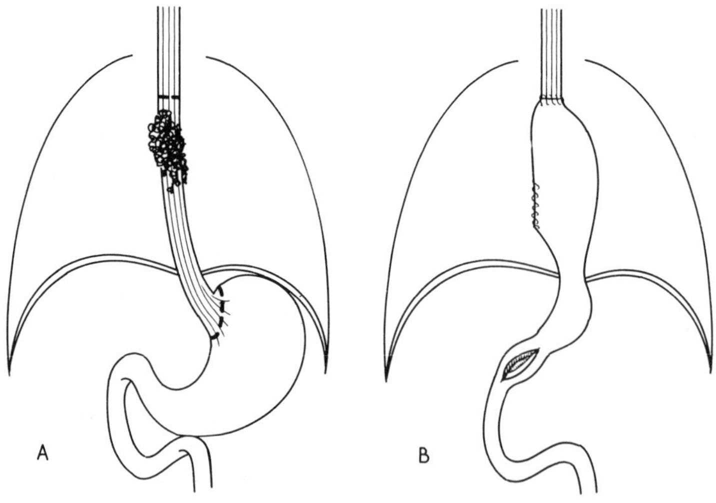

Fig. 24.11 *An oesophagectomy.*

those patients in whom the tumour is too far advanced for surgery.

Intubation may be carried out to keep the oesophagus open. A special funnel-shaped plastic tube (Celestin or Mousseau–Barbin) is inserted into the narrowed oesophagus and anchored to the stomach wall (Fig. 24.12).

A gastrostomy tube may be introduced into the stomach via the abdominal wall and the patient fed by this.

Specific preoperative preparation for an oesophagectomy Following a chest x-ray, a barium swallow, oesophagoscopy and biopsy will be carried out. Oesophageal washings may be taken to examine the contents for malignant cells. The intake of the patient will be monitored closely. Further tests will be carried out to assess the patient's general state of health. These will include blood tests for haemoglobin, electrolytes, blood grouping and cross-matching. The main aim is to ensure that the patient is in the best state for a major operation. The patient's nutrition is of prime importance and if he is unable to take sufficient nutrients by mouth, other means will be used. Vitamin and iron supplements will be necessary. Otherwise the preparation is the same as that for a lobectomy, although abdominal surgery may also be involved and therefore the patient will have additional preparation for this. A washout above the stricture may be required and specific attention must be paid to oral hygiene, any carious teeth being removed.

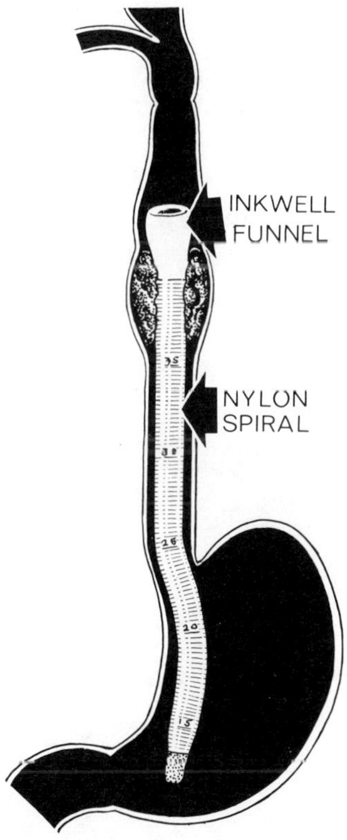

Fig. 24.12 *Celestin tube.*

Specific postoperative care The patient will return from the recovery ward with an intravenous infusion in progress (invariably blood) and a nasogastric tube. He is usually shocked, requiring quarter-hourly observations. The nasogastric tube is aspirated hourly to prevent regurgitation of acid and therefore irritation of the suture line, and between aspirations may be attached to a small drainage bag. Nothing is given by mouth for at least 24 hours and many surgeons prefer longer.

Because removal of the tumour is usually via the thoracic cavity, the patient will require the same aftercare as that for a lobectomy. If entry has been through the abdominal cavity as well, he will also require the same care as that given following an abdominal operation.

Strictures of the oesophagus may occur due to fibrosis following inflammation or the swallowing of caustic substances. This may be overcome by the use of oesophageal bougies to dilate the lumen, or by surgery.

Foreign bodies are usually passed along the gastrointestinal tract but may become impacted in the oesophagus, in which case they will be removed by means of an oesophagoscope and forceps.

Oesophagitis

A small part of the oesophagus lies below the diaphragm and is subject to abdominal pressures. However, because there is a sharp angle between the stomach and the oesophagus, which is encircled by the diaphragm and the muscles are arranged around the cardiac sphincter, reflux of stomach contents into the oesophagus is normally prevented. If the pressures are lowered due to reduced activity of the vagus or the effects of hormones, drugs and substances such as coffee, tea, nicotine or alcohol, reflux will occur. This also happens in a sliding hiatus hernia. The lining of the oesophagus is not able to withstand the acid and thus oesophagitis occurs which may lead to ulceration and fibrosis.

The patient presents with a burning sensation behind the sternum (heart burn) which more frequently occurs when he has been lying down or bending over. There may also be a return of gastric contents into the mouth.

A barium swallow and meal and oesophagoscopy with a biopsy, will diagnose the condition. Medical care will follow, the patient being advised to sleep with several pillows and to take antacids. If a hiatus hernia is present and the treatment is ineffective, surgery will be necessary.

Diaphragmatic hernia

In a true diaphragmatic hernia there is a congenital defect in the diaphragm through which the abdominal organs pass into the thorax. A gunshot or crushing injury may also have the same effect, but these causes are not common.

There are two types of hiatus hernia which, although usually congenital, do not give rise to symptoms until adulthood. More than 85% are of the type termed sliding or oesophagogastric (Fig. 24.13a) and occur when the junction between the stomach and the oesophagus rises above the diaphragm through an enlargement of the oesophageal opening. This results in a reflux of gastric juice into the lower end of the oesophagus. In the rolling or para-oesophageal hernia (Fig. 24.13b) the junction between the oesophagus and stomach remains in the abdominal cavity and there is no reflux.

Treatment

Operative treatment is only necessary in 30% of cases and may be carried out through either the chest or the abdomen. The aim is to return the organs to the abdomen and to carry out procedures which help to prevent reflux—these may include a vagotomy and repair of the defect in the diaphragm. The preparation and care will depend upon which route is taken.

Achalasia

Absence or damage to the nerve plexus in the lower part of the oesophagus causes failure of the oeso-

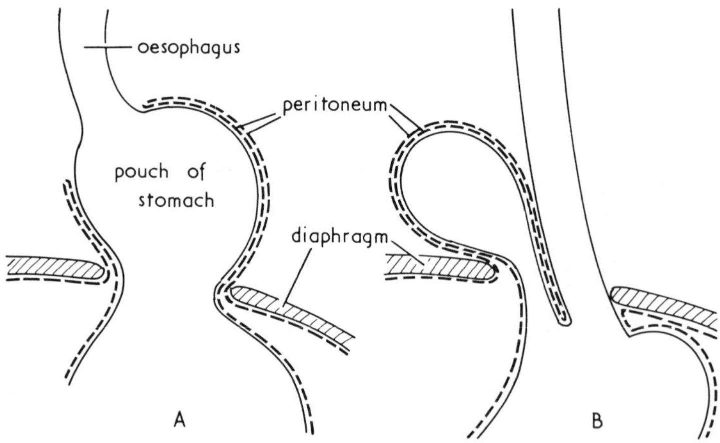

Fig. 24.13 **A.** *Sliding hiatus hernia.* **B.** *Rolling hiatus hernia.*

phageal sphincter to relax. This means that the oesophagus does not empty its contents into the stomach but becomes grossly dilated with stale food which may be regurgitated and therefore aspirated into the lungs.

The patient, who may be in his 40s, complains of a long history of dysphagia, pain or discomfort behind the sternum, recurrent attacks of pneumonia and bad breath.

Treatment

The condition is diagnosed on barium swallow. If it is not treated, it could become malignant. One method is to use dilators in order to overcome the obstruction. At a later stage Heller's operation can be done in which a longitudinal incision is made through the muscular coats of the lower oesophagus and cardiac end of the stomach down to, but not including, the mucosa (Fig. 24.14). Entry through the thoracic cavity will require the same pre- and postoperative care as for a lobectomy. Following surgery, antacids may be necessary to treat reflux oesophagitis.

Oesophageal atresia (Fig. 24.15)

This is a congenital defect in which the oesophagus is a blind-ended tube. There may also be a fistula into the trachea (tracho-oesophageal fistula). Soon after birth the baby produces an excessive amount of mucus and becomes cyanotic, particularly after taking a little feed. The condition urgently requires operation, but until this is carried out the airway has to be kept clear by frequent aspiration and tipping of the infant. If fluids are required, they are given intravenously. Body temperature is controlled by nursing the baby in an incubator. The baby must also be protected from infection. Antibiotics are given to prevent respiratory complications and vitamin K to prevent bleeding.

Initially a temporary operation may be performed such as a gastrostomy. Later, part of the bowel may be used to refashion the missing part of the oesophagus, joining it at one end to the oesophageal pouch and at the other end to the stomach (Fig. 24.16). The gastrostomy is left in until the child is taking adequate nourishment by mouth, which may be for several months. It may be necessary for the child to return to hospital each month for dilatation of the oesophagus.

SUGGESTED WORK

1. Look at the notes of those patients suffering from carcinoma of the lung and find out whether smoking was a significant factor. Do these patients

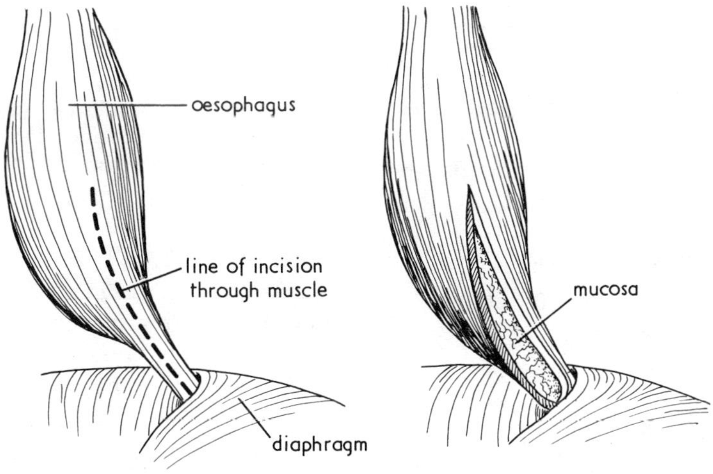

Fig. 24.14 *Treatment of achalasia.*

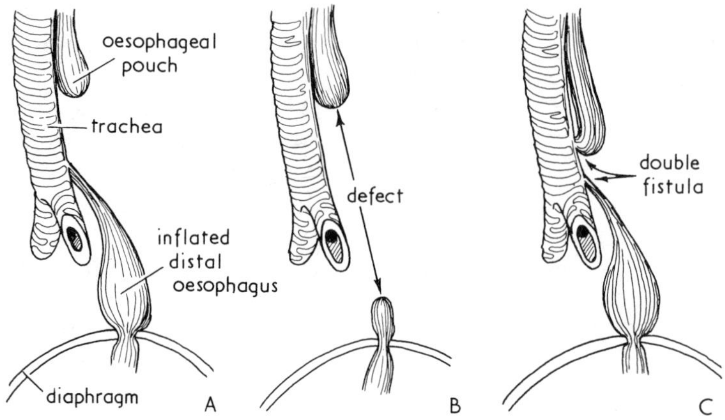

Fig. 24.15 *Types of oesophageal atresia.*

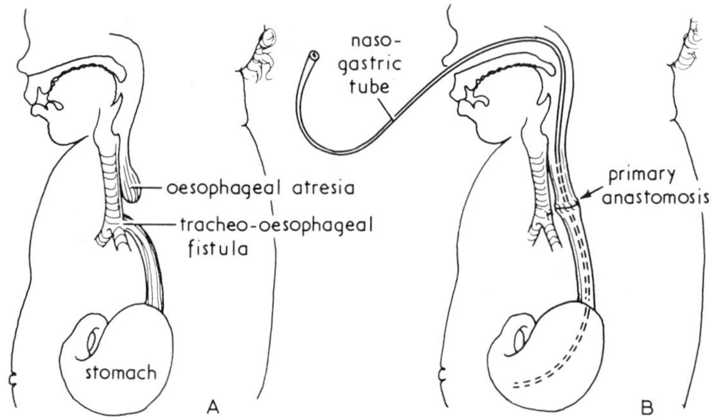

Fig. 24.16 *Management of an oesophageal atresia.*

have anything in common in their social back-grounds?

2. Find out the procedures for changing and removing the underwater seal drain in your hospital.

3. Find out whether hypothermia is used in your hospital and, if so, for which patients. How is it done?

SUGGESTED READING

Egger G. *et al.* (1983). *British Medical Journal*; **287** (6399), 1125–8.

Hansen M., Lavendero R. (1981). A multidisciplinary education programme for patients undergoing cardiovascular surgery. 7 (5): 19–24.

* * *

Mr JAMES CARTER (aged 60) is married with two children with families of their own. He has been admitted with a suspected carcinoma of the bronchus, which has now been confirmed by sigmoidoscopy. He is a heavy smoker and has become progressively more breathless in recent months. He has also lost some weight.

Prior to admission he had chest x-rays and tomograms. He had been prescribed ferrous gluconate for anaemia and advised to stop smoking and go to the dentist. His sputum had shown malignant cells.

Medical plan
Lobectomy and bone scan.

Identification of the patient's needs and problems once the immediate postoperative period is over and action arising from these

Expansion of the lung and removal of secretions
Keep the patient sitting up once he has fully recovered from the operation and his blood pressure is stable. Encourage him to do the breathing exercises and to cough every 2 hours holding his wound. Continue a high concentration of oxygen as prescribed. Encourage fluids. His family may be able to supply drinks he enjoys. Encourage him to move, and explain why this is important. Discourage smoking and explain why.

Pain
Administer prescribed analgesia as required. Make sure that he is not suffering unnecessarily. Ensure analgesia is given before the physiotherapist attends the patient. Check with the patient how effective it is.

Anaemia
Monitor and regulate the rate of the blood transfusion. Observe the patient's temperature, pulse and respiration half-hourly for adverse reactions.

Drainage tubes and wound
While the patient remains in bed ensure that the drainage tube is led out through a gap in the pillows and pinned to a pillow to prevent it sticking into the patient or dragging. Support the wound when the patient coughs and teach him how to do this. Check that the tubes are patent and not blocked and that the fluid level is swinging. Note the amount and type of drainage in the basal drainage bottle; record and report if abnormal. Empty the drainage bottle as necessary with an aseptic technique and check that the clamps are readily available. Ensure that the patient has been x-rayed and that the x-rays are available for the doctor to examine when the drainage tube is to be removed. Explain to the patient what the removal of the tube will be like and that the doctor will ask him to take a deep breath in and hold it, immediately before taking the tube out. Ensure that analgesia has been written up; this may be prescribed as a premedication.

Check the wound and remove the sutures on the 10th to 14th day as ordered if the wound is healthy. If the wound is red or a stitch abscess is present, arrange for the doctor to see it first. Remove stitch from stab wound 5 days after removing drainage tube. If Vaseline gauze had been applied to stab wound on removal of the drainage tube, this should be replaced by a dry dressing within 48 hours.

Prevention of deep vein thrombosis
Place a cradle in the bed and encourage the patient to move his legs and flex his muscles when in bed. Administer subcutaneous heparin as prescribed. Observe for a rise in the temperature and regularly examine the calf for pain. Start mobilisation the first postoperative day if possible.

Prevention of infection
Ask any members of the family with a cold not to visit until clear. Administer antibiotics as prescribed. Monitor temperature carefully and note any increasing difficulty in breathing.

Mobilisation
Help the patient to sit out of bed for bedmaking and again in the afternoon for half an hour on the first postoperative day if his condition is satisfactory. Make sure that no tubes are dragging. Gradually increase this period if there are no adverse effects. Once all tubes are out he can be assisted to the bathroom. The physiotherapist will be teaching him exercises to encourage him to move his arm, which the nurse may supplement.

Nutrition
Discuss with him his diet and the importance of building him up. Discover what food he can manage and enjoy. His wife and family might be able to help in providing some titbits. 'Build Up' and other high-protein supplements can also be provided.

Hygiene
Initially Mr Carter will require a bedbath. As he improves, encourage him to do as much as possible

for himself but do not allow him to become too tired. When attending to his pressure areas turn him on to his operated side.

Excretion
He will require an aperient about the 3rd day postoperatively, depending on his condition. A commode will probably be most suitable.

Psychological
He will want to know what was found at the operation and what his prognosis is. He should be told as much as he wants to know and is able to bear if the outlook is not good. He may find the visit of a minister of religion helpful. The ward team caring for him must liaise and be kept informed of what he has been told.

Relatives
His wife and other members of the family will need support and an opportunity to talk freely. The general practitioner will need to be kept up to date as he also will be supporting the wife and family.

25

Conditions of the Breast

The breast is an essential part of the femininity of women. Its possible or actual loss will therefore have a significant effect on a woman's feelings about herself and her relationship with men. Thus the nurse will have to play a very supportive role, enabling the patient to come to terms with her changed body image. The nature of the surgery will mean that emphasis will have to be placed on encouraging the patient to exercise her arm and take other measures to prevent gross oedema occurring.

Specific emphasis in the nursing history

Skin. Observe for discharge from the nipple, changes in the skin of the breast and any other abnormalities of the breast.

Sexuality. The relationship of the patient to her partner and the effects she feels the operation will have on this.

Breathing. Evidence of smoking, or respiratory problems.

Pain. The presence of pain anywhere in the body, particularly in the back.

DISORDERS OF THE NIPPLE

Painful cracks and fissures of the nipple may develop during breast-feeding if the nipples are not prepared adequately in the later stages of pregnancy, and care taken when the baby is suckling. Once they have occurred, breast-feeding must be discontinued on the affected breast and the milk expressed. Local antiseptics are applied to prevent infection.

Acute and chronic eczema can affect the nipples in the same way as other parts of the body, and is usually associated with fissures. Paget's disease of the nipple is a condition of eczema associated with malignant disease and must therefore be distinguished from ordinary eczema. It spreads from the nipples to the surrounding skin, causing the nipple to disappear and the surface of the skin to become bright red and weeping. It is usually found in women aged 40 to 60 years and is confined to one breast, whereas simple eczema affects the younger woman and both breasts. The treatment is as for carcinoma of the breast. Abscesses and sebaceous cysts of the areola, and syphilitic ulcers (primary sores) of the nipple are occasionally seen.

INFLAMMATORY CONDITIONS OF THE BREAST

Acute mastitis and acute mammary abscesses are the most common of these conditions. Infection of the breast is most likely to occur during lactation, the usual infecting organisms being the *Staphylococcus* and *Streptococcus*. The breast or part of it becomes swollen, red and tender and the lymph nodes in the axilla become enlarged. The condition is treated with antibiotics, the baby being allowed to empty the breast of milk or this is done with a breast pump. If pus forms, drainage will be required. In some patients suppression of lactation will be necessary and an oestrogen derivative such as ethinyloestradiol may be given. Chronic abscesses may develop due to the infection of a pre-existing cyst or tuberculosis, and these require incision and drainage. If the breast is very nodular on examination, it should be examined again at a different time in the menstrual cycle.

Fibrocystic dysplasia (chronic mastitis)

Single or multiple cysts of various sizes may occur in the breast due to the stagnation and retention of secretions. The latter arises because of the increase of glandular tissue, epithelial cells lining the ducts and fibrosis in the breast. The condition may affect women of any age, married or unmarried, but is most common in those in their late twenties or thirties without children.

The breasts are painful and tender, particularly during menstruation and when moving the arms. They feel lumpy and nodular, are red and there may be a clear serous discharge from the nipple. The lymph nodes in the axilla may be enlarged and tender. A biopsy is taken to exclude carcinoma and the patient advised to wear a firm supporting brassiere. Cysts may occur as a result of chronic mastitis or occasionally with benign tumours. They are aspirated under a local anaesthetic.

BENIGN TUMOURS

Although less common than malignant tumours, the most frequently occurring are the fibroadenomas. These are usually painless, freely movable, hard nodules found in the woman under the age of 30 years. Some of them are larger, forming cysts and growing more quickly, and these may ulcerate onto the skin. Either type will be removed by excision—lumpectomy. Duct papillomata cause a bloodstained discharge from the nipple, coming from the affected duct. A very fine probe is passed down the affected duct, and the duct with the papilloma inside are removed through the incision.

CARCINOMA OF THE BREAST

This is one of the most malignant conditions occurring in women. As many as 10 000 women die each year from this condition and yet, if treated in time, it can be cured. It is uncommon in men but if it does occur it spreads at an early stage and so usually presents in an advanced condition. It is most likely to affect women over the age of 35 with a maternal or family history of breast cancer, particularly if a mother or sister was affected, and especially so if it occurred in them before the menopause. Those women who have not had children or have borne them after the age of 30 appear more likely to be affected.

The most common form is *scirrhous* carcinoma, which usually presents as a hard irregular mass and can be removed in the early stages. It soon becomes fixed to the overlying skin and later to the underlying muscles. As it progresses there are skin changes with dimpling and puckering of the skin over the site of the tumour. The skin takes on the appearance of an orange skin (peau d'orange) and there may be nodules and ulceration with more extensive infiltration of the skin. The axillary nodules become palpable, and later enlarged and hard.

The tumour not only spreads to the adjacent skin and muscle but also via the lymphatics and bloodstream. Malignant cells spread via the lymphatics to the axillary nodes and internal mammary chain, eventually reaching the nodes of the neck, the pleural and peritoneal cavities, and may therefore affect the opposite breast, the ovaries and pelvis. The cells spread via the bloodstream causing secondary deposits in the bones which may lead to pathological fractures, and paraplegia if the vertebrae are affected. Metastases are also common in the liver, sometimes causing jaundice.

There are four stages of carcinoma of the breast (Fig. 25.1). In stage I the tumour is limited to the breast tissue; in stage II it has spread to the axillary nodes or underlying fascia but is still confined to the immediate vicinity of the breast; in stage III local spread is more advanced; and in stage IV it has spread to distant organs and tissues which may only become evident on x-ray.

Early recognition is therefore important and, with wide publicity regarding the need for regular examination of the breast by the woman herself, it should be possible to detect carcinoma of the breast at an early stage while there is a 100% cure rate. Examination of the breast is usually carried out at

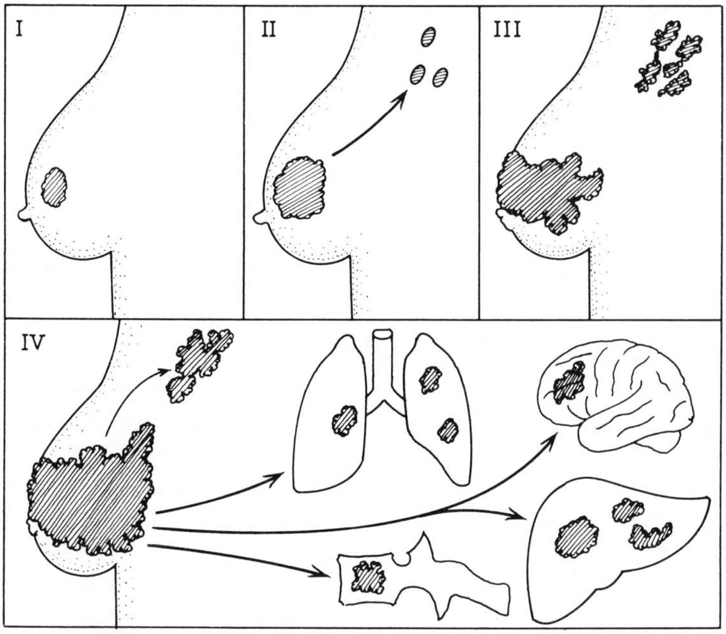

Fig. 25.1 *Stages in carcinoma of the breast.*

the same time as a cervical smear. If a lump is present, thermography may be done in which a heat-sensitive device is used to detect abnormal circulation in the area. Mammography and xerography involve the taking of special x-rays of the breast which detect abnormal tissue. A biopsy of the lump may be taken by aspirating tissue with a syringe. If discharge from the nipples is present, pressure is applied and a sample smeared onto a slide for cytology—this is called aspiration cytology (Fig. 25.2). The patient will be examined for any evidence of enlarged lymph nodes in the axilla

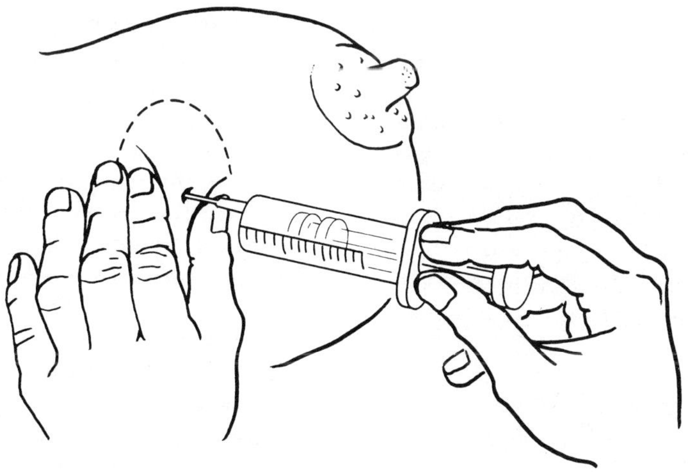

Fig. 25.2 *Aspiration cytology.*

and questioned about any back pain. The abdomen will be felt for an enlarged liver or ascites, and frequently the patient is taken to theatre for a biopsy of the lump. A frozen section is taken while the patient is on the operating table, and if it is positive the surgeon will then proceed to a mastectomy.

Management

Surgeons vary as to the operative procedure they use but if the tumour is in stage I, a simple mastectomy, in which the tumour and breast tissue only are removed, is preferred. If required this may be followed up by irradiation of the axillary and other lymphatic drainage areas. However, if the carcinoma is more advanced, the surgeon may do a modified radical mastectomy, in which the nipple and skin surrounding it, the complete breast and connective tissue, and the lymph nodes in the axilla are removed. Some surgeons will also remove the pectoralis minor (Patey operation), and in a radical mastectomy the pectoralis major muscle will be removed. These operations are frequently followed by radiotherapy to control the local metastases. If the skin edges cannot be brought together, a skin graft will be necessary in order to prevent tension on the wound leading to sloughing. In stages III and IV, radiotherapy, hormone therapy and cytotoxic drugs will be used rather than surgery.

Specific preoperative preparation

The situation is explained to the woman and her husband, with details of the treatment she is to receive. If she is to have a frozen section which if positive will be followed by a mastectomy, she will be reassured that as soon as possible after the operation she will be told the result. It may reassure her at this stage to see some of the prostheses or to meet a patient who has recovered from the operation. Her husband may need some guidance as to how he may best support his wife following the operation.

The physiotherapist will visit the patient and show her the exercises she will be required to do postoperatively, including deep breathing, gentle arm exercises and movement of the legs. Both axillae are shaved. Blood is grouped and cross-matched. A bone scan may be carried out prior to the operation or at a later stage to look for secondaries.

Specific postoperative care

The patient usually returns from theatre with a pressure bandage over the wound and one or two drainage tubes (such as a Redivac) in position. As soon as she is sufficiently conscious and her blood pressure is satisfactory, she is gradually sat up in bed with her arm supported on a pillow to encourage drainage. The drainage bottles must be kept vacuumed and changed as required, there being a fair amount of blood and serum lost. The patient should be observed carefully for shock, reactionary haemorrhage, pneumothorax and surgical emphysema. Any chest pain or a raised temperature may indicate a chest infection or a pulmonary embolism. Analgesia will be required and possibly a sedative later on. An intravenous infusion is generally in progress and will require the usual care.

At a fairly early stage postoperatively the patient will want to know the outcome of the operation. A simple, matter-of-fact statement of what has been done by the surgeon should be given. The patient may want to weep quietly on her own and the nurse should be sensitive to her requirements, if necessary drawing the curtains round her. The husband should also be told before he goes in to visit her. Later she should be given the opportunity to discuss her feelings and the problems that she is concerned about so these can be dealt with.

The dressing is not usually touched for the first few days, but when it is taken down the wound is inspected for any sloughing or the formation of a haematoma which will need to be evacuated. The drainage tubes are removed 24 hours after the drainage is minimal, and the stitches removed in 10 to 14 days.

The physiotherapist will visit the patient and encourage deep breathing, gentle arm exercises and leg exercises. She will emphasise good posture and, once the wound is healing satisfactorily, encourage the patient to comb her hair and touch the small of her back. The exercises are particularly important for the patient who has had a radical mastectomy.

Even if the arm is elevated, some patients develop oedema at some stage which persists despite further elevation and arm exercises. In this case an elastic stockinette sleeve may be prescribed either for wear at night only or, if necessary, in the daytime as well. If this is insufficient, it may be possible for the surgeon to re-establish lymphatic channels.

While in hospital the patient will be fitted with a light-weight prosthesis which is more comfortable at this stage. A mastectomy nurse specialist or appliance officer will be able to discuss the most suitable permanent type. Prostheses may be made of a variety of materials containing liquid, ceramic particles, silicone gel, moulded silicone elastomer, fluid and air. They may be round, elliptical or tear-drop in shape and in some types a nipple is provided. Some are more suitable for a simple and others for a radical mastectomy. The activity and age of the patient, and the size of the breast all have to be taken into consideration. The majority of prostheses may be obtained on a National Health prescription.

If a bone scan has not been done before, it will be carried out after the operation. The patient's haemoglobin will also be checked for anaemia. On return home the mastectomy nurse specialist may visit and help her with problems that arise. Another source of help is the Mastectomy Association.

Some breast cancers are hormone dependent and therefore if metastases are present the surgeon may remove the ovaries and later the adrenal glands or pituitary. These cases will require permanent steroid replacement therapy, or, alternatively, hormones—the androgens to premenopausal women and oestrogens to postmenopausal women.

Radiotherapy is frequently given following surgery, once the wound has healed, to the skin and lymph nodes into which the breast drains. However, there is some evidence that radiotherapy following a simple mastectomy diminishes the immune response of the body to malignant cells and may therefore be best used only where there is known spread of the cells. It is also used where the carcinoma is too advanced to operate, when it may relieve oedema. If the disease has already spread to other organs and tissues, radiotherapy may be useful in reducing pain, as in bone metastases. Radioactive isotopes such as gold or yttrium or cytotoxic drugs such as mustine hydrochloride may be injected into the pleural or peritoneal cavities if effusions are present due to metastases. Cytotoxic drugs such as mustine hydrochloride or cyclophosphamide may be given intravenously in the advanced case.

SUGGESTED WORK

1. Find out which prostheses are available on the NHS. How much guidance are the patients in your hospital given on what is available? What are the advantages and disadvantages of the different types of prostheses?

2. Contact the branch of the Mastectomy Association in your area and find out if they have any comments about the way these patients are treated in hospital and what improvements they would like to see.

3. What type of treatment for cancer of the breast is most commonly used in your hospital?

SUGGESTED READING

Bullough B. (1981). Nurses as teachers and support persons for breast cancer patients. *Cancer Nursing*; **4**(3): 221–5.

Bullough B. (1982). Emotional support for the patient with breast cancer. *Health Values*; **6**(2): 19–22.

Dostal E. R., Elder L. E. (1979). Breast cancer: special nursing considerations. *Journal of Practical Nursing*; **29**(4): 16–18.

Emotional aspects of mastectomy, planning a caring programme (1980). *Nursing Mirror*; **150**(3): 35–7.

Health Education Council (1979). *Living with the Loss of a Breast: a Booklet for Mastectomy Patients*. London: Health Education Council.

Marchant J. (1978). *Rehabilitation of Mastectomy Patients*. London: Heinemann.

Robinson N., Swash I. (1977). *Mastectomy: a Patients' Guide to Coping with Breast Surgery*. Wellingborough: Thorsons.

* * *

Mrs BETTY WALLEN (aged 35) is married with no children. She has been admitted with a lump in her breast which was discovered on attendance at the cervical cytology clinic. As a result of a fall when a child she lost her two front teeth and has a small dental plate which she is very self-conscious about. Her husband is a business executive and travels a great deal.

Medical plan
A frozen section of the lump is to be taken in theatre and this is to be followed by either a lumpectomy or a mastectomy depending on the diagnosis. She is to have a bone scan.

Identification of the patient's needs and problems on admission to hospital and action arising from these

Distress at the possible diagnosis
Give Mrs Wallen the opportunity to discuss her fears and allow her privacy if she is weepy. Explain that the mastectomy will only be done if it is essential and she will be told the result as soon as she is ready to receive it. It is also important to stress that surgical removal of the tumour and the surrounding tissue is sufficient to stop its spread if it is caught early enough. She may wish to discuss her relationship with her husband and how the operation might affect this. Discuss with her husband her fears and how he can help to overcome these. Speaking to someone who has had the condition may help her to realise that even if she does have the operation she can still look attractive. Arrange for the mastectomy nurse to visit her.

Worry about her reaction when she is given the result
Reassure her that whatever the result she will probably have a little weep as a reaction from the strain. Explain that she may have the curtains drawn before she has the news. Her husband will be informed before he visits her, unless she would prefer to explain to him.

Worry about the longer term effects if it is a cancer
Make sure that there is a nurse with the doctor when he is explaining the prognosis. Help Mrs Wallen to realise that even if the lump is a cancer there are many treatments available according to the stage it has reached.

Prevention of respiratory complications
Arrange for the physiotherapist to come and show her how to deep breathe, and the exercises she will be required to do after the operation to ensure good movement of the arm.

Worry about the operation and the anaesthetic
Reassure her that she will quickly go to sleep and that the injection beforehand will help to relax her and make her sleepy. Give her the opportunity to talk to a patient who has had an operation and who would be helpful.

Embarrassment about not wearing her denture
Make sure the denture is easily available for her on the locker top so that she can put it in as soon as she feels ready. If she has not already put it in, do this before she has any visitors or the doctor sees her.

Operation on the correct breast
Check the operating list with the notes, and the latter with the patient. Check whether the correct breast has been marked. If any discrepancies, report. Go through the checklist to see if all the preparations have been carried out correctly.

26

Neurological Conditions

The contents of the cranial cavity are closely packed together, leaving little room for an increase in their size. Any operation results in some degree of oedema but if this is more than minimal or if haemorrhage occurs, increased pressure will be present within the cavity which will cause damage to its contents, the patient becoming comatose and eventually dying. The nurse's role in making the neurological observations accurately and reporting changes promptly is therefore vital. She will also need to provide particular support for the patient's relatives.

Specific emphasis in the nursing history

Mental. Alertness. Any behaviour out of character. The presence of headaches, drowsiness, fits or vertigo.

Nutrition. Nausea, vomiting and when it occurs.

Communication. Any difficulties the patient has in expressing himself, or lack of understanding.

Mobility. Any loss of movement, abnormal movements or ataxia.

Skin. Any loss of sensation.

Vital signs. Raised blood pressure, slow pulse and respirations.

Special senses. Alterations in sight, hearing, smell or taste.

Neurosurgery may be required for various types of space-occupying lesions of the brain, and for lesions of the spinal cord or the peripheral nerves.

SPACE-OCCUPYING LESIONS OF THE BRAIN

Anything which takes up space in the cranial cavity comes under this heading, including benign and malignant growths, abscesses, hydrocephalus and haemorrhage.

Cerebral tumours

At least 50% of tumours arise from the neuroglia, the connective tissue of the nervous system, and are called *gliomas*. They grow slowly, but by the time they are diagnosed it is often only possible to remove part of the tumour to relieve intracranial pressure. The *astrocytoma* is the most common of these tumours and frequently has small cysts. If it is diagnosed early enough, it may be excised with a good prognosis. An *ependymoma* is a tumour of the lining of the ventricles and is usually treated with radiation.

Meningiomas form 15% of brain tumours and are tumours of the meninges. They sometimes occur after trauma in the region of a scar and do not usually spread. However, they may develop at a site where surgery is not possible. The prognosis is good if the complete tumour is removed.

Carcinomatous metastases (secondary growths) comprise 20–30% of all brain tumours, the primary being elsewhere in the body. They mainly develop in the cerebrum but do arise in the cerebellum as well. The most common site of the primary growth is in the bronchi, but it may be in the breast, kidney, gastrointestinal tract or from a melanoma in the skin, the malignant cells being spread via the bloodstream. Treatment depends on the prognosis of the primary growth: if this is good, the secondary growth in the brain will be treated as any other tumour of the cerebrum or cerebellum.

Neuromas are tumours which develop from the Schwann cells, either on their own in the middle aged or as part of a generalised neurofibromatosis (Von Recklinghausen's disease) in the younger individual. The *acoustic* neuroma is the most common form, and develops on the vestibular branch of the eighth cranial nerve. It grows very slowly and can be removed if discovered early enough, although there is always facial paralysis after the operation.

Vascular tumours

Angiomas are benign tumours and only cause problems because of pressure or particularly if they rupture. Haemangioblastoma may be associated with similar tumours in other parts of the body and cause polycythaemia. Some of these tumours are cystic and can be drained, in which case the prognosis is good. However, if they are solid, they are difficult to remove because of the danger of haemorrhage.

Abscesses

Infection most commonly spreads from diseases of the middle ear but may also arise from the mastoid, sinuses or as a result of a compound fracture of the skull. The infection may originate from some other part of the body such as the lungs, travelling in the bloodstream. As well as a mild degree of raised intracranial pressure, the signs will depend on what the abscess is pressing on. Because of its proximity to the ear, the temporal lobe is most commonly affected, although abscesses do occur in the cerebellar region as well. The abscess is aspirated through burr holes; antibiotics are given and the underlying disease treated. Some abscesses have to be excised and antibiotics injected into the space.

Hydrocephalus

The production of cerebrospinal fluid (CSF) by the choroid plexus in the ventricles is balanced by its absorption in the arachnoid villi. If anything obstructs the flow of CSF out of the ventricles or more distally so that it cannot reach the arachnoid granulations and be absorbed, the amount of CSF in the ventricles will increase so causing hydrocephalus in children and raised intracranial pressure in adults. This may be due to a congenital abnormality or infection such as a meningitis. A bypass operation is carried out to drain the cerebrospinal fluid from the ventricles into the jugular vein, by means of tubing with a one-way valve (Fig. 26.1).

Trauma

Brain damage can occur even when their is no fractured skull. The latter is only serious if the bone is depressed or there is a compound fracture, but it may indicate the extent of the brain damage. Damage to the brain is in most cases the result of the brain moving within the cranial cavity. The older the individual, the greater the degree of movement. This may cause damage to the cells themselves or to the blood vessels, and the resulting oedema or haemorrhage will cause compression of the brain. The injury may be on the side of the blow or on the opposite side (contre coup, Fig. 26.2). Concussion varies from a state of unconsciousness which persists until death to a short loss of consciousness, but it is associated with diffuse contusions and lacerations of the brain and leads to some degree of amnesia.

Haemorrhage (Fig. 26.3)

Extradural haemorrhage

Haemorrhage occurring between the skull and the dura mater is most frequently due to damage to the middle meningeal artery. It develops rapidly, associated oedema aggravating the situation. It must be relieved promptly or coning will occur.

Subdural haemorrhage

This type of haemorrhage occurs between the dura and arachnoid mater. In the young person it requires a severe blow and is therefore usually

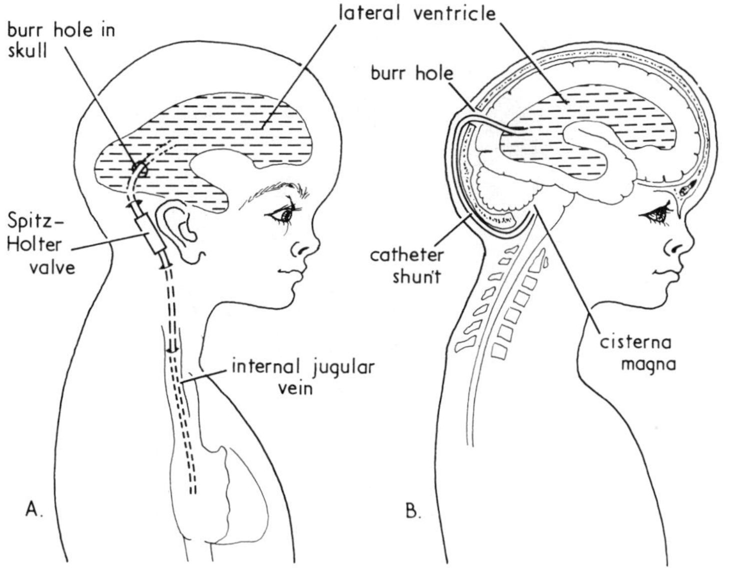

Fig. 26.1 *Methods of treating a hydrocephalus.*

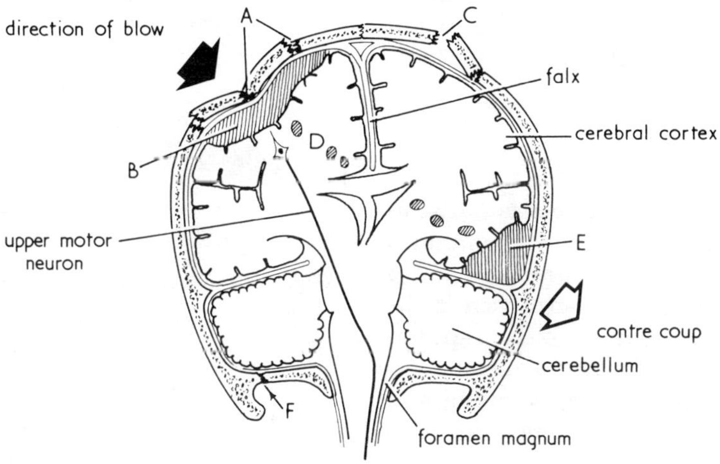

Fig. 26.2 *The contre coup effect.* **A.** Depressed fracture. **B.** *Subdural haemorrhage.* **C.** *Fracture by bursting.* **D.** *Line of small haemorrhages.* **E.** *Contre coup.* **F.** *Fracture of base.*

associated with a fractured skull. It occurs more easily in the elderly. The symptoms are similar to those of extradural haemorrhage but develop over a period of 2 to 3 weeks after the injury and tend to fluctuate. The patient complains of a headache which increases in severity and he becomes increasingly drowsy. As with an extradural haemorrhage, the clot must be removed.

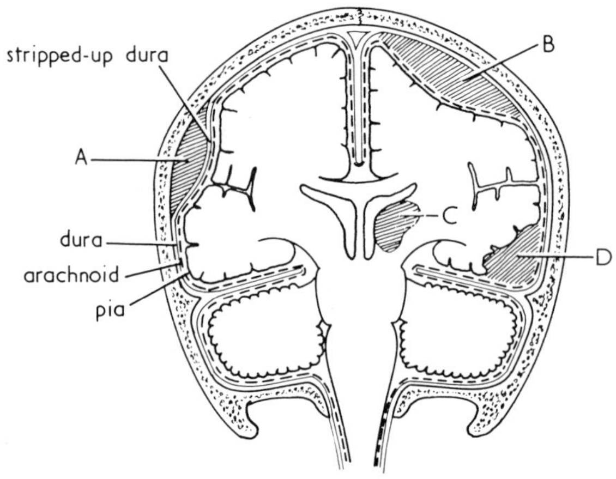

Fig. 26.3 *Types of brain haemorrhage which may occur.* **A.** *Extradural* **B.** *Subdural.* **C.** *Intracerebral.* **D.** *Subarachnoid.*

Intracranial haemorrhage

This is associated with severe head injuries, particularly if there is a depressed fracture of the skull and a penetrating wound. Patients usually remain deeply unconscious for a long period of time, and if they do recover, have some degree of physical and mental handicap.

Traumatic subarachnoid haemorrhage

More commonly, this condition does not arise as the result of trauma, but due to the combined effects of an increasing blood pressure and a weakness in the form of a berry aneurysm in the blood vessels of the brain which ruptures (Fig. 26.4). Evidence of a raised intracranial pressure with headache, photophobia, vomiting and neck stiffness will be present. There may also be an increasing degree of drowsiness.

Damage to the brain stem

Fractures of the base of the skull and those injuries caused by rapid acceleration or deceleration will probably involve the brain stem. A deep coma and death are frequently the outcome, and may be due to damage to the reticular formation, the vital centres, or coning.

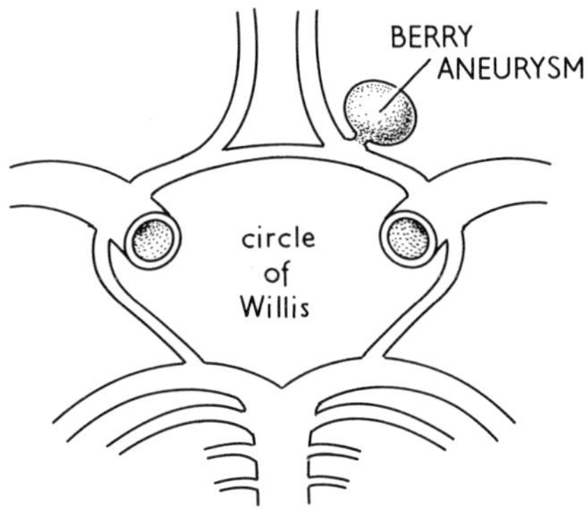

Fig. 26.4 *Vascular abnormalities of the blood supply to the brain.*

RAISED INTRACRANIAL PRESSURE

Any space-occupying lesion will cause some degree of raised intracranial pressure although the rate at which it develops and its severity will vary according to the condition.

Headache

A subarachnoid haemorrhage may cause a sudden severe headache at the back of the head which gradually becomes more diffuse. In a slowly developing tumour the headache is usually worse in the morning, gradually disappearing during the day. It is a throbbing type of headache made worse by anything that increases intracranial pressure still further, such as coughing or bending, but is usually reduced by mild analgesics.

Papilloedema

Raised intracranial pressure affects the blood vessels in the retina and these can be seen with an ophthalmoscope. It may lead to frequent, intermittent loss of vision for a few seconds, especially when the individual gets up in the morning or stoops down.

Vomiting is frequently present, and when tumours are present, it occurs in the morning before breakfast and may not be accompanied by nausea.

Alteration in level of consciousness

This may vary from a slight drowsiness to a profound coma. Tumours may lead to mild personality changes or dementia. Usually there is a progressive change in the level of consciousness which is most noticeable with a haemorrhage.

Epileptiform fits

These may be associated with a focal lesion such as temporal lobe epilepsy in which the aura may indicate to the doctor where the lesion is. They may include disturbances of vision, hearing or smell and Jacksonian attacks which indicate a lesion of the motor area of the brain.

Disturbances of language

The patient may have some difficulty in understanding commands, in naming objects or in saying what he wants, depending on the site of the lesion.

Hemiplegia or hemiparesis

Paralysis or weakness will be present if the lesion is in the region of the pyramidal tracts, therefore affecting motor function.

Disturbance of the cranial nerves

If the cranial nerve is near the lesion, it may become damaged from pressure. A lesion in the region of the optic nerve may cause a hemianopia with loss of half the visual field in each eye or blindness in one eye. Damage to the olfactory nerve will cause a loss of smell. Involvement of the facial nerve causes pain in that region, whereas damage to the trigeminal nerve will result in anaesthesia of the face. Deafness and vertigo indicate a lesion in the region of the auditory nerve.

Disturbance of sensation

If sensory nerve pathways are interrupted, this will lead to a lack of information being fed into the brain so that the individual is unable to recognise the position of his body if his eyes are closed, and to a lack of sensation.

Blood pressure, pulse and respirations

As intracranial pressure rises, the pulse becomes slower and the blood pressure increases in an effort to supply the brain with sufficient blood. The respirations become slower and irregular.

Parkinsonism

This normally develops as a result of degeneration of the basal ganglia, the cause being unknown. However, the characteristic symptoms of rigidity, tremor and poverty of movement may be produced by a tumour in the region of the basal ganglia.

Nystagmus

A movement of the eyes from side to side, this may be present if the lesion is in the cerebellum or sometimes following a head injury.

Ataxia

This is a staggering, drunken type of walking which is present in lesions of the cerebellum.

Investigations

1. Plain x-rays may show some displacement of structures.

2. Electroencephalogram (EEG), in which electrical currents in the brain are measured by attaching electrodes to the head.

3. Lumbar puncture or cisternal puncture. This is not done if there is evidence of raised intracranial pressure as it will result in herniation of the brain and pressure on the vital centres.

4. Echoencephalography to the upper part of the brain above the tentorium.

5. Brain scanning following an intravenous infusion of the isotope technetium.

6. Computerised axial tomography (CAT scan). This is a way of x-raying the brain at varying depths but requires the patient to remain still for some time and therefore a child or confused patient would require sedation.

7. Angiography. The injection of a radio-opaque substance into the carotid artery followed by x-rays.

8. Ventriculography. Air or a contrast medium may be introduced directly into the ventricles by means of burr holes.

9. Air encephalography. The introduction of air into the ventricles by means of a lumbar puncture.

Management of patients with a space-occupying lesion

Raised intracranial pressure may be reduced by means of hypertonic intravenous solutions such as mannitol 20% or corticosteroids.

Surgery to the brain

Surgery may be carried out to remove a tumour or part of a tumour or, as in hydrocephalus, as a short-circuiting procedure to bypass an obstruction. Great care has to be taken if a general anaesthetic is used to prevent a lowering of oxygen level or a further increase in the intracranial pressure. Therefore a local anaesthetic may be preferred. If the operation is carried out under a general anaesthetic, hypothermia may be used, reducing the body temperature to 28°C, chlorpromazine being administered to overcome shivering.

Specific preoperative preparation

The head is shaved over the area specified by the surgeon. The patient needs to be reassured that the hair will soon grow again and that immediately following the operation he will have a dressing and a cotton cap covering his head. Once the wound has healed he can be supplied with a wig if desired. Following the shave, the head is covered with a tubular cotton cap. Baseline neurological observations are taken immediately prior to the operation. The doctor may commence an intravenous infusion. A booster dose of steroids will be required if the patient is already receiving steroid treatment.

Specific postoperative care

The patient is kept in the recovery room until he has fully recovered from the anaesthetic because of the difficulty of monitoring the neurological signs in the anaesthetised patient.

He will be nursed in a recumbent position for operations of the cerebrum, but operations below the tentorium may require the patient to be nursed sitting up. Simple analgesics such as aspirin are usually sufficient to control the pain.

Neurological observations are made every quarter of an hour until the signs they are stable. These include an assessment of the level of consciousness and particularly any deterioration in it, in which case the doctor must be informed immediately. The pupils are examined to see that they are equal and of normal size. Enlargement of the pupil on the side of the operation indicates a haemorrhage in that area. Any increase in the blood pressure or fall in the pulse rate will also reveal a rising intracranial pressure. Abnormalities of respiration such as noisy, stertorous breathing or slow irregular breathing will also be looked for. The presence of fits, rigidity or hemiplegia will be noted.

Local and systemic antibiotics are usually given to prevent infection. Corticosteroids will be given if the patient had been receiving them prior to operation, or to reduce cerebral oedema. A rise in the temperature may indicate damage to the hypothalamus and will require active measures to reduce it. If it occurs after a few days, it will be due to infection and may require further antibiotic treatment. Mannitol or frusemide may be given intravenously to reduce raised intracranial pressure.

The wound is inspected by the surgeon and if any blood or CSF has collected, he will aspirate it. The stitches are usually removed on the third day.

If the operation is in the frontal region, there will be some degree of swelling of the eyelids which can be reduced with cold compresses.

THE PITUITARY

The pituitary gland (no bigger than a pea) lies in a bony cavity at the base of the skull known as the sella turcica. The gland is connected to the hypothalamus by the pituitary stalk. It consists of two parts, the anterior lobe (or adenohypophysis) and the posterior lobe (the neurohypophysis). Although the two parts are closely related anatomically, they are functionally quite separate. The anterior pituitary controls the activity of the thyroid and adrenal glands, the gonads, growth and the production of milk. The posterior pituitary produces antidiuretic hormone, which controls urinary output, and oxytocin, which stimulates contraction of the voluntary muscles.

Tumours of the pituitary gland

These only arise in the anterior lobe and are called adenomas because they develop in glandular tissue. They are also named according to the particular cells in which they are found. The most common are the *chromophobe* adenomas which do not secrete but destroy the normal tissue. They may cause a loss of sexual activity and interference with water metabolism, i.e. polyuria. *Acidophil* adenomas produce disturbances of growth which in the child cause gigantism. In the adult there is an excessive growth of the bone and soft tissue, particularly of the face, hands and feet—acromegaly. *Basophil* adenomas cause a disturbance of metabolism—Cushing's syndrome—which in women leads to the development of virilism and in boys precocious puberty. An enlarging tumour will also cause the signs of raised intracranial pressure and may press on the optic chiasma causing visual disturbances.

Pituitary tumours may be removed (hypophysectomy), or radioactive yttrium or gold may be implanted via a cannula through the sphenoid sinus.

Hypophysectomy

Specific preoperative care The approach is either through the inner angle of the eye or through the nose. Prior to the operation, skull x-rays and tomograms will be taken to demonstrate the bony structures. If gross nasal infection is present, the operation will be postponed. Injections of cortisone and hydrocortisone are commenced the day before the operation and continued during and after it. A piece of muscle will be taken from the thigh during the operation to be used as a graft in the space left. An appropriate site on the leg must therefore be shaved. The nose is plugged with 10% cocaine and 1 in 1000 adrenaline. If the approach is via the orbit, the eyebrow may have to be shaved as well.

Specific postoperative care The patient will be cared for as for any intracranial operation. The blood pressure is taken quarter-hourly and must be very carefully watched. If the blood pressure falls and the pulse rises, the amount of hydrocortisone will have to be increased. The patient is therefore on an intravenous infusion to facilitate this. Antibiotics are continued for at least a week postoperatively. The fluid balance chart must be kept accurately as any increase in the urinary output may indicate diabetes insipidus and will require the administration of Pitressin tartrate by injection. Occasionally hypoglycaemia may arise due to the sudden reduction in the growth hormone. It must be recognised and treated promptly. A rise in temperature or other evidence of infection may indicate the development of meningitis, a rare complication. The stitches from the orbital incision are removed on the fifth day and those in the leg on the seventh day. The sphenoidal packing is removed after 9 days. Following removal of the packing there may be cerebrospinal rhinorrhoea, leaking of fluid via the nose. If it persists for longer than 48 hours, the surgeon usually returns the patient to theatre to replace the muscle graft, again packing it in position. This pack is left in for 7 to 10 days.

The patient will be discharged on cortisone and thyroxine, the dose carefully tailored to his needs. If polyuria has not subsided before discharge, he will require pitressin snuff as well. He should be advised to avoid stressful situations and infection and always to carry a steroid card on him.

SUGGESTED WORK

1. Compare the effects of a cerebral vascular accident with those of a brain tumour.
2. How much recovery is obtained following surgery for a brain tumour? Is any support required on discharge?

SUGGESTED READING

Bickerton J., Small J. (1981). *Neurology for Nurses.* London: Heinemann.

Eareckson J., Estes S. (1978). *A Step Further.* London: Pickering Inglis.

Hearn D. (1972). *Crash Tackle.* Arthur Barder.

* * *

Miss HELEN PRIOR (aged 58) has just bought a cottage in the country to which she intends to retire. After a weekend of gardening she suddenly became aware of a severe headache at the back of her head and started vomiting. She was admitted to hospital with a provisional diagnosis of subarachnoid haemorrhage which was confirmed by an arteriogram.

Medical plan
Clipping of the ruptured arteries under a general anaesthetic.

Identification of the patient's needs and problems on admission and action arising from these

Headache
Keep in a quiet darkened room, lying flat. Administer prescribed analgesics as required. Handle the patient gently when carrying out nursing procedures. Be sensitive to those things which irritate the patient and deal with them quickly. Record the presence of headaches and any change in their intensity.

Vomiting
Keep the vomit bowl emptied. Give Miss Prior a mouthwash after vomiting and wash her face. Remain with her while she is vomiting. Record the amount and type of vomit and report any increase. Administer prescribed antiemetics as required.

Neurological state
Monitor and record her blood pressure for any rise, and any associated fall in pulse rate. Check the level of consciousness half-hourly, recording this and reporting any deepening of unconsciousness. Check the size and reaction of the pupils. All the neurological observations should be done half-hourly until stable, and immediately before going to theatre.

Psychological
Ensure that Miss Prior knows that the nurses are easily available, putting the bell in her hand. Give her the opportunity to discuss the risks of having the operation and of not having it. Find out if she has any worries regarding the cottage or her work and arrange for the social worker to see her if necessary.

General hygiene
Bedbath her, being very gentle when moving her. Help her to clean her teeth. Attend to her pressure areas, particularly heels, elbows and sacrum; if she is not too hot, a sheepskin may be a useful preventative measure.

Nutrition
Once the vomiting is under control a light diet may be commenced. Initially she will require feeding,

but as she improves one pillow may be given, thus allowing her to feed herself. A plastic straw can be used for fluids, although she will probably prefer tea out of a cup. Fluids should be encouraged.

Excretion
A slipper bedpan may be used as this may be more comfortable if the patient is not allowed to sit up. Two nurses should lift her onto the bedpan. A bowel action will be avoided in the first few days, but once her condition begins to improve aperients will be necessary to prevent constipation.

Social
Arrange for the social worker to come and discuss where she will go on discharge and if there are any relatives or friends who will be available. If she wishes to make a will, arrange for a member of the administrative staff to come and see her.

Immediate specific preparation for the operation
Explain the need for shaving the head and reassure her that it will be kept covered until the hair has grown again. Shave the head and cover with a cotton tubular cap.

27

Injuries to Bones and Joints

The presence of a fracture always implies an emergency situation with disruption to the patient's normal life. Many of these fractures will only be met in the accident and emergency department. The nurse's role will therefore be to ensure that patients will be able to return home and that they understand any instructions that they have been given.

Specific emphasis in the nursing history

General appearance. Any abnormality in the position of the limbs, or shortening. The presence of shock.

Pain. Position and if related to movement. The presence of tenderness.

Skin. The presence of swelling or bruising and any alteration in sensation.

Mobility. Loss of movement in a limb or abnormal mobility.

Social. The availability of help. Problems of accommodation related to the disability.

FRACTURES

A fracture is a break in the continuity of a bone and is inevitably accompanied by damage to the surrounding tissue. The most common cause is sudden force applied to the bone. A direct force will result in a fracture at the point of impact, and usually results in a transverse or comminuted fracture. An indirect force may be of a twisting nature, causing an oblique or spiral fracture. Violent contraction of muscle may sometimes fracture the bone to which it is attached.

Types of fracture

Bones which are weakened through disease—tumours, cysts or infection in the bones, or more generalised diseases such as osteoporosis and Cushing's syndrome—or drugs are easily fractured. Prolonged use of steroids also leads to osteoporosis and pathological fractures, which are more common in the vertebrae, femur and humerus.

Greenstick fractures (Fig. 27.1) occur in children who still have a large amount of cartilage. They are usually incomplete, the bone bending or buckling. buckling.

Simple or closed fractures (Fig. 27.2) are those in which, although the bone is broken, there is no connection between it and the surface of the skin.

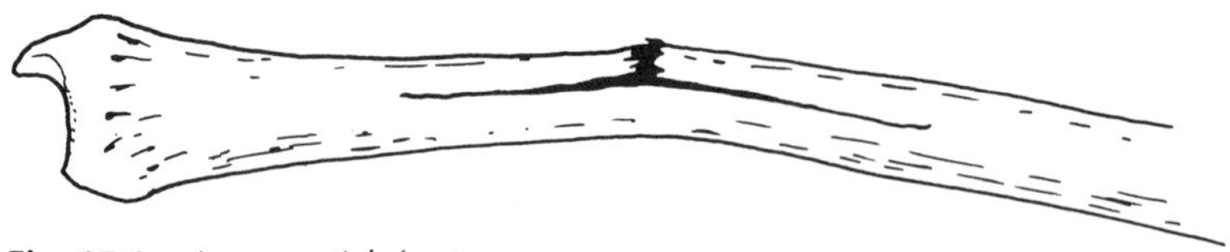

Fig. 27.1 *A greenstick fracture.*

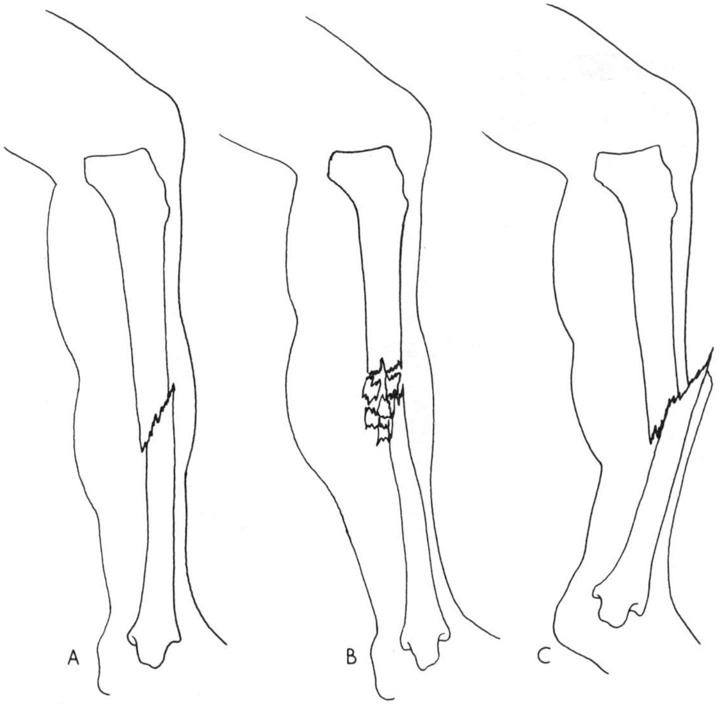

Fig. 27.2 *Types of fracture. (a) A simple fracture. (b) A comminuted fracture. (c) A compound or open fracture.*

Compound or open fractures communicate with an outside wound and therefore infection may be introduced.

Comminuted fractures are those in which the bone at the fracture site is broken into many fragments.

Complicated fractures involve important structures such as joints, blood vessels and nerves.

Impacted fractures occur when the bone ends are driven into one another.

Fatigue or stress fractures are caused by repeated stress such as prolonged marching and usually occur in the lower limbs.

Recognition of a fracture

Following a recent injury, the presence of localised pain, tenderness and deformity and later swelling and bruising suggests that a fracture is present. This is confirmed if there is a sensation of crepitus (grating of the bone ends), abnormal mobility or shortening of a limb. The diagnosis is confirmed by x-ray.

Repair of fractures

If the two broken ends of bone are held together and immobilised, healing takes place in the following way (Fig. 27.3). Bleeding from the broken ends forms a haematoma around the fracture site which gradually becomes organised and converted into fibrous tissue by the leucocytes and fibroblasts which remove the dead tissue and lay down the fibrous tissue. At the same time new blood vessels grow into this tissue from the adjacent capillaries. A provisional callus is formed as the cells of the periosteum, at the ends of the bones, increase forming a bony network which bridges the gap between the two bones. Osteoblasts are also laying down bone on the inside of the bone. Remodelling

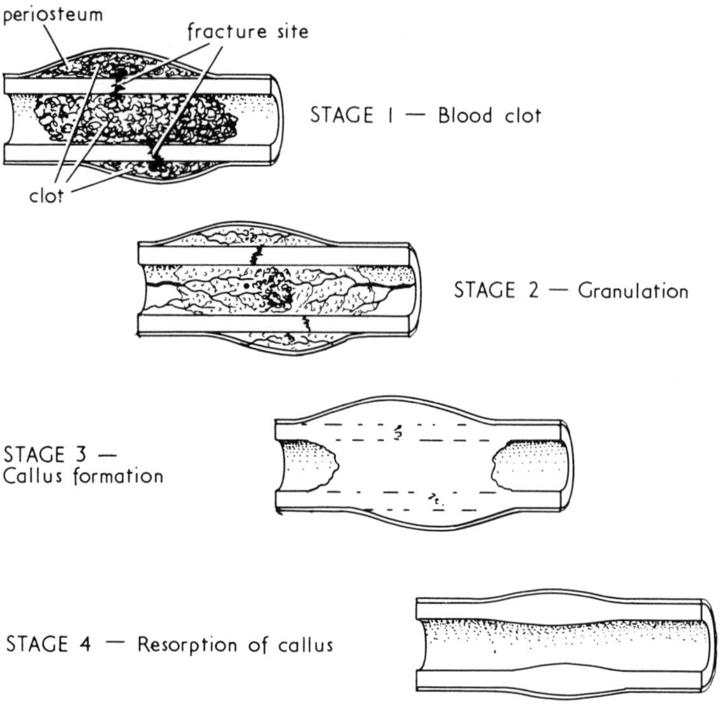

Fig. 27.3 *Repair of fractures.*

then takes place, in which excess callus is reabsorbed, the typical lamellar bone structure reformed, and the medullary canal refashioned. Eventually the bone is either completely or partially restored to its original state. This may take several months.

Complications arising from fractures

Although most fractures heal without problems, there are inevitably some which lead to complications either associated with the fracture itself or due to the associated injuries. There is usually a high degree of shock because of the considerable loss of blood into the tissue.

Nonunion or delayed union of the bones may arise as a result of a poor blood supply, infection, or if the bones are separated by soft tissue. A bone graft is used from some other part of the body to encourage healing.

In *malunion* the fracture unites in a deformed position and may result in shortening of a limb. Refracturing will be necessary if there is marked disability.

Infection is most likely to arise in compound fractures, although operative procedures may also be a cause despite every effort being made to avoid this. Infection of the bone is called osteomyelitis and results in persistent discharging sinuses (Fig. 27.4). Part of the bone dies, forming a sequestrum (dead bone) which acts as a foreign body. This needs to be removed surgically, the infected bone being drained and antibiotics given. Bone chips may be required if the condition becomes chronic. The patient is cared for as with any infection.

Avascular necrosis (due to death of the bone) occurs if the blood supply to the bone is cut off, which sometimes happens in a fractured neck of femur (Fig. 27.5). The part is removed and an arthroplasty or arthrodesis performed, depending on the site of the fracture.

Severing or crushing of blood vessels may occur, cutting off the blood supply to a part and so causing

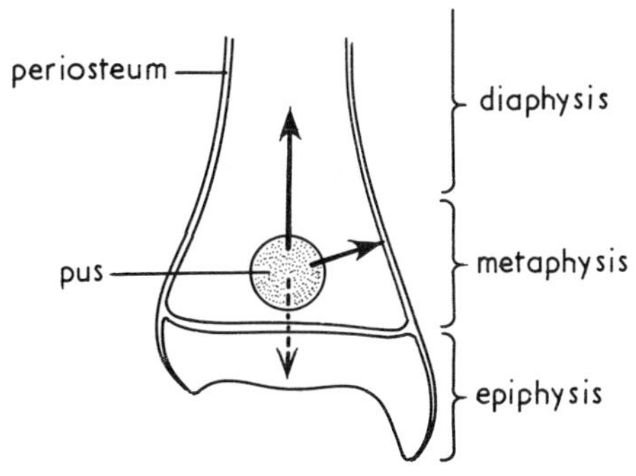

Fig. 27.4 *The spread of acute osteomyelitis.*

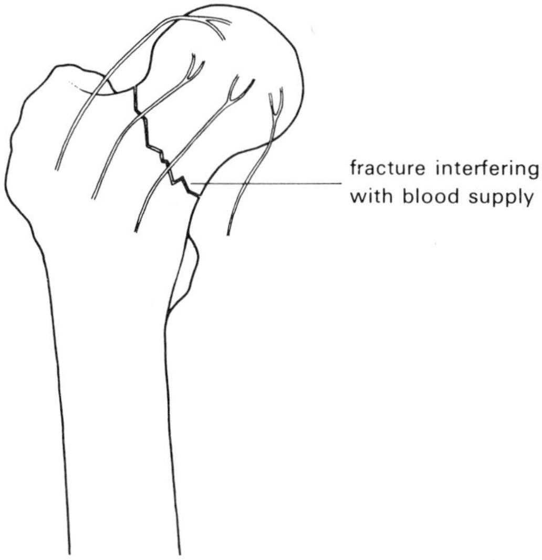

Fig. 27.5 *Blood supply to the head of the femur.*

gangrene. Emergency surgery is required if manipulation does not restore the circulation.

Damage to nerves may be temporary, but if the nerve cell itself has been damaged, paralysis will be permanent.

Damage to underlying organs may occur following fracture of the ribs or pelvis. Treatment of the resulting conditions may be more urgent than that of the original fracture.

Injury to joints, tendons and muscle will result in loss of power and function. Many years later osteoarthritis may develop.

Crush syndrome occurs if the tissues suffer a crush injury or a tourniquet is left on too long. The cells become damaged and so release their contents into the circulation. These substances block the kidney tubules and the patient suffers from acute renal failure, which may result in death.

Severe damage to a limb will cause it to swell, the fluid being lost from the general circulation. This results in the blood pressure falling and therefore the blood supply to the kidney being reduced. If the blood supply to the kidney is not restored quickly, this will also lead to death of the patient through renal failure.

Fat embolism. In severe injuries, especially of the femur and tibia, fat molecules may escape from the marrow of a broken bone into the general circulation (Fig. 27.6). These emboli will travel in the circulation until they are too big to pass along the blood capillaries, and will thus obstruct them. They may travel to the brain, lung or any other organ or part of the body. The effects will depend upon which vessels are obstructed.

If the embolus reaches the lungs, the patient will become dyspnoeic and cyanotic with chest pain. An embolism in the brain will cause mental confusion and loss of consciousness with a raised temperature. An embolism in the systemic circulation will lead to petechiae on the skin of the chest and shoulder.

Treatment is to ensure that the fracture is adequately immobilised and that the patient receives a high concentration of oxygen, by ventilator if necessary. Clofibrate is given to reduce the lipaemia and Trasylol to reduce pulmonary oedema and congestion. General nursing care is aimed at reducing the temperature.

Principles of treating fractures

In the first-aid situation, fractures may not require such urgent treatment as other injuries. The main aim, however, is to move them as little as possible in order to prevent further injury, therefore some type of splint is applied. Management of shock is of great importance.

In hospital the fracture is reduced by manipulation, usually under a general anaesthetic, and

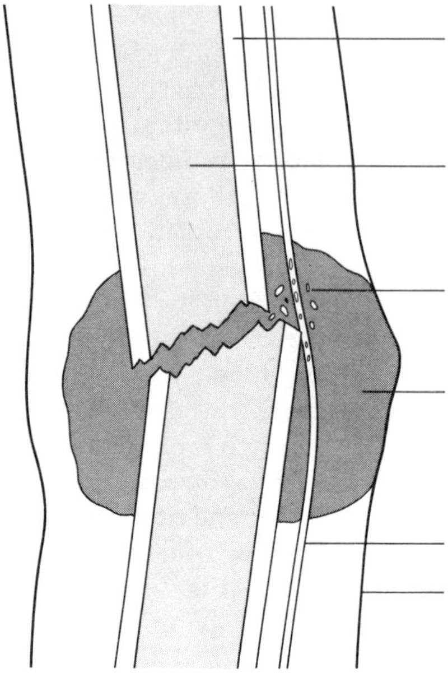

Fig. 27.6 *The release of a fat embolism.*

then held in position by some means. Open reduction is required for some fractures where direct vision of the bones is needed. Plaster of Paris, traction and internal fixation are the main methods of immobilisation. The age of the patient, the severity of the fracture, and involvement of other structures will influence the type of immobilisation used.

Plaster of Paris

This may be applied as a complete cast or in the form of slabs or gutters. The latter are used when a large amount of oedema is expected, when they are bandaged on with a cotton bandage.

Following the application of a plaster, the limb is kept elevated for 24 hours. If the patient is going home, a checklist of those things he needs to report to the doctor or hospital is either given to him or stuck on the plaster. If the patient remains in hospital, the nurse should check for any pain, which always requires attention to the plaster and not analgesia. Both limbs should be compared for temperature, the presence of pulses and any discoloration of the skin or nails. Loss of movement or numbness will also suggest interference with the nerve supply. The presence of any of these signs must be reported to the doctor immediately.

Hexcelite

This is a mesh-like plastic bandage which can be used instead of plaster of Paris. It is soaked in hot water and applied as a bandage, being moulded afterwards. It is particularly useful if the plaster will have to remain on for a long time. The padding and stockinette are of a man-made material which can be dried easily. Hexcelite is strong but light and allows free circulation. It is not damaged by water so the patient can bath, and generally it is comfortable.

Traction

This involves the application of a pulling force on the long axis of a limb in order to reduce a fracture and so prevent shortening. It will overcome muscle spasm and the overriding of the two ends of the bone, particularly where there are powerful muscles, as in the leg.

Fixed traction The cord from the strapping or pin is fixed to a splint on the limb in order to provide traction between two fixed points.

Balanced or sliding traction The cord is attached to a weight over a pulley on the bed. The foot of the bed is raised, thus allowing the patient's own body to exert counter-traction. The traction is therefore between two movable points.

Skin traction This may be used where a large weight is not required, as in the elderly or very young, or where temporary immobilisation is necessary prior to operation. Adhesive plaster or Ventfoam is applied to the leg and either fixed or balanced traction is used (Fig. 27.7). If the patient has this type of traction applied, it is important to check that the extension plaster has not slipped or become unstuck and that the patient has not developed an allergy to it. The skin is checked regularly for pressure over the ankles and Achilles tendon; the presence of foot drop is also noted. Exercises of the muscles are essential to prevent wasting.

A Gallow's traction is used in infants and small children (Fig. 27.8). Extension plaster is applied to both legs from above the knees, the knees being kept slightly flexed with plastic splints, and cords from the spreaders are fixed to a cross-bar above the bed in such a way that the legs are vertical and the buttocks lifted off the bed. The weight of the body supplies the counter force.

Skeletal traction In this type of traction a metal pin is inserted through a bone, such as the tibia for a fractured shaft of femur or the calcaneum for fractures of the tibia and fibula (Fig. 27.9). For a fractured shaft of femur a Steinmann or Denham pin or Kirschner wire (Fig. 27.10) is inserted in theatre. The leg is supported in a Thomas' or Fisk splint with a knee flexion attachment. The Thomas' splint is suspended from the overhead beam by cords and weights. A stirrup is attached to the pin and this has a cord passing from it over a pulley attached to the foot of the bed. At the end of the cord are weights to exert traction.

For some conditions of the hip a metal 'U' loop is attached to the pin so that the loop protrudes beyond the foot, a cord and weight going from the end of this over a pulley at the end of the bed. In both types of traction the foot of the bed is elevated to provide counter-traction. The feet must be checked for sensation, colour and movement. All weights must be hanging free. If a Thomas' splint is being used, the skin under the ring must be moved regularly to relieve pressure. The site of the pin and wire is checked for infection. Exercises are essential to prevent muscle wasting and foot drop.

Internal fixation of fractures

Many fractures are managed satisfactorily by manipulation and immobilisation in a plaster of Paris splint or by traction. However, in certain patients or particular types of injury the fracture is openly reduced and then fixed internally.

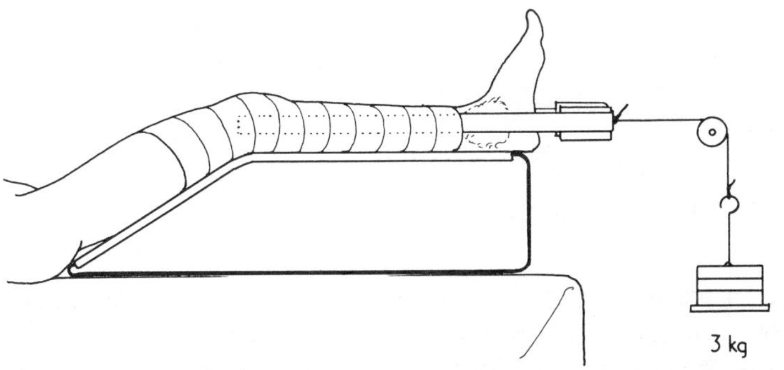

Fig. 27.7 *Skin traction.*

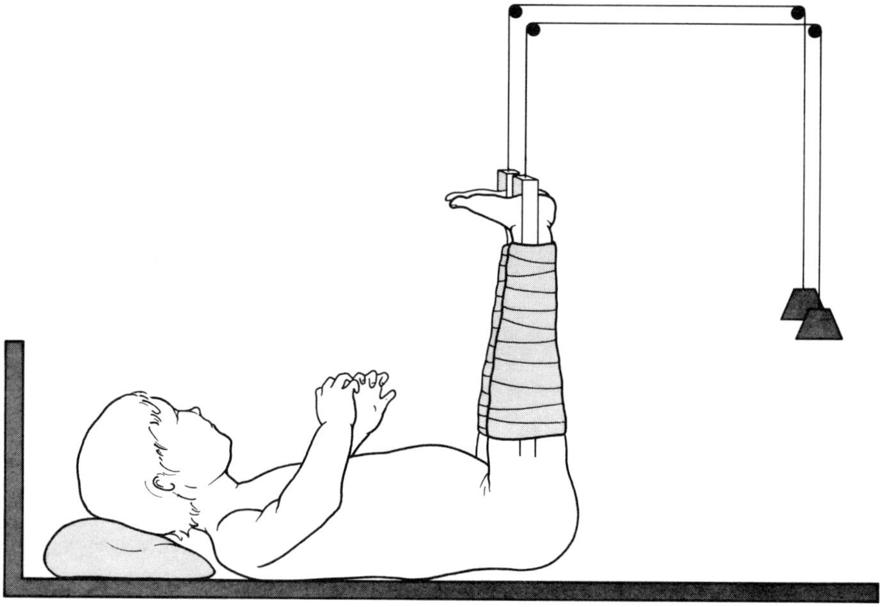

Fig. 27.8 *A Gallow's traction.*

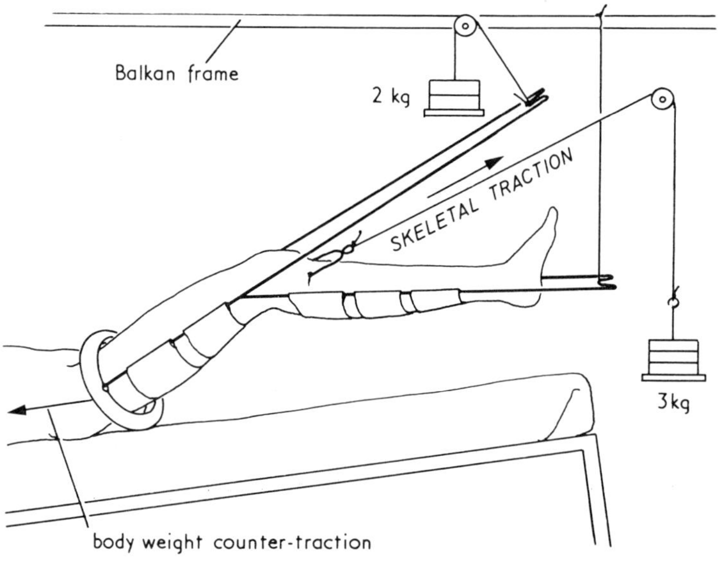

Fig. 27.9 *Skeletal traction.*

Elderly patients with a fracture of the femur usually have internal fixation to allow early mobilisation and to prevent the development of hypostatic pneumonia or deep vein thrombosis. In some fractures, such as those involving the elbow or knee joint, open reduction is essential to get a good result. Fractures in the radius and ulna are frequently unstable and therefore require internal

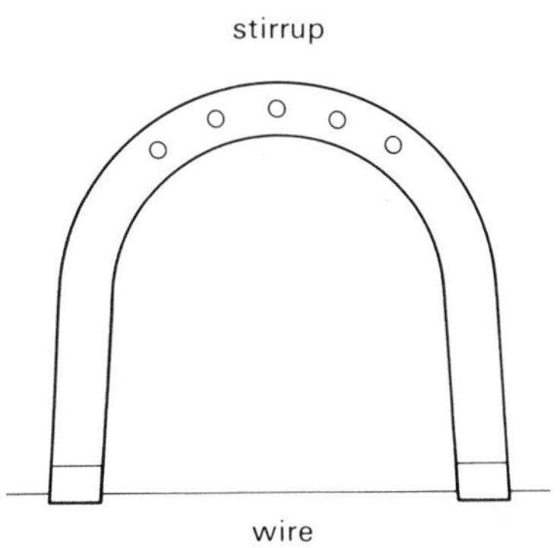

Fig. 27.10 *Kirschner wire and stirrup for skeletal traction.*

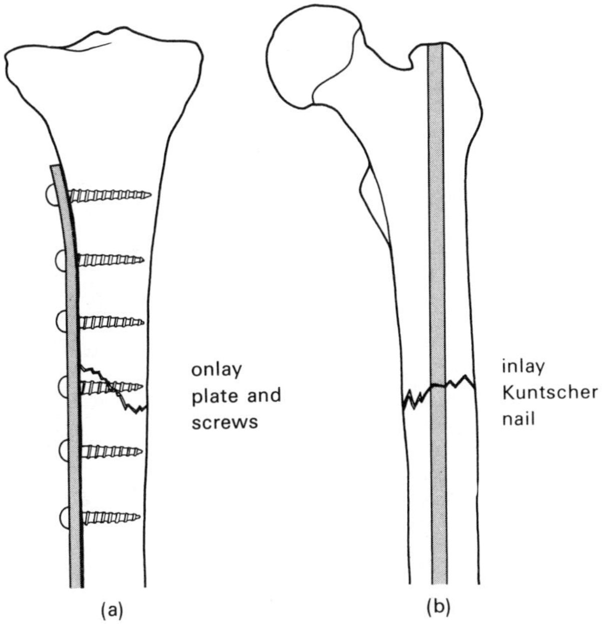

Fig. 27.11 *(a) Onlay (plate and screws). (b) Inlay (Kuntscher nail).*

fixation. If closed reduction cannot be done because muscle or soft tissue is between the fracture ends, or where there is injury to blood vessels or nerves, open reduction will be necessary. Multiple fractures and pathological fractures are other examples in which internal fixation is used.

Methods of internal fixation There are two types of internal fixation: inlay, in which nails, pins or screws are introduced into the bone; and onlay, which is achieved by plates on the surface of the bone or very occasionally wires around the bone (Fig. 27.11a).

Inlay fixation. Intramedullary nails (Kuntscher) may be used for fractures of the middle third of the femur or humerus and Muller's in the tibia (Fig. 27.11b). They are not used if the fracture is comminuted.

A guidewire is inserted first and the canal is then made bigger, after which the nail is inserted. In the femur it is inserted through the greater trochanter. A pin, such as the Smith–Peterson pin, is used to immobilise fractures of the neck of the femur. Again a guidewire is inserted first. The pin has a central hole which enables it to be inserted over the guidewire. It may be used alone or with a plate if more strength is required.

Screws may be used to keep small pieces of bone in position or to apply compression to a fracture. In the latter case the plate is secured to the shorter part of the bone with screws. The compression device (Fig. 27.12) is then secured to the longer part of bone and fixed with one screw. The hook of the compression device is then inserted into a small hole at the end of the plate, and the nut is then tightened to bring the two bone ends together.

Onlay fixation. Plates of stainless steel or vitallium are attached with screws on either side of the fracture for strength, or the plates may be used with pins. This method is used for fractures of the arm, tibia and fibula or the lower end of the femur.

External wires are very occasionally used to hold a fracture in place but they may interfere with the periosteum and therefore the blood supply to the bone, so causing necrosis of the bone.

DISLOCATIONS AND SUBLUXATIONS

A dislocation has occurred when the articular surfaces of the joint have been displaced to such an extent that there is no contact between them. In

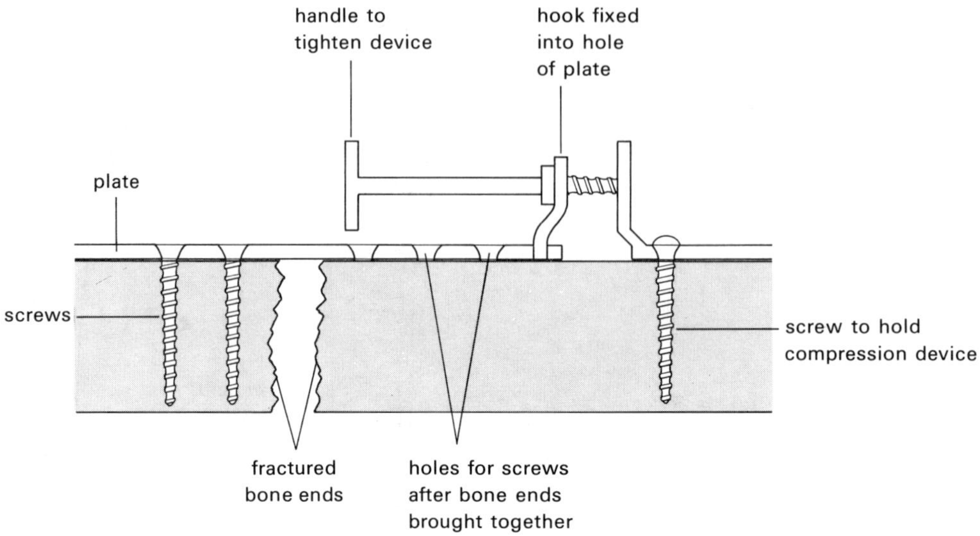

Fig. 27.12 *Compression device.*

subluxations there is some contact between the articular surfaces although displacement has occurred. If the articular surfaces are also fractured, this is called a fracture dislocation.

Dislocations are mainly traumatic, with tearing of the joint capsule and considerable damage to soft tissue. They may also occur because of disease or congenital abnormalities. In some joints, particularly the shoulder, the dislocation (originally due to severe violence) may recur following minor injuries. This is called recurrent or habitual dislocation.

The dislocation is reduced and the joint rested to allow the swelling and pain to subside, after which active movements are encouraged.

SUGGESTED WORK

1. Find out which fractures are dealt with in accident and emergency and then sent home and which require admission.
2. Which are the most common fractures seen in accident and emergency? Does the situation of your hospital influence this?

SUGGESTED READING

Crawford Adams J. (1978). *Outline of Fractures.* Edinburgh: Churchill Livingstone.
Hull Isaacs (1980). *Healing of Fractures. A Programmed Text.* Sheffield: National Health Service Learning Resource Unit.
McRae R. (1981). *Practical Fracture Treatment.* New York: Churchill Livingstone.
Stewart J. D. M., Hallett J. P. (1983). *Traction and Orthopaedic Appliances.* Edinburgh: Churchill Livingstone.
Understanding Traction (1967). London: Nursing Times.

* * *

PAUL WALLACE (aged 17) has been admitted as an emergency following a road traffic accident with a fractured shaft of femur. His girlfriend, Lorraine, has also been admitted with suspected head injuries. His parents have been informed by the police.

Medical plan
Skeletal traction using a Denham pin has been applied.

Identification of the patient's needs and problems and action arising from these

Pain
Administer prescribed analgesics as required. Inform the doctor when something milder would be more appropriate.

Traction
Check that weights are hanging free and that the pin is straight. Inspect the leg where the pin is inserted for any pus. If present, take a swab, clean aseptically and report.

Mobility
As Paul is confined to bed, a 'monkey pole' should be provided to enable him to lift himself regularly and to aid him getting on to bedpans. Encourage regular exercise of his good leg and static exercises of the affected leg. Arrange for the physiotherapist to teach him these. Exercise of his upper limbs is also important. Check the movement of the foot on the fractured side.

Hygiene
Enable the patient to wash as much as he is able, giving him help with his legs and back. Apply preventative measures to those pressure areas at risk, particularly the heel of his good leg and his elbows. Protect the bed and position his pillows so that he is able to clean his teeth. Check the skin on his fractured leg where it is vulnerable.

Nutrition
Check that he is being given sufficient to satisfy his appetite, and that he is eating a well-balanced diet and not a lot of biscuits or crisps. Advise him to avoid choosing heavy indigestible meals. Help to position him so that he can eat comfortably.

Elimination
Encourage Paul to drink plenty, emptying his urinal as required. When using a bedpan, help him to get into a comfortable position; a pillow in his back may give the support necessary. Encourage plenty of fruit and vegetables and fluids to prevent constipation. If it does occur, give him an aperient as prescribed.

Psychological
Keep Paul informed on the state of his girlfriend. Once she has recovered sufficiently, enable messages to be sent between the two. As soon as she is fit to visit him, arrange for her to be brought to the ward. Boredom will be Paul's main problem. Encourage his family and friends to bring in games and hobbies and to spend time talking and playing games with him. Place him next to another youngster if possible, perhaps on a balcony. He might have his own television brought in. Encourage him to do something constructive for the ward.

28

Injuries to the Upper Limbs and Chest

Injuries to the upper limb do not usually require the individual to be admitted to hospital unless they are associated with other injuries. The nurse will therefore be mainly responsible for ensuring that any instructions are clearly understood. If, however, she discovers that the patient could not manage at home, then an admission would have to be arranged.

Specific emphasis in the nursing history

General appearance. Observe for any evidence of shock such as pallor, weak rapid pulse, low blood pressure. Note any abnormality in the position of the limbs or alteration in the length.

Pain. Where is the pain? Is it increased by movement?

Skin. Note the presence of any swelling or bruising and whether the sensation of the extremities has been affected.

Mobility. Is the patient able to move the affected part normally?

Social. If the patient is likely to be returned home, is there anyone there to care for him if necessary?

Fractures of the clavicle

These commonly occur due to a fall on the outstretched hand. Reduction is not usually necessary, neither is it possible to immobilise the fracture. Although the subclavian vessels and brachial plexus are near the bone, they are rarely trapped. Healing is good although there is usually some permanent degree of irregularity in the bone.

The arm is rested in a collar and cuff and active exercises are started once the pain has been relieved. If for cosmetic reasons an overgrowth of the bone is to be avoided, the patient is nursed flat on his back, with a small pillow placed between the shoulders.

Dislocation and subluxation of the acromioclavicular joint

These injuries are common. In a subluxation the joint capsule is torn, but the ligaments holding the clavicle to the coracoid process of the scapula remain intact. In a dislocation the ligaments are also torn. The outer end of the clavicle becomes prominent and in a dislocation tenderness and bruising are present over the shoulder.

Dislocation and subluxation of the sternoclavicular joint

These are uncommon injuries and are due to a fall on the outstretched hand. A posterior dislocation is rare, but may involve the great vessels or trachea and may therefore lead to death.

These conditions are treated by reduction by manipulation and a sling or strapping. Surgery may be necessary to repair torn ligaments.

Fractures of the scapula

These are uncommon, and do not require reduction. A sling is worn and active exercises are encouraged early.

Dislocation of the shoulder joint

Dislocation of the shoulder is a very common injury, most frequently seen following severe trauma. Most commonly the dislocation is anterior, the head of the humerus being displaced forwards to lie below the coracoid process of the scapula. There is obvious deformity, severe pain and inability to move the shoulder in any direction. A posterior dislocation rarely occurs.

Treatment is by reduction under a general anaesthetic, either by Kocher's method in which the humerus is externally rotated, so causing it to return to the glenoid cavity, or by the Hippocratic method in which traction is applied in a downward and outward direction, the surgeon placing his stockinged foot in the axilla to provide counter-traction.

After reduction the limb is rested in a sling, and abduction and external rotation of the shoulder are restricted for 3 weeks, after which active movements are encouraged. Damage to the axillary nerve may arise as a result of the dislocation or efforts to reduce it. This will cause deltoid paralysis which usually recovers spontaneously. Recurrent dislocation may occur after a very severe injury or repeated injuries and will require surgery to repair the torn ligament.

Fracture of the neck of the humerus

Fracture of the neck of the humerus most commonly occurs in the elderly as a result of a fall on the arm. Many of these are impacted fractures and therefore do not require immobilisation. The emphasis is on exercises to restore as much movement as possible to the arm. If the fracture is not impacted, immobilisation with a bandage will be necessary until the pain has subsided, after which intensive exercise will begin.

A similar fracture occurs in children about the age of 12 following a fall from a height in which there is fracture separation of the upper humeral epiphysis. The treatment is the same as for the older patient.

Fracture of the shaft of the humerus

This is a very common injury, transverse fractures being caused by direct injury, and spiral fractures by a fall on the outstretched hand. Reduction is not usually necessary. A collar-and-cuff sling is applied with the arm flexed and the elbow hanging freely. Alternatively, a shaped plaster of Paris slab is applied to the upper arm from the axilla down the inner side of the arm, under the elbow and up the outer side to finish on top of the shoulder. This is kept on for 6 to 8 weeks. In either case the unsupported weight of the arm provides the traction required. Internal fixation may be necessary in some cases. Occasionally the radial nerve which winds round the humerus is damaged, causing 'wrist drop' (Figs. 28.1 and 28.2). This usually recovers spontaneously.

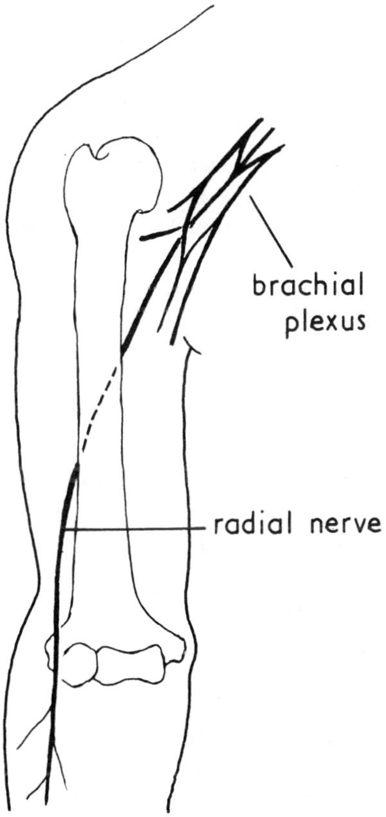

Fig. 28.1 *The position of the radial nerve.*

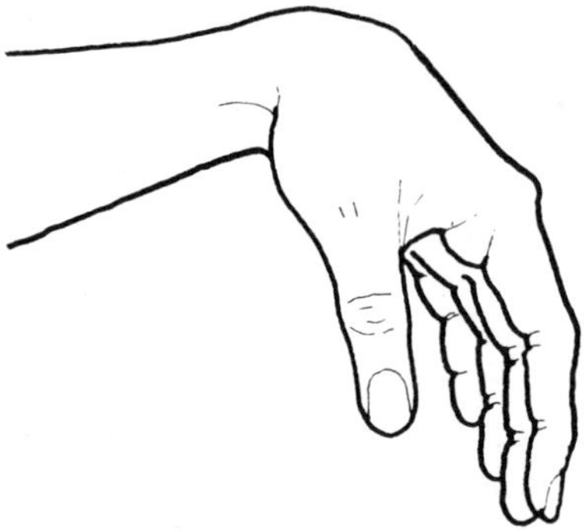

Fig. 28.2 *Wrist drop due to a damaged radial nerve.*

Supracondylar fracture of the humerus

This fracture is most commonly found in children and arises due to a fall on the outstretched hand. It may cause injury to the brachial artery, so damaging the muscles of the forearm with fibrosis and shortening, the wrist and fingers being held in flexion (Volkmann's ischaemic contraction). In severe cases the hand may become gangrenous.

The fracture is reduced and immobilised in a plaster with a window at the wrist to check the radial pulse. The temperature and colour of the limb are carefully noted. For some patients a collar-and-cuff bandage may be all that is required.

Dislocation of the elbow

This is another common injury arising due to a fall on the outstretched hand. The ulna and radius are displaced backwards and outwards in relation to the humerus. It may be associated with fractures of the arm. The injury is reduced by manipulation and rested in a collar-and-cuff sling for 3 weeks, after which active exercises are commenced.

Fracture of the olecranon

A transverse fracture of the olecranon with separation of a fragment will occur if the elbow is violently flexed when falling on the hand. The fragment requires internal fixation with a nail, lag screw or wiring. A plaster of Paris is then applied from the axilla to the wrist with the arm flexed at the elbow. Comminuted fractures which are often compound are caused by a direct blow. If the patient is still able to extend the arm, a sling or plaster is applied and active exercises commenced. If the tendon has been torn, it is reattached to the ulna, the fragments of the bone being removed.

Fracture of the radius

In adults, fracture of the head of the radius arises as a result of a fall on the hand causing the head of the radius to be driven against the condyle of the humerus, resulting in a vertical split (Fig. 28.3). If there is little displacement, a collar-and-cuff sling is applied and elbow flexion increased daily as the swelling subsides. After 10 days active movements are encouraged. If there is gross displacement or comminution, the head of the radius is removed.

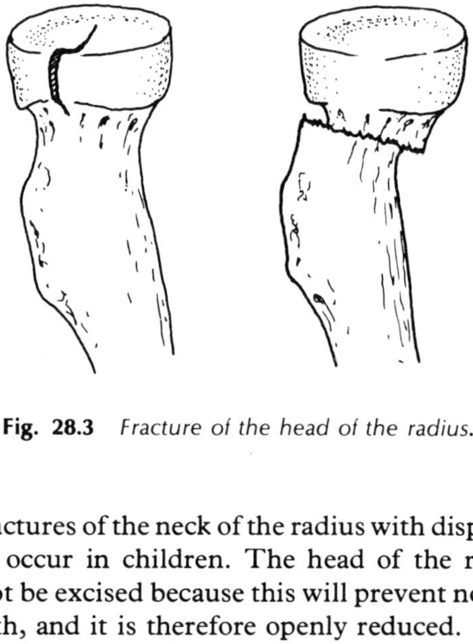

Fig. 28.3 *Fracture of the head of the radius.*

Fractures of the neck of the radius with displacement occur in children. The head of the radius cannot be excised because this will prevent normal growth, and it is therefore openly reduced.

Fractures of the shaft of the radius are treated by open reduction and a plate or an intramedullary nail.

Fractures of both radius and ulna shafts are reduced by manipulation, after which a plaster is applied from the axilla to the hand over padding to allow for swelling. A band of plaster across the palm between the thumb and index finger prevents rotation. The fingers are left free to allow movement. The plaster remains on for 6 weeks in children and 10 to 12 weeks in adults. It is sometimes necessary in adults to use metal plates or an intramedullary nail.

Colles fracture

This is a fracture of the lower end of the radius, usually associated with a fracture of the styloid process of the ulna (Fig. 28.4). The displacement is characteristically described as a 'dinner fork deformity'. It is caused by a fall on the outstretched hand.

The fracture is reduced by manipulation under a general anaesthetic (Fig. 28.5). Initially a plaster slab is applied and secured by a cotton bandage to allow the swelling to subside. The arm is then supported in a sling. The following day a full below-elbow plaster is applied which remains on for 5 to 6 weeks. The patient is encouraged to move his fingers, elbow and shoulder. On removal of the plaster further exercises are necessary to strengthen the muscles.

Fracture of the ulna

This injury is associated with a dislocation of the head of the radius. The fracture is reduced by manipulation under a general anaesthetic and a plaster applied from the axilla to the hand which is retained for 6 weeks.

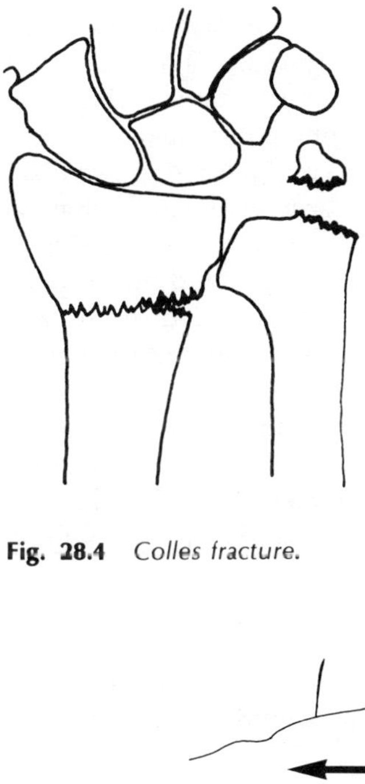

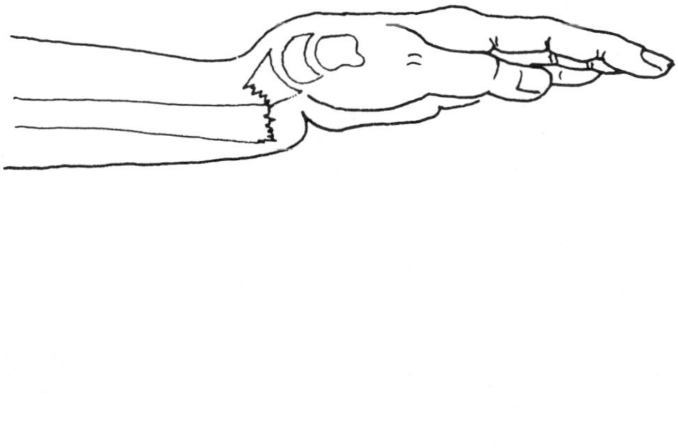

Fig. 28.4 *Colles fracture.*

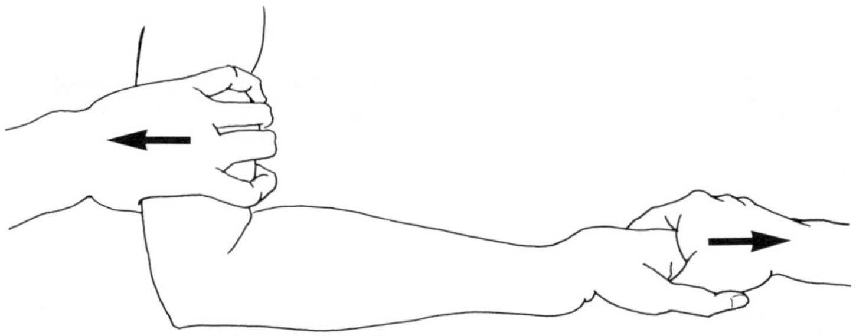

Fig. 28.5 *Manipulation of a Colles fracture.*

Fractures and dislocations in the hand

The commonest of these is a fracture of the scaphoid bone, which occurs after a heavy fall on the hand in which the wrist is forcibly bent back. Treatment is by immobilisation in a below-elbow plaster which includes the thumb joint. This is kept on for 10 to 12 weeks.

Dislocation of the lunate

This injury usually compresses the median nerve affecting sensation in the thumb, index and middle finger. It must therefore be reduced promptly by manipulation or, if necessary, open reduction.

Bennett's fracture

This is a fracture–dislocation of the joint between the first metacarpal and the trapezium (Fig. 28.6).

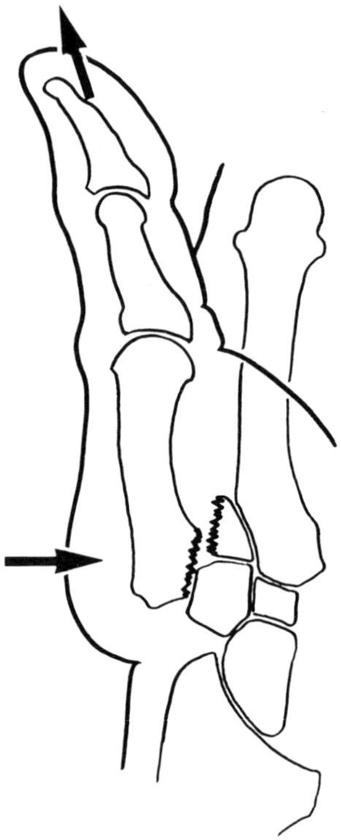

Fig. 28.6 *Bennett's fracture of the thumb. (The arrows show the forces necessary to reduce it.)*

Reduction is usually easy but retention in plaster difficult.

Fractures of the phalanges

These are accurately reduced and splinted in a position of semi-flexion. They are not immobilised for longer than is necessary. If a haematoma forms under the nail, the latter has to be perforated to release the blood and relieve the pain. In some fractures an intramedullary wire is required for internal fixation.

Fractures of the ribs

Indirect violence, such as a crushing injury to the chest wall, will cause several ribs to fracture but the lung is not usually penetrated. A direct blow to the chest wall will cause a fracture of the rib which receives the impact. Occasionally severe coughing will also cause a fracture. These types of fracture are much more likely to damage the pleura and the lung, causing a pneumothorax.

If several ribs are fractured in two places (stove-in chest), a flail chest will result so that paradoxical respiration will occur in which this section is sucked in on inspiration and blown out on expiration. Treatment will be centred on maintaining respiration with either an endotracheal tube or a tracheostomy being used to maintain adequate ventilation of the lungs, and occasionally a respirator. Drainage of the pneumothorax may be necessary with an underwater seal drain. If necessary, the ribs may be wired. The patient will rest in bed.

Fractures of the sternum

These are rare and follow a blow on the chest. They are associated with multiple injuries of the chest wall and spine.

SUGGESTED WORK

1. Find out from a patient who has had a Colles fracture what difficulties she found in trying to manage at home.

SUGGESTED READING

Roaf F., Hodkinson L. J. (1980). *Textbook of Orthopaedic Nursing*. London: Blackwell Scientific.

* * *

Mrs IRENE LONG (aged 76) is a widow living on her own in a third-floor flat. Her relatives are in Australia and her only companion is her cat. While shopping she slipped and fell, sustaining a Colles fracture.

Medical plan
Reduction and manipulation under a general anaesthetic. Plaster slab until the swelling has subsided, then a full below-elbow plaster for 5–6 weeks.

Identification of the patient's needs and problems and action arising from these

Social
Admit Mrs Long overnight. Inform the social worker about the cat and request her to investigate whether Mrs Long would be able to manage on discharge. She will need to arrange for someone to keep an eye on Mrs Long for the 6 weeks, and for her shopping to be collected. A home help or meals on wheels may be arranged. A neighbour may be able to give some assistance. She may require the district nurse to help her have a bath.

Psychological
Explain the arrangements which have been made for her cat. Reassure her that once her plaster is taken off she will be restored to her full independence, but that accepting help now may prevent accidents which could prolong her dependence on others.

Care of the arm
Support the arm in a sling. Observe for abnormal pain and altered sensation, swelling and colour in the fingers. (Other structures may have been affected.)

Pain
Administer prescribed analgesics as required. Night sedation may also be necessary.

Effects of the general anaesthetic
Give all the general care required following anaesthesia. Particularly observe for any confusion.

Hygiene
Give the patient aid with washing and cleaning her teeth.

Preparation for transfer home
Contact the social worker to ensure that Mrs Long can manage at home and that there is a supply of food. Arrange transport for the patient to go home after her lunch. Arrange an OPD appointment with transport. Explain to the patient the need to exercise her fingers, elbow and shoulder.

29

Injuries to the Lower Limbs and Pelvis

As with any other fracture, injuries in these areas constitute an emergency situation with all that implies for the patient in the disruption of his normal life. A large proportion of these patients will be elderly and female, and emphasis will be on early mobilisation. The nurse will therefore have to enable the patient to be as independent as possible but at the same time to guard against further accidents. Another significant group of patients are the young men who enter hospital after road traffic accidents. They will require different skills in order to prevent them from becoming bored and frustrated with their long stay in hospital. Co-operation with the physiotherapist will be a major part of the nurse's care for the patient.

Specific emphasis in the nursing history

General appearance. Observe for any evidence of shock such as pallor, weak rapid pulse, low blood pressure. Note any abnormality in the position of the limbs or alteration in the length.

Pain. Where is the pain? Is it increased by movement?

Skin. Note the presence of any swelling or bruising and whether the sensation of the extremities has been affected.

Mobility. Is the patient able to move the affected part normally?

Social. If the patient is likely to be returned home, is there anyone there to care for him if necessary?

FRACTURES OF THE FEMUR

The upper end of the femur can be divided into the head, neck and trochanteric areas, and fractures at each of these sites present different problems.

Fracture of the neck of the femur (subcapital)

The neck of the femur is the narrow wedge of bone joining the head to the trochanteric region. As the individual ages so osteoporotic changes take place in the bone and a minor fall may fracture the neck of the femur or the trochanteric area. The main blood supply to the head is via blood vessels from the nutrient artery and passing up the neck of the femur. If these are damaged, as happens in a fractured neck of femur, the blood supply from the ligament and capsular blood vessels may be insufficient and the area will die—avascular necrosis—a process which can take many months to occur. If there is no danger of this occurring, a Smith–Peterson nail or nail and plate will be used to immobilise the fracture. If there is a likelihood of avascular necrosis, the femoral head will be removed and a prosthesis inserted—arthroplasty (Fig. 29.1).

Arthroplasty

Replacement of the femoral head is also required for patients with osteoarthritis and rheumatoid arthritis if the hip joint is very painful. In this case a

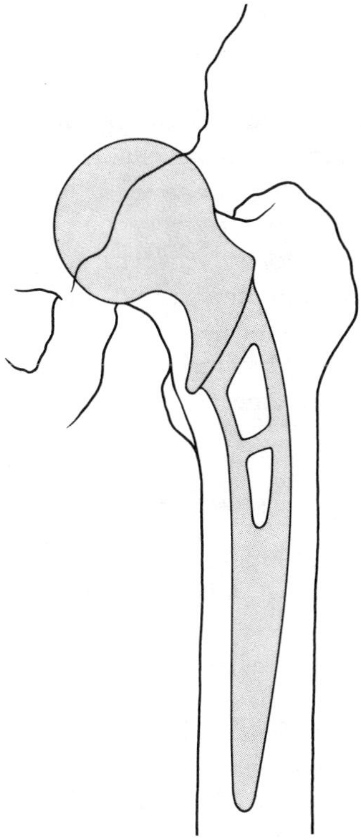

Fig. 29.1 *Replacement of the head of the femur with an Austin Moore hip prosthesis for avascular necrosis.*

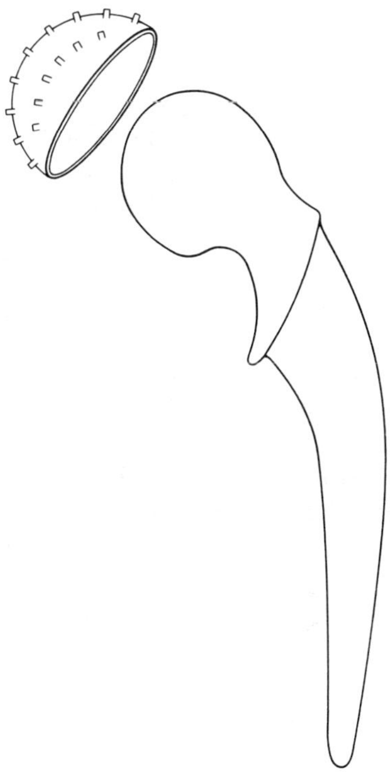

Fig. 29.2 *McKee Farrer total hip replacement.*

total hip replacement will be required in which a metal cup is inserted into the acetabulum following removal of the articular cartilage (Fig. 29.2). The cavity is deepened with a reamer, and holes may be drilled to provide a key for the cement. The head of the femur is excised and a cavity is reamed to fit the stem of the prosthesis. If cement is used, this is then introduced into the cavity and the prosthesis placed in position and held until the cement is set. The prostheses are made of stainless steel, vitallium, titanium or polypropylene, but only one metal is used in each case, they are never combined as they will react with one another.

Trochanteric fracture

This is treated with a nail and plate. The nail passes up the centre of the femoral neck and the plate is attached to the outer aspect of the femur (Fig. 29.3).

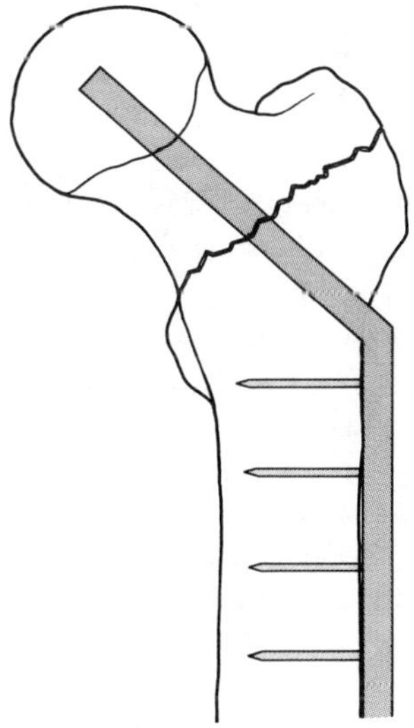

Fig. 29.3 *Fracture of the trochanter fixed with a nail and plate.*

Specific care of a patient undergoing an arthroplasty or nail and plate of the neck of the femur

The fracture may be immobilised with Ventfoam traction and 5-pound (2.2-kg) weights until the next day. Preoperatively the correct side is marked and the trochanteric area shaved. The pelvis is x-rayed for other injuries.

Postoperatively following an arthroplasty the patient may return with a plaster of Paris cylinder or traction to prevent hip and knee flexion. This remains on for about 4 days. On arrival back to the ward the patient will be nursed with one or two pillows for 24 hours. An abduction pillow is positioned to prevent the leg internally rotating, and vacuum drainage tubes will be in position for the first 48 hours. The operated leg is placed on a pillow and the foot must be checked for sensation and movement, especially dorsiflexion. The patient should not be rolled onto the operated side. The aim is early mobilisation to prevent pressure sores, retention of urine and deep vein thrombosis. Antibiotics are given to prevent infection.

Although some surgeons may keep the patient in bed for up to 6 days postoperatively, the majority get them up on the first postoperative day to stand and later in the day to walk, partial weight bearing being effected with crutches and a frame. Straight leg raising is avoided, as is crossing of the legs. By the fourth or fifth day the patient can sit out in a high chair but the leg must not be put on a stool. A pillow may be placed between the legs to maintain abduction. By the eighth day the patient may have progressed to walking sticks and managing the stairs, initially one step at a time. Eventually straight leg raising and quadriceps exercises can be started but the patient should still not put the leg on a stool when sitting, or cross the legs. Patients are usually discharged after 2 or 3 weeks, continuing physiotherapy as out-patients. The prosthesis lasts from 10 to 20 years. If it is rejected, it has to be removed and a girdlestone operation carried out.

Excision arthroplasty (girdlestone operation, pseudoarthrosis)

This operation is used if an arthroplasty is not successful. The head and neck of the femur and upper edge of the acetabulum are excised, and muscle and soft tissue are then brought between the shaft of the femur and the pelvis. This allows some movement, and removes the pain, but the limb is shortened and less stable than before.

Specific care Postoperatively the patient is put on skeletal traction for 4 to 6 weeks. All movements of the hip, knee and foot are encouraged including quadriceps exercises. The patient is gradually mobilised when the traction is removed and may require a raised shoe.

Fracture of the shaft of the femur

These fractures are usually the result of a road traffic accident in which there has been considerable force, unless it is a pathological fracture. The patient is very shocked and will need attention before being taken to theatre. In the young male patient with powerful muscles, a Steinmann or Denham pin is inserted into the upper part of the tibia and traction applied, using 15 to 20 pounds (7–9 kg). In the elderly, who need to be mobilised as quickly as possible, a Kuntscher intramedullary nail is used. In children skin traction using weights up to 10 pounds (4.5 kg) is used. A specific type of gallows skin traction is used for the young child. The care of a patient on traction has been dealt with in Chapter 27.

The specific care of a patient following insertion of an intramedullary nail

As early as possible, a blood transfusion will have been commenced to combat blood loss and shock. Postoperatively traction may be applied or sandbags to immobilise the leg and prevent external rotation. Vacuum drains will be in position for 48 hours. While the patient is on traction, contraction exercises of the quadriceps and gluteal muscles are carried out. The first day postoperatively the patient can sit up in bed and, if his general condition is satisfactory, the intravenous infusion is removed. He is usually allowed to start walking, but not fully weight bearing until after 2 or 3 weeks.

Dislocation of the hip joint

This injury is the result of considerable violence such as may occur in a road traffic accident where there has been a head-on collision. The dislocation is reduced by manipulation under a general anaesthetic and traction is applied for 6 weeks. Active movements are commenced as soon as possible. There is a danger that the blood supply to the head of the femur will be cut off and so cause an avascular necrosis, and if this happens, it will have to be removed and an arthroplasty done. The other particular complication which may arise is damage to the sciatic nerve, and any pressure must be relieved promptly.

INJURIES TO THE PELVIS

Isolated fractures of the pelvis involving the pubic or ischial rami, or the wing of the ilium, do not require special treatment. The patient is kept in bed for 2 to 3 weeks and active exercises are encouraged. Analgesics are given as required. Internal organs are not usually involved.

Fractures interfering with the stability of the pelvic ring

In these injuries there is fracture or dislocation at two points. There is likely to be damage to internal organs if there has been much displacement of the bone. If there is not much displacement of the bones, the patient is nursed in bed for 4 to 6 weeks to allow the bone to unite. If there is much displacement, it will be corrected by manipulation and immobilised by nursing the patient in a pelvic sling. Rupture of the bladder or urethra will also need attention.

INJURIES TO THE KNEE

In the knee joint there are two semilunar cartilages or menisci. On the inner side is the medial cartilage and on the outer side the lateral cartilage. They are 'C' shaped and attached to the surface of the tibia by ligaments (Fig. 29.4).

Injuries to the cartilages of the knee typically occur in a football player when he turns with his foot fixed on the ground and his knee bent. There is

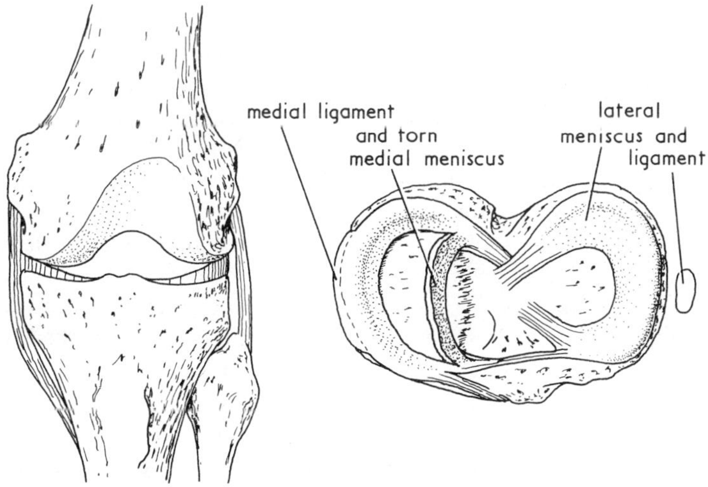

Fig. 29.4 *Injury to the semilunar cartilages.*

pain and within a few hours the joint swells. The pain subsides in 10 to 14 days. Following this injury the joint is weak and gives way under the individual. In a bucket-handle tear the cartilage becomes displaced and trapped in the joint, so locking it by preventing full extension. On examination the doctor will find wasting of the quadriceps and tenderness over the joint. The medial cartilage is more commonly affected than the lateral. As the cartilage will not heal it is removed (meniscectomy).

Specific care

An arthroscope may be used under a general anaesthetic to look at the interior of the knee joint. The patient is taught the quadriceps exercises he will be expected to carry out postoperatively. To prevent infection a povidine compress may be applied to the knee. In theatre an Esmarch's rubber bandage is applied to the leg and a pneumatic tourniquet high up around the thigh to create a bloodless field.

Postoperatively either a plaster of Paris cylinder or a Robert Jones bandage will have been applied to prevent bleeding following the removal of the tourniquet. The latter consists of a domestic bandage applied firmly over a layer of wool, on top of which another bandage is applied over a second layer of wool. The bandage is applied from the ankle to the upper thigh. The joint must be rested for the first few days postoperatively to allow the synovial effusion to subside. If severe pain, pyrexia and swelling of the foot occur, there is bleeding into the joint, and this will have to be aspirated and the joint rested. The foot of the bed and the leg are elevated to reduce any swelling or bleeding. Any complaint of pins and needles suggests that the bandage is pressing on the popliteal nerve and it needs to be released. Once the patient is conscious, foot and quadriceps exercises are started to prevent permanent weakness of the joint. To do these the patient is asked to tighten the muscle and maintain this for a count of 10 and then to relax for a count of 10. He should continue to do these exercises for 10 minutes in every hour. The patient will also be asked to lift the straight leg off the bed. A weight may be placed on the foot to develop the muscles, and this is continued for 10 days. If the patient has a plaster of Paris on, it is removed on the tenth day, after which he may bend his knee and walk with sticks. He will continue to have daily physiotherapy, practising on the stairs, and can return to work within a month and to football in 2 to 3 months.

The cruciate ligaments are two strong ligaments holding the femur and tibia together. Injury occurs as a result of considerable force in which the knee is hyperextended (Fig. 29.5). The joint is very painful, unstable and by the following day has become swollen. Treatment is frequently conservative, the knee being immobilised in a plaster cylinder for 6 weeks; intensive quadriceps exercises are done to strengthen the muscles. Some surgeons suture the ligament and then apply a plaster cylinder for 6 weeks.

Fracture of the patella

The patella is a sesamoid bone which is formed in the tendon of the quadriceps muscle and is part of the knee joint. Fractures of it cause bleeding into the joint.

Fractures of the patella are of two main types. *Transverse* fractures, which may or may not be displaced, are due to the sudden flexion of the knee combined with a violent contraction of the quadriceps muscle (Fig. 29.6). This may happen if an individual tries to stop a fall backward. *Comminuted* fractures are those in which the patella is separated into fragments and are due to a direct blow. Movement of the knee joint is painful and the patient cannot hold it in full extension. If the joint is full of blood (haemarthrosis), it will be swollen, and aspiration will be necessary.

In either type of fracture if there is no displacement, a plaster cylinder is applied with the knee in extension. In a displaced transverse fracture internal fixation with screws or wires will be necessary before applying the plaster cylinder. Sometimes a patellectomy is necessary, and this is always the case for displaced comminuted fractures. The care of this patient is similar to that of a patient with a meniscectomy.

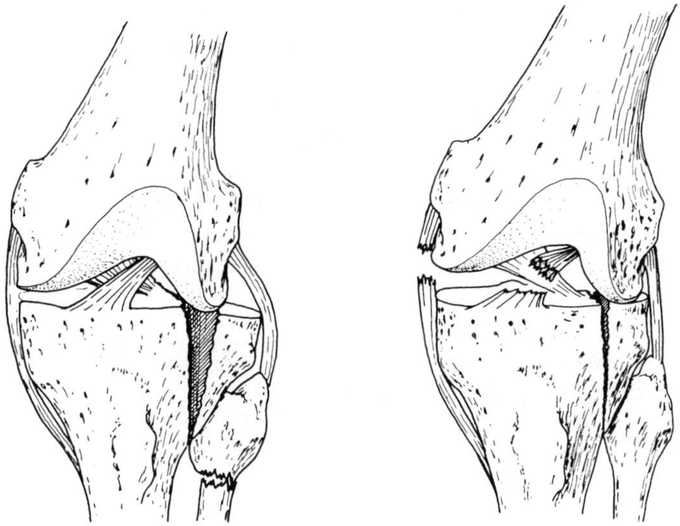

Fig. 29.5 *Damage to the cruciate ligaments.*

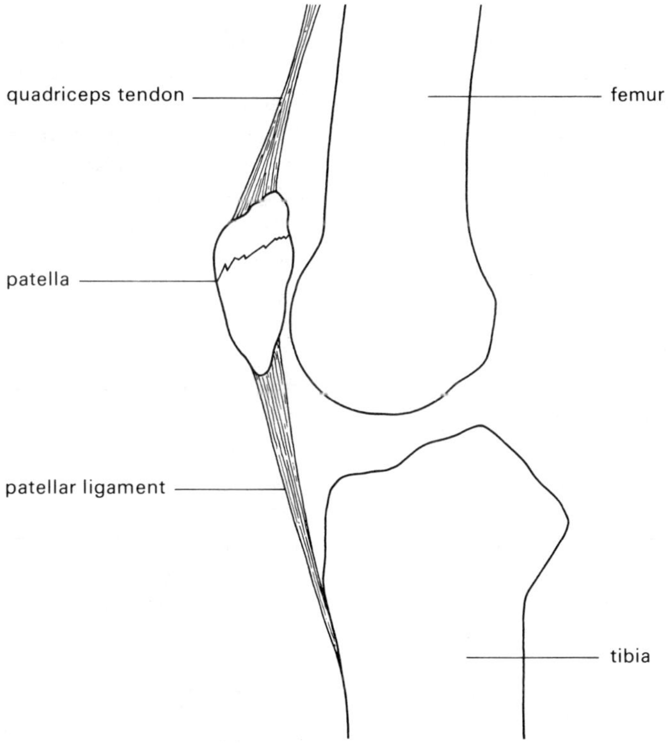

Fig. 29.6 *Transverse fracture of the patella.*

FRACTURES OF THE TIBIA AND FIBULA

These are very common and are frequently compound, which may interfere with the healing process. They also take some time to heal, even if not infected. Stable transverse fractures are reduced by manipulation and traction and then immobilised in an above-knee plaster with the knee in slight flexion. Internal fixation is required if the fracture is an unstable one, and this will be done with a metal plate and screws or an intramedullary nail. In some patients a Steinmann pin is passed through the calcaneum and traction is applied for 3 weeks, after which a plaster of Paris cylinder is applied. It will take at least 12 weeks before healing will take place so the splinting must remain on for at least this length of time. Even then, full weight bearing may not be safe.

POTT'S FRACTURE–DISLOCATIONS OF THE ANKLE

This is a term given to all fracture–dislocations of the ankle joint (Fig. 29.7). The commonest type is due to an external rotation and abduction force causing a spiral fracture of the external malleolus, and either a transverse fracture of the internal malleolus or a rupture of the internal lateral ligament. The talus and foot may be displaced outwards and backwards.

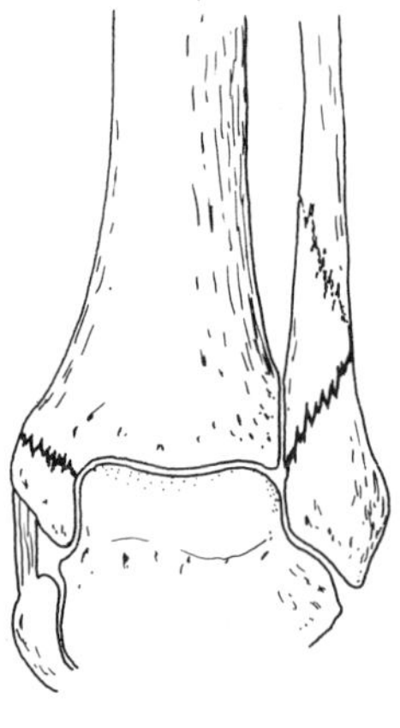

Fig. 29.7 *Pott's fracture.*

The fracture is reduced by manipulation under a general anaesthetic and a plaster applied from below the knee to the beginning of the toes which remains on for 4 to 6 weeks—10 weeks if there is displacement of the bones. Internal fixation will be used in the form of screws if the fracture is unstable. Following removal of the plaster, exercises will be encouraged to restore movement, and if oedema is a problem, an elastic sock can be worn.

FRACTURE OF THE CALCANEUM

This most frequently arises from a fall from a height and is therefore associated with other injuries, particularly of the spine. Even after treatment the pain persists for a considerable time. The patient remains in bed with the foot elevated to reduce swelling. Initially a pressure bandage may be applied. Once the swelling has subsided, the patient is mobilised, although not weight bearing.

FRACTURE OF THE TALUS

Fracture of the neck of the talus or dislocation of the bone occurs in injuries in which there is forced dorsiflexion. These fractures are reduced under anaesthetic, using a Kirschner wire if the fracture is unstable. A below-knee plaster is used to immobilise the fracture for 12 weeks, but weight bearing is avoided.

METATARSALS AND PHALANGES

The metatarsals may suffer a stress fracture in prolonged marching, otherwise crushing injuries are the most common. A plaster is only required if there is severe pain. Damage to soft tissue is the most serious problem in fractures of these bones and of the phalanges.

SUGGESTED WORK

1. Compare the specific nursing care given in your hospital for an internal fixation of fractured

neck of femur with that described in this chapter. Does it vary significantly? If so, what are the advantages?

2. Discuss with a patient who has had an arthroplasty what problems arose postoperatively and whether these were dealt with adequately.

SUGGESTED READING

Roaf F., Hodkinson L. J. (1980). *Textbook of Orthopaedic Nursing*. London: Blackwell Scientific.

* * *

Mrs JANE BROWN (aged 72) is a widow of 2 years. Her elder son lives 40 miles away from her and has a family of three teenagers. Her younger son has emigrated. She lives in an old house which is rented, amongst very friendly neighbours. The pain in her left hip has become progressively worse when she walks but is eased after rest. She is slightly overweight, due to an unsatisfactory diet. Her toenails are overgrown and, although she does not admit it, she obviously has some difficulty in hearing. She also has a tendency to constipation. She has been diagnosed as having osteoarthritis of the left hip, which has been treated with indomethacin and paracetamol.

Medical plan
Arthroplasty to left hip.

Identification of the patient's needs and problems during the continuing postoperative period

Pain
Administer prescribed analgesics as required. Take care in moving the patient.

Fluid and electrolyte balance
Encourage fluids by mouth. Maintain a fluid balance chart. Note any confusion or lethargy and report.

Nutrition
Guide the patient in choosing food which is nutritious. Make sure that she is sitting in a comfortable position prior to the meal. Arrange with the dietitian to devise with Mrs Brown a nutritious diet, which will not increase her weight and is easy to prepare and not too expensive. Talk with her son about the possible involvement of her neighbours or the necessity of a home help.

Elimination
Provide a commode or sani-chair. If no bowel action by the third day, administer an aperient. Encourage fluids and a high-roughage diet.

Prevention of chest infection
Arrange for the physiotherapist to help the patient with deep breathing. Mobilise early.

Prevention of dislocation of the hip
While in bed the patient will have an abduction pillow to prevent adduction. Mrs Brown should not be rolled on to the operated side but lifted for bedpans and pressure area care. Explain to the patient why she should not cross her legs.

Prevention of pressure sores
Move the patient every 2 hours, paying particular attention to the buttocks, shoulders and heels. Use a sheepskin. Ensure that Mrs Brown has plenty of fluids and a good diet.

Prevention of infection
Use a strict aseptic technique when dealing with the wound and removing the Redivac drain and stitches.

Hygiene
Bedbath for the first few days, allowing the patient to do what she is able. Gradually help her to progress to a shower or general bath. Provide facilities for cleaning her false teeth. Help her to do her hair. She may need to go to the occupational therapy department to gain confidence in using the bath or shower. Arrange for the chiropodist to attend to her toenails.

Mobility
On the first postoperative day stand Mrs Brown at the side of the bed. In the afternoon walk her with a frame. She may rest on the top of the bed. On the fourth day she may sit out in a high chair with a

pillow between the legs and no stool. By the eighth day sticks may be used and the stairs attempted.

Social
Arrange for the social worker to come and see her and possibly her son as well with a view to looking at any alterations to her house that may be required, and also ways in which she might go out more.

30

Injuries and Conditions of the Vertebral Column

The vertebral column carries the spinal cord within the neural canal, therefore any condition affecting it may also cause damage to the spinal cord. The vertebral column is also a very mobile series of small joints involved in posture and the many movements of the body. Thus surgery in this area will require some degree of immobilisation of the back, and the nurse must therefore be aware of what movements the patient is allowed to do and how to turn or assist the patient in getting out of bed without putting a strain on his back.

Specific emphasis in the nursing history

General appearance. Note the patient's posture and in particular the shape of the spine.

Mobility. Note the gait and the ability of the patient to carry out certain bending movements. Are other joints affected? Is there any associated paralysis?

Breathing. Is breathing affected in any way or is there any indication of a chest infection?

Pain. Note the presence of pain in the back or elsewhere in the body, and its character.

Skin. Is there any alteration in sensation, particularly in the feet?

Elimination. Are there any abnormalities of micturition or bowel action such as retention?

Sexual. Is sexual activity interfered with?

Social. Will there be some assistance available initially on return home? Are there any young children or elderly people requiring lifting? Does coal have to be brought in?

Employment. Is lifting part of the job, if so, is it possible for the patient's employer to reallocate this part of his job?

The fetus develops in a curled-up position in the uterus and therefore when a baby is born the spine is slightly curved in the thoracic and pelvic regions. These are called primary curves. Once the baby begins to lift his head and stand upright, further curves develop in the cervical and lumbar regions. These are called secondary curves.

Kyphosis

If the curve in the thoracic spine is exaggerated or there is a posterior curve in any other part of the spine, it is known as a kyphosis, and if it is associated with an exaggeration of the normal lumbar curve, it is a kypholordosis. Kyphosis may arise due to any of the following.

1. *Changes in the bone of the vertebral bodies* as a result of:

(a) congenital conditions in which some vertebrae are fused together;

(b) inflammatory conditions, such as tuberculosis or osteomyelitis, destroying the vertebral bodies;

(c) neoplastic destruction of the vertebral bodies;

(d) bone rarefaction in conditions such as osteoporosis, osteomalacia or rickets.

2. *Changes in the intervertebral discs.* Senile kyphosis arises as a result of degeneration of the intervertebral discs as well as of the bodies of the vertebrae.

3. *Loss of tone or faulty development of the supporting muscles in the spine.* This may be due to faulty posture or Scheuermann's disease, a condition which mainly affects boys. In the latter condition the growth of the thoracic vertebral bodies is interfered with and they become wedge shaped.

Treatment

The cause is treated and attention paid to the general health. Remedial exercises are given to develop muscle control. It may be necessary for the child to wear a spinal brace or be confined to a plaster bed if the condition is severe.

Lordosis

This is an exaggeration of the normal anterior curve in the lumbar spine. It may be associated with other deformities such as kyphosis or be the result of bad posture.

Treatment

Lordosis is dealt with in a similar manner to kyphosis, other deformities being treated at the same time.

Scoliosis

This condition is found more often in girls and consists of a lateral curvature of any part of the spine. There may be one curve affecting a large section of the spine, or two or more curves in opposite directions. At the same time there is a rotation deformity causing gross disfigurement.

Idiopathic scoliosis is the most common type but is not usually evident until the child is about 10 years old.

Postural scoliosis may develop due to bad sitting habits.

Compensatory scoliosis may arise in an effort to compensate for other abnormalities such as a short leg on one side.

Paralytic scoliosis may develop in a mild form of anterior poliomyelitis.

Treatment

Postural scoliosis is treated by attention to general health, remedial exercises and, if necessary, a plaster bed. If the deformity is fixed (structural), treatment is difficult. Any contributing cause is removed if possible. Remedial exercises are carried out and a Milwaukee brace worn until the child is about 10. Harrington rods may be inserted surgically to correct the deformity, after which a plaster jacket is worn.

Alternatively, a special corrective jacket may be made in order to exert a corrective force over a long period. This may be associated with spinal fusion to maintain the corrected position.

Spinal fusion This is done with bone grafts from adjacent ribs or the iliac crest. If the approach is through the thoracic cavity, an underwater seal drain will be inserted to drain the inevitable pneumothorax. The patient is nursed in a plaster bed which was made before the operation. Turning is achieved by using an anterior shell. The nursing care is the same as that for an osteotomy. The patient may suffer considerable pain from the donor area.

Spondylolisthesis

In this condition the body of the vertebra does not fuse with the neural arch during development, the two parts being joined only by fibrous tissue. This defect is known as spondylosis.

If this fibrous union is weak, or subject to sudden or continuous strain, it may give way and stretch, allowing the affected vertebral body to slide forward on the vertebra below, carrying with it the whole of the vertebral column above. This is known as spondylolisthesis and occurs in the lumbar region at the level of the fifth or occasionally the fourth vertebra.

There may be no symptoms or some degree of back pain, depending on how much displacement has taken place. Treatment is by the provision of a lumbosacral corset. If symptoms are severe, a spinal fusion may be necessary.

Spina bifida

This is a congenital abnormality in which the spinal processes of one or more vertebrae have not fused together to form the neural arch (Fig. 30.1). It most commonly occurs in the lumbar region. The contents of the spinal canal may prolapse through this opening.

Spina bifida occulta is the mildest form of the condition in which there is a bony defect but the meninges and nervous tissue are not involved. Although it may be associated with other congenital abnormalities, it does not normally require treatment.

Meningocele occurs when the meninges only prolapse through the bony defect. It can be treated surgically with no complications.

Meningomyelocele or spina bifida cystica occurs when the cord as well as the meninges prolapses and the spinal nerves become stretched. This leads to a loss of sensation and paralysis of those areas supplied by the spinal nerves, that is the lower limbs. There are usually other associated abnormalities.

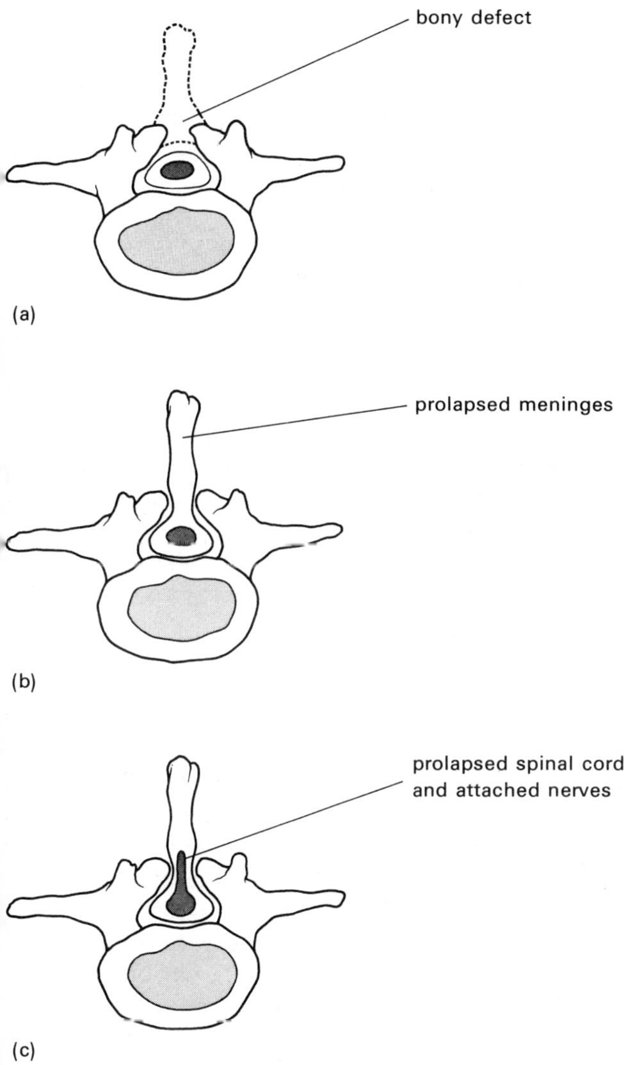

Fig. 30.1 *(a) Spina bifida occulta. (b) Meningocele. (c) Myelomeningocele.*

Treatment

The sac is excised and the gap closed with muscle flaps, but the mortality is high. Antibiotic cover is required and the infant is handled as little as possible postoperatively. Frequently an ileal conduit is necessary to control urinary incontinence. Orthopaedic operations will be carried out to correct deformities of the lower limbs such as talipes equino varus, and muscle transplant operations to overcome the imbalance between antagonistic muscles.

Ankylosing spondylitis (rheumatoid spondylitis)

Ankylosis (fixation) means a diminished range of movement of a joint due to arthritis. It may be bony, in which case the joint surfaces are fixed together by bone or fibrous tissue with strong fibrous adhesions which fix the joint incompletely, allowing some painful movement.

In ankylosing spondylitis the ligaments of the spine are gradually replaced by bone, so that the spine becomes rigid with the head bent forward and there is limitation of chest expansion (Fig. 30.2). It starts in the sacroiliac joints but arthritis is often present in other joints such as the hip. Other organs may have associated changes.

The treatment consists of specific exercises, swimming, a firm bed and high chair to prevent the

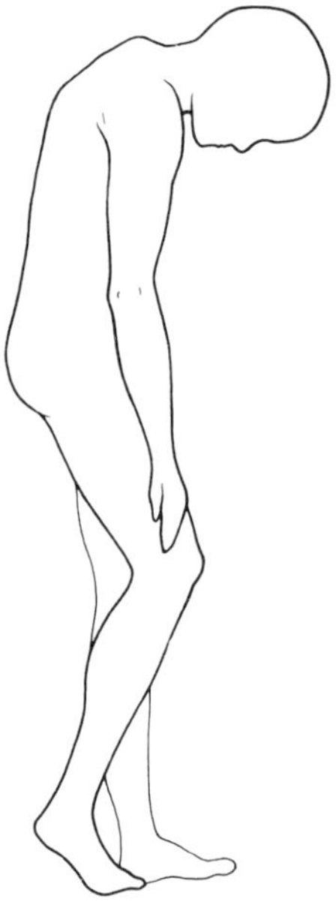

Fig. 30.2 *Ankylosing spondylitis with rigid back and bent head.*

spine becoming fixed in a flexed position. Medication is aimed at relieving the pain and the inflammation. Flexion deformity may be corrected surgically by a posterior spinal osteotomy, usually in the lumbar region.

Specific care of a patient having a spinal osteotomy

The patient usually has a nasogastric tube passed in theatre and this is aspirated hourly. Fluids are commenced once bowel sounds are heard and the tube is removed when adequate fluids are being taken. An intravenous infusion will be in progress. If possible the patient is nursed in a Stryker bed to aid turning. He will return from theatre with a back plaster, the anterior shell being provided the next day. The patient will lie on his back in the shell and his limbs should be checked for movement, sensation and foot pulses. Once the anterior shell has been provided he will be turned prone and will remain in this postion while a new back plaster is made and dried. He will continue to lie in a prone position each day for as long as he can tolerate, increasing the amount of time in this position each day. Care should be taken to prevent sores on the knees. On the third or fourth day the patient is stood out of bed for a few minutes, with the back plaster on. By the fourteenth day he should be ready to have a plaster of Paris jacket applied.

Tumours

Benign or malignant tumours may arise from the bones forming the vertebral column, the spinal cord, the nerve roots, or the membranes covering the spinal cord. Malignant tumours are usually secondary growths, having spread from a primary growth in the breast, prostate, lung or other organ, and mostly affect the vertebrae. Primary growths are rare. The tumour causes damage by pressing on the spinal cord, so interfering with sensory information passing up the cord and motor information coming down the cord. There is therefore weakness or paralysis below the point of the lesion, and diminished sensation. The clinical picture will depend upon the level of the lesion. If it is above the level of the fourth cervical vertebra, it is incompatible with life. One immediately below this level in the neck will result in paralysis of the respiratory muscles and a quadriplegia. Growths in the lumbar region lead to a paraplegia with a loss of reflex emptying of the bladder and bowel and sexual function. As the growth presses on the nerve roots there is also aching pain which radiates round the trunk (girdle pain).

Diagnosis will be made on a full neurological examination in which muscle power, reflexes and sensation are tested. X-rays may show evidence of bone disease. A lumbar puncture will show a very low CSF pressure and yellow discoloration of the fluid due to stagnation. Queckenstedt's test is negative, i.e. pressure in the manometer does not rise if pressure is applied over the jugular vein. A myelogram will demonstrate the level of the lesion by obstructing the flow of the radio-opaque fluid up or down the subarachnoid space. A cisternal puncture may be necessary if the tumour is high.

Many of the benign tumours of the spinal cord can be surgically removed. Secondary growths of the vertebral column may be partially removed to relieve pressure, and then treated with radiotherapy.

Prolapsed intervertebral disc

Between each pair of vertebral bones is an intervertebral disc. Each of these consists of a central semifluid gelatinous mass, known as the nucleus pulposus, enclosed in a fibrous envelope, the annulus fibrosis. The disc acts as a cushion between the vertebrae, allowing movement. When an intervertebral disc prolapses the outer fibrous ring becomes torn and the central nucleus bulges through it (Fig. 30.3). This most commonly occurs in the lumbar region.

A prolapsed disc may press on nerve roots or on the spine itself. In the former case it will produce pain and weakness in the area supplied by that nerve, and in the latter, paralysis below the level of the lesion. Lesions in the lumbar region produce severe back pain and sciatica, where the pain radiates down the leg to the foot. The ability to raise the leg when extended is also limited. Disturbance of sensation with numbness of the outer side of the leg and sole of the foot is also present. The knee and ankle reflexes are lost. Thoracic lesions (which are rare) may press on the spinal cord causing paraplegia. Cervical lesions are more frequently due to degeneration, but if a prolapse does occur, the patient will have difficulty in moving his head and will also have pain radiating along his arm with an associated weakness, loss of sensation and reflexes.

Diagnosis is confirmed by a myelogram, which will also demonstrate where the lesion is. Treatment is by rest on a firm bed for 4 to 8 weeks which may enable the disc to shrink back. Pelvic traction may be applied with a corset and weights of 15–25 lb (7–11 kg). If necessary after this, or as a primary form of treatment in mild cases, a plaster jacket or steel corset is worn. Analgesia will be required.

Laminectomy

If the patient's symptoms do not respond to conservative treatment, they recur frequently, or there are severe neurological symptoms, a laminectomy will be carried out. The operation is most easily done with the patient in the prone position. The pelvis is elevated 38 cm off the table and the abdomen allowed to sag to prevent venous congestion. The lamina, or lamina and spinous process, is removed from one or sometimes two vertebrae and the disc is removed.

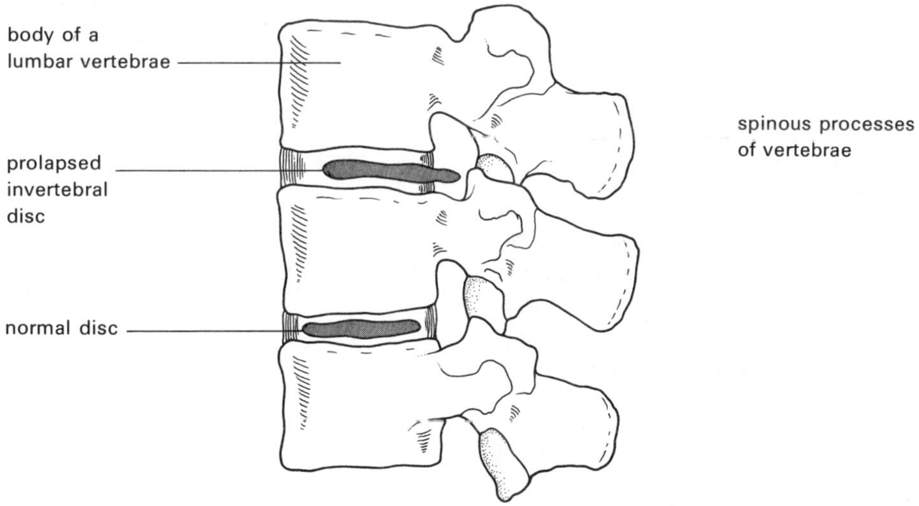

Fig. 30.3 *A prolapsed intervertebral disc.*

Specific care

Preoperatively the affected side should be marked with a cross on the buttock. The female patient is taught how to use a slipper bedpan or suitable urinal. The patient is also taught how to stabilise the spine before moving, avoiding flexion and twisting movements. Back-raising exercises may also be taught.

Postoperatively the patient may lay on the back or side, but the spine and thighs should be kept straight and there should be adequate support. Pain is severe and will require analgesics. The dressing is inspected and the usual observations maintained. The patient's feet and legs are examined regularly for any change in temperature, sensations or movement. Fluids are encouraged once they are tolerated. When turning the patient 2-hourly, the spine must be kept straight. If using an ordinary bedpan, a pillow can be folded lengthwise under the back.

Some surgeons start extension, flexion and rotation exercises on the second day, and these are continued for several weeks. Mobilisation begins about the fifth day but usually the patient should not sit on a chair but should stand or walk. Sometimes the patient wears a corset for a while; muscle exercises are important. The patient will be discharged 3 to 4 weeks after the operation.

Patients may require advice regarding their occupation, and can return to work 5 to 8 weeks after the operation. They may also need to be taught to lift correctly.

Fractures of the vertebral column

The important distinction between fractures in this region is whether they are stable and therefore require little treatment or whether they are unstable due to rupture of the ligaments, and therefore offer a threat of injury to the spinal cord. Pathological fractures frequently occur in the spine.

Compressed wedge fractures are a common form of injury and are caused by a fall from a height or when the spine is forcibly flexed. The vertebral body is compressed in front causing it to become wedge shaped. The associated ligaments are rarely ruptured. This type of fracture may occur either in the cervical or thoracolumbar region. Extension injuries may cause the posterior part of the vertebral body to become compressed. There is not usually any damage to the spinal cord, although persistent backache may be troublesome, and arthritis may develop later.

Burst fracture of the vertebral body is caused by a compression force on the vertebrae when the spine is straight. The intervertebral disc is forced into the vertebral body which is broken into fragments. One of the fragments may press on the spinal cord causing pressure symptoms. This type of fracture is not common.

The above are stable fractures and are treated by rest in bed for 2 to 3 weeks until the pain is relieved and then by muscle-strengthening exercises.

Fracture–dislocations are not as common as the stable fractures but when they do occur they are more common in the neck than in the lower spine. The stabilising ligaments are ruptured and the pedicles and laminae are fractured so that the upper part of the vertebral body is displaced forward in relation to the lower (Fig. 30.4). The lower vertebrae may be crushed. This occurs as a result of a fall in which the head is flexed or there is severe flexion of the lumbar region. The cord may be partially or completely severed. If damage to the spinal cord has occurred, it must be relieved promptly or permanent damage may result.

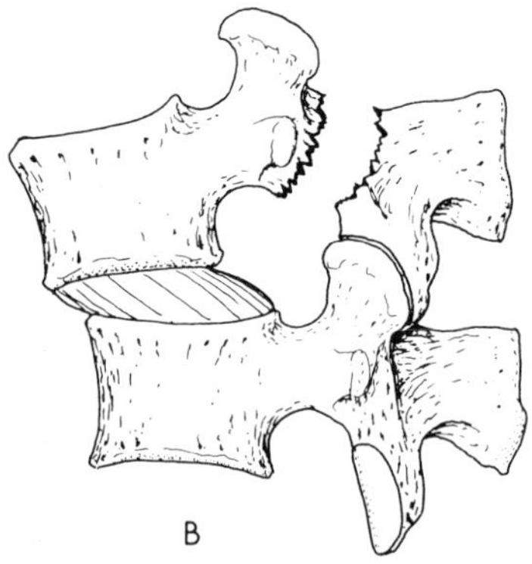

Fig. 30.4 *Fracture–dislocation of the spine.*

Treatment

In *cervical* fracture–dislocations traction is applied by skull calipers (Fig. 30.5) or tongs, the ends of which have been introduced through small holes which have been made in the parietal bones of the skull. The weights applied to the traction are increased up to 22 or more pounds (10 kg or more) until x-rays show reduction has taken place. Once this has happened the weights are gradually reduced to 12 lb (5 kg) or less to prevent damage to the cord. The lighter traction is maintained for 3 weeks, after which a plaster jacket is applied. Some surgeons prefer to put a plaster jacket on once reduction has taken place.

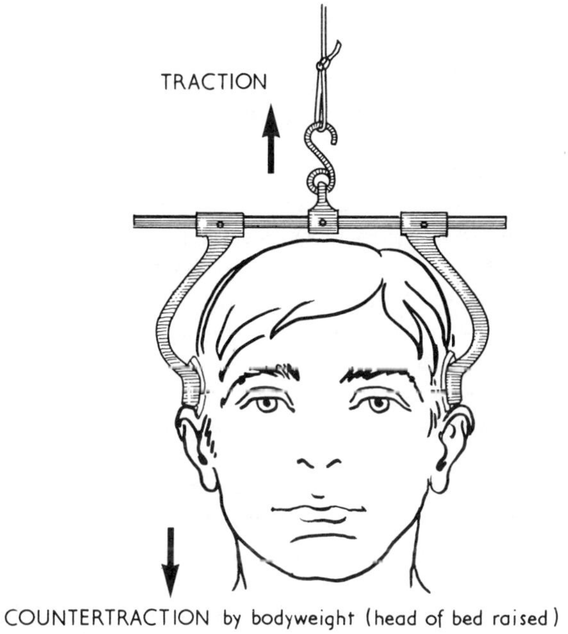

Fig. 30.5 *Caliper traction of the skull for cervical fracture–dislocation treatment.*

Internal fixation may be done, if reduction is unstable, by anterior cervical fusion of the bodies of the vertebrae or posterior wiring of the spinous processes.

In *lumbar* fracture–dislocations, if the spine is not involved, the patient may be nursed prone, after a closely fitting plaster jacket has been applied if this is necessary. Traction may be required to maintain reduction. An operation may be necessary to immobilise the fracture with a plate or wire if fusion does not take place.

The patient is nursed on a Stryker frame which enables him to be turned every 2 hours, or, failing this, on sorbo mattresses and pillows. The major aim in nursing care is to prevent complications from arising. Pressure sores will develop due to the lack of sensation and inability to move if adequate precautions are not taken. All the nursing care required for a paraplegic patient is necessary.

Spinal shock in which the muscles are flaccid lasts up to a fortnight, although if the cord is completely severed it may be longer than this. Eventually it wears off and is followed by spastic paralysis. Contractures of the limbs must therefore be prevented by passive movements.

The patient may want to discuss the effects of the damage on his or her sexual function. A male patient can be told that erection can still be achieved as a reflex after stimulation, but that ejaculation and orgasm are unlikely and he may be infertile. The female patient will be able to take a passive role in sexual intercourse but will not have an orgasm. Her fertility is not affected and she may therefore become pregnant. If so, the pregnancy will be able to continue up to term and a normal vaginal delivery take place.

SUGGESTED WORK

1. Find out from a patient what effects the presence of back pain has had upon his or her life, both socially and in employment.

2. Do a survey of a group of nurses in your hospital to find out the incidence of back pain and the effects it has had on their careers.

SUGGESTED READING

Consumers Association (1978). *Avoiding Back Trouble.* London: Which?

Hart G. (1981). Spinal cord injury: impact on client's significant others. *Association of Rehabilitation Nurses*; **6** (1): 11–15.

Hollis M. (1981). *Safer Lifting for Patient Care*. London: Blackwell Scientific.
Pratt R. (1971). *Nursing Care of Paraplegic Patients*. A Nursing Times Publication. London: Macmillan.
Schuler M. (1982). Sexual counselling for the spinal cord injured: a review of five programmes. *Journal of Sexual and Marital Therapy*; **8** (3): 241–52.
Webb P. (1982). Self help groups for back pain sufferers. *Health Visitor*; **55** (9): 487–90.

* * *

Miss MARGARET WELLS (aged 24) is a nurse who has been suffering from a prolapsed intervertebral disc. She is resident at the hospital, her home being 120 miles away.

Medical plan
Laminectomy

Identification of the patient's needs and problems in the continuing postoperative period and action arising from these

Pain
Administer prescribed analgesics as required, evaluating their efficacy.

Mobility
Nurse Margaret on her back, keeping her spine and thighs straight. Get her to stabilise her spine before being turned. Explain why she must not twist her spine. On the fifth day help her to get up slowly and watch out for faintness. Help her to stand with two nurses. After instruction from the physiotherapist, Margaret may be walked with assistance but should return to bed afterwards. Find out from the physiotherapist what muscle exercises are to be done and encourage the patient to do them.

Wound
Inspect the dressing. Remove the stitches on the third day.

Possible interference to the blood or nerve supply
Examine the feet and legs for sensation, movement, colour and temperature.

Nutrition
While being nursed on her back she will need food that is easily handled. Make sure that everything is to hand and cut the food up if necessary. Advise her to avoid choosing large indigestible meals. Encourage fluids.

Hygiene
Wash the patient while she remains in bed. She may lie on her side to clean her teeth. Once up, she will need help in washing her lower limbs.

Excretion
Use a slipper pan if possible, or place a pillow under her back. Take care when inserting the bedpan. An aperient is not usually given until the patient is up and can use the commode or go to the toilet.

Prevention of pressure sores
Attend to her pressure areas, particularly her heels and elbows. She may appreciate a sheepskin until she is allowed up.

Psychological
She may be very frustrated at the length of time treatment has already taken, and will continue to take. She may need to discuss with the nursing administration the possibility of moving to a less strenuous area. Boredom will be a problem as it is difficult to do very much lying on one's back. Visitors should be encouraged and one of them might like to read to her. The wireless and television will also help to pass the time. Prismatic glasses may also be used.

31

Deformities, Congenital and Acquired

Most of the conditions mentioned in this chapter are related to children, and the reader should refer to Chapter 40 for the approach to nursing care. Some of these conditions require the child to have repeated admission to hospital which may interfere with education or, even more importantly, the relationships within the home. The nurse must therefore be careful to foster these relationships and not in any way usurp them.

Specific emphasis in the nursing history

General appearance. Note the posture and the comparison of the patient's progress with the normal physical and mental milestones.

Mobility. Is there any loss of power in muscles, limping, limitation in the movement of joints or shortening of a limb?

Pain. Note the presence of this in the joints or the extremities.

Social background. The number of children in the family and their age. Work commitment of both parents. Financial situation. Distance of the home from the hospital.

Skin. Alteration of sensation or change in colour of the extremities.

Nutrition. The type of diet the child is on.

Elimination. Note normal habits and language used.

Torticollis (wry neck)

This may be a congenital condition or may arise due to bony or inflammatory lesions. The congenital form develops as a result of injury to one sternomastoid muscle at birth. Some of the muscle fibres are replaced with fibrous tissue, so shortening them and causing the head to be tilted to one side. Over a period of time the face becomes asymmetrical and scoliosis may develop.

In the first few weeks of life, daily stretching of the affected muscle may be all that is required. In older children in which the condition has persisted the muscle and associated fascia are divided surgically by a subcutaneous tenotomy and the head is immobilised in the opposite position to the deformity by plaster of Paris. In severe cases an open operation is necessary to correct the condition.

Cervical rib syndrome

A cervical rib is an extra rib arising from the seventh cervical vertebra. A fibrous band in a similar position causes the same problems. The condition may not produce any effects, or there may be compression and irritation of the nerve root supplying the brachial plexus, the sympathetic nerves or the subclavian artery. This will result in sensory disturbance along the inner border of the arm and forearm. There may be wasting and loss of power in the muscles of the hand. The hand may also be cold, blue and have a diminished pulse due to effects on the artery.

The patient is given exercises to develop the muscles of the shoulder and is advised to avoid lifting heavy articles. Occasionally division of the scalenus muscle is required.

Genu valgum (knock knee)

This is a common deformity in young children, often without apparent cause, although mild rickets may be present. It usually disappears spontaneously by the age of 10 years. If necessary, the child's shoes may be wedged on the inner side. However, the child should be seen at least every 6 months and if the condition appears to be getting worse, metal staples are inserted at the lower end of the femur, at the epiphysis on the inside. These inhibit growth on that side. Once the deformity is corrected the staples are removed.

Slipped upper femoral epiphysis (adolescent coxa vara)

In this condition the epiphysis of the upper end of the femur slips downward and backwards. It appears to be due to a deficiency in hormones and occurs mainly in boys between the ages of 10 and 15. The chronic form is more common than the acute.

The child will have a limp, limitation of hip movement and pain in the hip or knee. If there is only a slight slip, the epiphysis is pinned to the femur. The hip is non-weight bearing for 12 weeks. If the slip is marked, an osteotomy will be necessary. The same condition may occur in the other hip and will also require treatment.

Congenital dislocation of the hip

In this condition there is a lack of development of the acetabulum and deformity of the femoral head. The cause is unknown, although there is a familial incidence. It is more common in girls and usually affects one hip, most often the left, although in one-third of cases it is bilateral. Laxity of the joint or dislocation is present at birth but there are a small number of cases which are not discovered until the child starts walking. It is essential to diagnose the condition early, and this is done by using Ortolani's or Barlow's test (Fig. 31.1).

With the child on his back, each flexed leg is held in the examiner's hands, the thumbs on the inner aspect of the thighs. The hips are then abducted and externally rotated and if one of the hips can be dislocated, there will be a click. By an extension of this test a lax joint may also be found, but this condition generally recovers spontaneously.

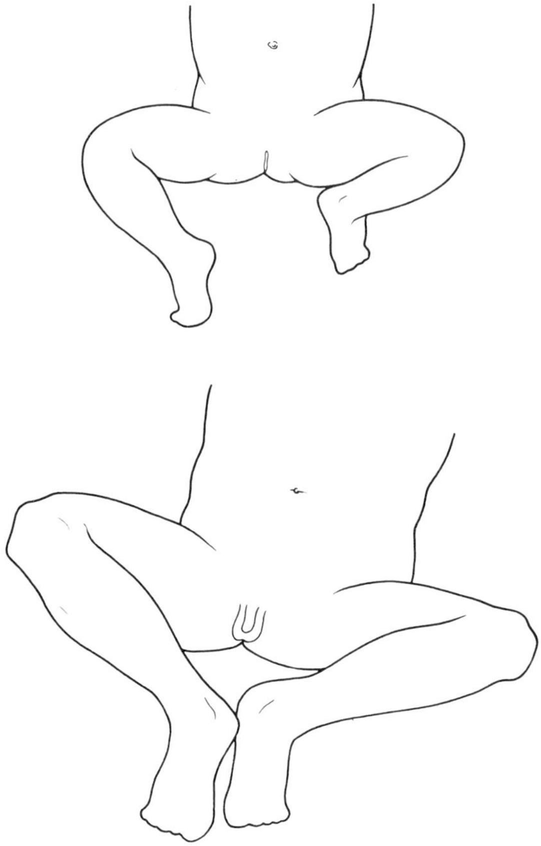

Fig. 31.1 *Ortolani's or Barlow's test showing limited movement (abduction) of the right hip.*

If the child is not diagnosed until he is walking, there will be shortening of the leg on the affected side causing a limp. On examination there is limited abduction of the flexed leg on the affected side. Diagnosis is confirmed by x-ray.

Management of the baby in the neonatal period is mainly by using a thick pad or napkin between the legs to keep them abducted. After 1 or 2 weeks, if the condition persists, a polythene splint may be applied to keep the legs in abduction. If there is no response to treatment, a tenotomy may be necessary to release the joint from a tight adductor muscle. Splinting will continue. For some children further treatment is required. After 1 year traction is applied for 3 to 4 weeks to reduce the hip, and if this is not successful, open reduction will be performed. The hip is held in a position of abduction by plaster of Paris splints, by a 'frog plaster' or Batchelor's knee splints (Figs. 31.2 and 31.3). The former consists of a plaster from the waist to the ankles with a piece cut away in the genital region. The latter are plaster cylinders on each leg and a metal bar holding the two legs apart.

If a congenital dislocated hip has not been diagnosed until the child is walking, it may not respond to this treatment and a Salter or Chiari-type osteotomy may be done (Figs. 31.4 and 31.5). In the former the pelvic bone is divided above the joint and a bone graft inserted, so directing the acetabulum in a downward direction. In older children a Chiari-type of osteotomy is done, in which the pelvic bone is divided above the joint and the acetabulum displaced inwards so that the pelvic bone forms an enlarged cavity.

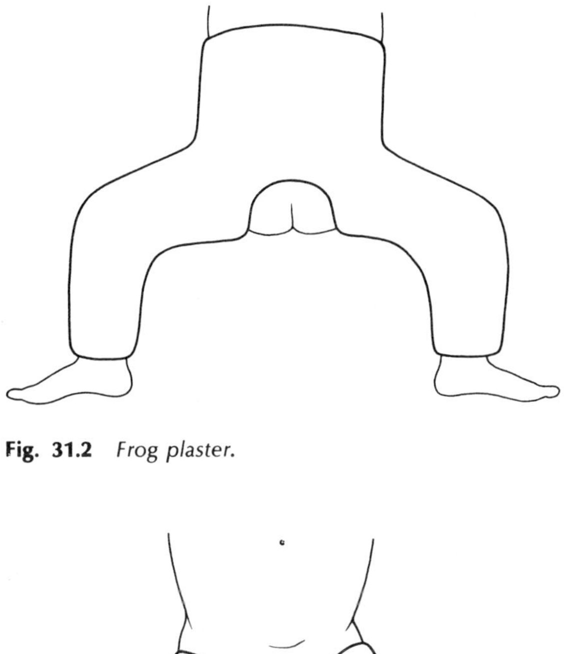

Fig. 31.2 *Frog plaster.*

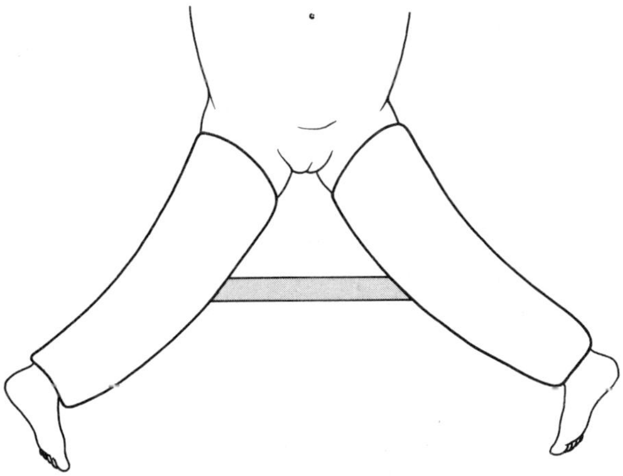

Fig. 31.3 *Batchelor's knee splints.*

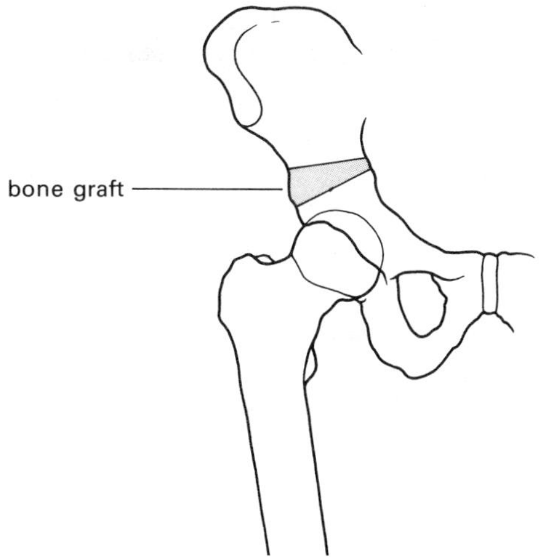

Fig. 31.4 *Salter-type osteotomy.*

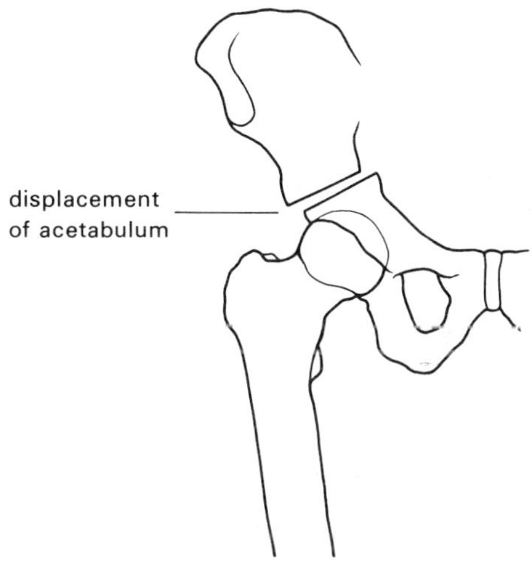

Fig. 31.5 *Chiari-type osteotomy.*

If the child is in a 'frog plaster', there is some difficulty in keeping this clean around the perineal area and the edge of the plaster is protected with waterproof adhesive plaster. The care is that for any plaster. The child may insert small items inside the plaster which if not removed will cause sores.

Talipes

Talipes is a congenital deformity of the foot and ankle (Fig. 31.6) which is often associated with other congenital abnormalities.

Talipes equinovarus (club foot)

This is a common congenital deformity in which the foot is twisted inwards and the heel is drawn up in relation to the forefoot and inverted.

Treatment is started as soon as possible after birth and consists of overcorrection of the deformity by manipulation and then holding the foot in the corrected position, until the muscles are strong enough to prevent the deformity recurring. A Denis Browne splint is frequently used (Fig. 31.7). Both feet are fixed to the splint by adhesive

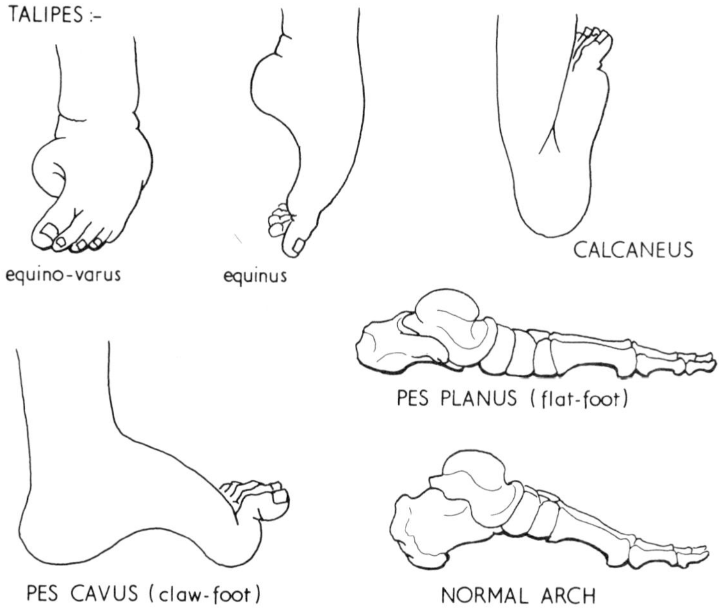

Fig. 31.6 *Abnormalities of the foot.*

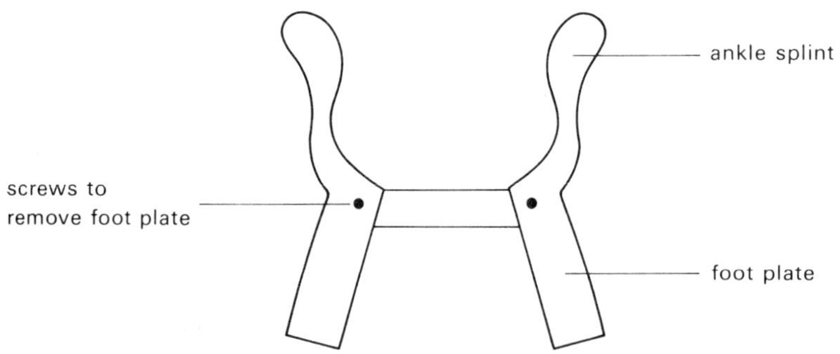

Fig. 31.7 *Dennis Browne splint.*

strapping. Manipulation and resplinting are repeated twice weekly. After 9 months, open-toed boots are fitted to the splints. During this time the child is encouraged to move his legs and so develop the muscles. Alternatively, serial plasters may be used to correct the deformity. Operative correction is occasionally necessary in the severely deformed or if the condition recurs.

Congenital talipes calcaneus

This is a less common condition in which the child is born with the foot dorsiflexed, the top of the foot being in contact with the front of the leg. It is corrected by stretching and a corrective splint.

Talipes valgus or talipes planus (flat foot)

The inner longitudinal arch of the foot is flattened and this may be a congenital or acquired condition, following debilitating illnesses or overweight. It is treated with remedial exercises and arch supports. Occasionally manipulation under a general anaesthetic is required followed by the application of a plaster of Paris for 6 to 8 weeks.

Pes cavus (claw foot)

The longitudinal arch of the foot is abnormally high. The toes become clawed and the transverse arch of the foot flattened. It arises due to weak muscles in the foot and becomes a painful condition because the heel is taking the body's weight.

Treatment in children is with a metatarsal bar which is attached to the sole of the shoe just behind the heads of the metatarsal bones, so relieving pressure on them. Surgery is required in the more serious form.

Hallux valgus

This condition mainly develops in women and is frequently due to the wearing of shoes with pointed toes. The big toe is bent in towards the other toes, so causing the metatarsophalangeal joint to become prominent. Because of the friction on this joint a bursa forms (bunion). Arthritic changes are also likely to occur.

The condition is treated by removing the excess bone formation (exostosis) and the base of the proximal phalanx—Keller's operation. The formation of fibrous tissue fixes the joint. Following the operation, passive toe movements are commenced after 2 to 3 days and the patient is discharged after 2 weeks.

In younger patients a reshaping operation with a osteotomy is done. Postoperatively the patient may have a plaster of Paris on the toe for 2 weeks. From the first day postoperatively the patient is encouraged to do foot and ankle exercises, and on discharge wears sandals and is measured for orthopaedic sandals.

Hallux rigidus

This condition is due to a congenital deformity of the metatarsophalangeal joint in which osteoarthritis develops. The joint becomes painful and limited in movement and a bursa may develop at this site. In younger patients an arthrodesis of the joint is done and in older patients a Keller's operation.

Hammer toe

This is a common condition which most frequently affects the second toe and may be associated with a hallux valgus. It may be congenital or develop due to faulty shoes. There is a fixed flexion deformity of the proximal interphalangeal joint, with hyperextension of the metatarsophalangeal joint. An arthrodesis of the joint with bone or a wire is the most satisfactory method of treatment. A plaster of Paris cap is applied postoperatively and this is changed on the tenth day.

Ingrowing toenail

Tight footwear and incorrect cutting of the nails may lead to this painful condition in which the toenail cuts into the soft tissue and causes infection. In mild cases the edge of the nail is cut away and the ulcer packed with pledgets of cotton wool. More severe cases require the removal of the nail and underlying tissue.

Dupuytren's contracture of the hand

The palmar fascia of the hand slowly becomes thickened and contracted, forming tight bands from the palm into the fingers. This causes the fingers to be drawn down into the palm. The condition is frequently bilateral and more common in males, there being a hereditary tendency to develop it.

Treatment is by excision either of the bands or of the palmar fascia. Severe contraction of the little finger may require it to be amputated. Postoperatively observation of sensation in the hand is essential in case the digital nerve has been damaged.

Carpal tunnel syndrome

The scaphoid, lunate and hamate bones of the hand (carpal bones) form a 'U'-shaped tunnel on their palmar surface (Fig. 31.8). The tunnel is completed by a sheet of tough inelastic fibrous tissue—the transverse carpal ligament—which stretches across the groove. If the space becomes narrowed due to arthritis of the carpal bones or thickening of the ligaments, the median nerve will become compressed. Swelling of the tissues in the tunnel will have a similar effect and is associated with hormonal changes such as occur at the menopause. A Colles fracture and dislocation of the wrist may also be causes.

The compression may affect the nerve directly or indirectly through reducing its blood supply. The patient suffers varying degrees of pain which is typically worse at night when the blood pressure is low. There may be altered sensation on the thumb side of the hand and sometimes wasting and weakness of the thumb. The compression is relieved surgically by division of the transverse carpal ligament.

SUGGESTED WORK

1. Discuss with a mother of a child admitted for correction of a congenital dislocation of the hip what effects this has had on the child and on the life of the family.

2. Do a survey on the shoes worn both on and off duty by the nurses in your intake and note the effects on their feet.

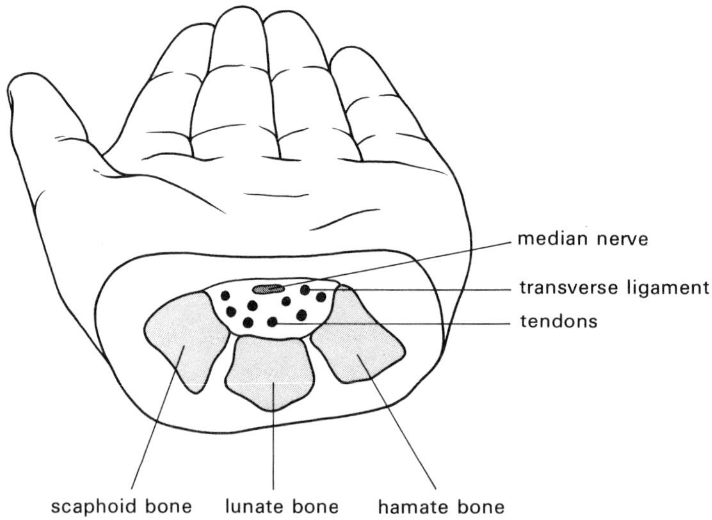

Fig. 31.8 *The carpal tunnel.*

SUGGESTED READING

Hale G., ed. (1979). *The New Source Book for the Disabled*. London: Heinemann.
Open University (1975). *Facing the Future*. Units 4–8. Milton Keynes: Open University Press.
Whitely J., Sandhu J. *Directory of Non-Medical Research Relating to Handicapped People*. Newcastle: Handicapped Persons Research Unit, Newcastle Polytechnic.

* * *

EMMA WALKER is an only child who was born 1 year ago with a congenital dislocation of the hip. Although she started treatment at an early stage, there was little response. She was admitted 4 weeks ago for traction but unfortunately this was not sufficient.

Medical plan
Open reduction with the application of Batchelor's knee splints.

Identification of the patient's needs and problems following the application of knee splints and action arising from these

Prevention of damage to the plaster
Ensure that the air can get to the plaster, and if necessary use a fan. Take care to handle the plaster with the flat of the hand. Observe the toes for colour and temperature.

Hygiene
Encourage the mother to wash Emma and attend to her toilet needs. Show her where everything is and what needs to be done. Show her how to check the top of the plaster for things inserted by Emma. Explain the importance of caring for the skin around the edge of the plaster casts and the buttocks. Ask her to report any redness or soreness. The nurse should also make regular checks.

Nutrition
Continue with the mixed diet Emma is already having. Encourage the parents to stay with her when she is attempting to feed herself if possible. Show the mother how to position her with pillows. When Emma is attempting to feed herself, protect the bed and reassure the parents about the mess. Her mother may want to bring Emma's own cup in.

Excretion
Emma may be content to soil a napkin, which should be changed as soon as possible.

Mobility
Normally Emma would either be crawling or walking with help. See if her father or some relative can make a platform with castors and buffers so that Emma can move around. Ensure that the environment is safe for this.

Boredom and separation from home
Discuss with the parents suitable toys and mobiles that can be used. Also look at ways of preventing them from slipping out of her reach. Ensure that during the day Emma is in a position where she can see plenty of activity.

32

Conditions of Bone

Many of the conditions described in this chapter are chronic, developing over a number of years and associated with varying degrees of pain. Persistent crippling pain has a demoralising effect on the individual, particularly as sympathy soon runs out. It may become central to people's lives, but if they want to maintain their social contacts, they have to learn to put it on one side. The nurse must be able to realise the effects on the personality of constant pain and make allowances for this. She must also do everything she can to minimise the pain and make the patient as comfortable as possible, which at times will require considerable patience. However, once the patient has had an operation the level of pain may actually have been reduced and the patient's attitude totally changed. These can therefore be very rewarding patients to nurse. The patient with a malignant condition will require all the skills at the disposal of the nurse.

Specific emphasis in the nursing history

Pain. At rest or related to movement? Which position does the patient find most comfortable?

General appearance. Has the ageing process been accelerated due to pain? Note posture, gait, weight loss, evidence of healed fractures, deformed, hot or swollen joints or the abnormal shape of bones. Is there any pallor or lethargy present? Stunting of growth in children?

Mobility. Is this limited by pain? How much can the patient do? Is there any difficulty in getting out of chairs or managing toilet requirements?

Skin. Note the presence of pressure sores or nodules.

Vital signs. Note the presence of a raised temperature.

Social. Will any adaptations be required in the patient's home or will he require rehousing? Are there family or friends who can support?

BENIGN TUMOURS

These may arise from cartilage cells (chondroma) or bone cells (osteoma, osteoclastoma). A chondroma or osteoma is only excised if it is affecting other structures. The osteoclastoma is locally destructive and may become malignant and is therefore completely excised, the cavity being filled with bone chips. Internal fixation may be necessary to prevent a pathological fracture, and radiotherapy may also be beneficial.

MALIGNANT TUMOURS

These are usually secondary, having spread from malignant tumours in other parts of the body. Spread may particularly occur from the breast, prostate, kidneys, thyroid and lungs. These tumours are associated with persistent, severe pain and are rarely treated by surgery.

Sarcoma is a less common tumour but has a very poor prognosis. It is a primary tumour of the bone-forming cells (osteoblasts) in which there is either an excessive formation of bone or destruction of it.

It most frequently affects young adults. It is an extremely malignant condition spreading locally through the bone and to the lung and other organs via the bloodstream, but not through the lymph nodes. Radiotherapy and amputation of the limb are the methods of controlling the condition.

OSTEOGENESIS IMPERFECTA (FRAGILITAS OSSIUM)

This is a hereditary condition in which all the bones are abnormally brittle. In severe forms the child will not survive infancy, and less severe forms require great care to reduce the number of fractures which lead to deformities and stunting of growth. Children with this condition frequently have blue sclera of the eyes. Some of the deformities will require surgical correction.

OSTEITIS DEFORMANS

This condition develops after the age of 40. There is an excessive production of bone and at the same time an excessive breakdown of it. The bone therefore becomes progressively thicker and softer, with an increased blood supply. Later the bones become more brittle and may fracture. The bones most commonly affected are the pelvis, skull, vertebrae and long bones of the leg. It may start in one bone and then spread to the others.

The head becomes enlarged, the legs bowed and there is a kyphosis. Deafness may arise due to pressure on the auditory nerve if that part of the cranium enlarges. Pathological fractures are common. The condition may lead on to sarcoma of one of the affected bones.

If no symptoms are present, treatment is not required, otherwise the hormone calcitonin from the thyroid is used to suppress bone reabsorption, so reducing the abnormal turnover of bone.

OSTEITIS FIBROSA CYSTICA (HYPERPARATHYROIDISM)

A benign tumour of the parathyroid glands will cause an excess secretion of parathormone. This hormone causes calcium to leave the bones, so raising the level of calcium in the blood. The bones become less rigid, with multiple cysts, leading to gross deformities and pathological fractures. The excess calcium is excreted by the kidneys and leads to renal calculi. Surgical removal of the tumour restores the balance of calcium to normal. Vitamin D is given in the postoperative period to aid bone repair.

RHEUMATOID ARTHRITIS

Rheumatoid arthritis is a chronic disease the cause of which is not yet known, although it is thought to be either an autoimmune or infective disease. It mainly affects the smaller joints such as the hands, but may also involve larger joints, particularly the knees. It is more common in women between the ages of 30 and 50. Still's disease is a particular form which attacks children.

The synovial membrane becomes inflamed and thickened, and this erodes the cartilage at the end of the bones. The inflammation causes fluid to accumulate and the joint to become swollen. Gradually the joints become deformed. Arthritis is a generalised condition, as well as affecting the bones it also involves the arteries, heart, lungs and nerves, and nodules may form in the subcutaneous tissue.

The patient may have a slight temperature, general malaise and weight loss, with pain and stiffness in the limbs. On examination the joints are found to be hot and swollen and the related muscles wasted. Nodules and anaemia may also be present.

Treatment of the condition is mainly medical, with rest, aspirin to control the pain, a good diet and physiotherapy once the acute stage has subsided. Anti-inflammatory drugs such as ibuprofen, indomethacin, and phenylbutazone are used to reduce the inflammatory process but they do have some unwanted side-effects. Injections of gold are given if these drugs are not able to contain the disease, but in many patients steroids are the only effective means of control. If an improvement is not achieved with any of the drugs mentioned, it may be necessary to use cytotoxic drugs such as cyclophosphamide or methotrexate.

The use of surgery in this condition is in order to improve the function and appearance of deformed joints and to relieve pain. This may be done by a synovectomy, arthrodesis, osteotomy or arthroplasty.

Synovectomy

This consists of removal of the inflamed synovial membrane (most commonly in the knee) at an early stage in the disease before degenerative changes of the cartilage have developed. Following the operation the patient may have a plaster cylinder which is removed on the tenth day. He is allowed to get up on the first postoperative day. Once the plaster has been removed the patient starts knee flexion exercises to prevent knee stiffness and partial weight bearing, gradually progressing to full weight bearing.

Arthrodesis

This process involves fusion of a joint with pins. It is used for smaller joints in place of an arthroplasty. A painful or unstable knee may be arthrodesed, but a total knee replacement is preferable as it retains function. Postoperatively the joint is enclosed in a plaster of Paris cylinder which remains on until the bones are seen to be united on x-ray.

Osteotomy

This is surgical division of the bone to correct a deformity, and is more commonly carried out for malunion in fractures.

Arthroplasty

This is the remodelling of a joint which may be performed on the elbow, knee and sometimes on a finger. The care of an arthroplasty of the knee is similar to that following a meniscectomy (see Chapter 29). (Also see Chapter 29 for the care of a total hip replacement.)

OSTEOARTHRITIS

This is a degenerative form of arthritis and occurs in the older age group. It is not a generalised disease, but the severe pain may have a debilitating effect on the individual.

Osteoarthritis usually affects the weight-bearing joints such as the hip, lumbar spine and knees, although other joints can be involved. Previous fractures, inflammation or surgery in the region of the joint may predispose to this condition. Perthes' disease, congenital dislocation of the hip, obesity, poor posture and abnormal stress are other predisposing factors.

The cartilage becomes soft and eroded and small bony growths develop at the edges of the articulating surfaces. Gradually the whole of the cartilage is destroyed. The exposed bone becomes thickened, and a degenerative cyst may develop in the underlying bone.

The patient suffers severe pain which is worse on movement but relieved by rest. However, lack of movement leads to stiffness. Gradually the joint becomes stiffer and deformed and the associated muscles waste.

Rest and analgesics may give some relief but the patient frequently needs surgical intervention in the form of an arthrodesis, osteotomy or arthroplasty. Osteoarthritis is the commonest reason for an arthroplasty of the hip.

TUBERCULOSIS OF THE BONE AND JOINTS

Tuberculosis is a chronic infection which initially infects the lungs and then travels via the bloodstream to bones or other organs. It most commonly affects the ends of long bones, spreading to the joints and causing a specific arthritis. The spine, hips and knee joints are those most commonly affected. It causes a chronic osteomyelitis which, unlike the acute form, is almost entirely destructive in character, no new bone being formed.

In a joint there is destruction of the synovial membrane and erosion of the cartilage with eventual destruction of bone. Cold abscesses may form and track to other tissues, eventually perforating.

The lesion may heal spontaneously but the tubercle bacilli remain dormant. The patient complains of pain in the bone or joint which is worse following activity but relieved by rest. Deformity and swelling may also be present and the patient will also be suffering from the general effects of the disease with a slight rise in the temperature, night sweats and a generalised malaise.

Treatment is by rest, both general and of the specific joint affected which may require the application of plaster of Paris. Initially three drugs, isoniazid, rifampicin and ethambutol, or streptomycin and pyrazinamide, are given for 8 weeks. This is followed by two drugs, one of them being isoniazid, which are continued for 6 to 18 months. In later life damaged joints may require surgical treatment with an arthrodesis or arthroplasty. Any cold abscesses are aspirated, not incised, in order to prevent a secondary infection.

SUGGESTED WORK

1. Find out how long patients have had to wait in order to be admitted for an arthroplasty. What effect has this had on the patient? Compare the waiting time for admission in your hospital with that in another, preferably in a different area.

2. Find out from a patient with rheumatoid arthritis how this condition has changed the way she would have liked to live her life.

SUGGESTED READING

Mattix M. W. (1979). Pre-operative education for the total hip patient. *Operating Nurses Association Journal*; **6**(6): 251–2.

Woodall C. (1980). *A Disjointed Life*. London: Heinemann.

33

Gynaecological Conditions

Gynaecological conditions may vary from the very minor disorders which nevertheless may cause considerable distress to the patient, to those which require major surgery. Inevitably these disorders are associated in the mind of the woman with her sexuality and her ability to bear children.

Specific emphasis in the nursing history

General appearance. Lethargy, pallor, weight loss, abdominal distension. Bent posture.

Menstruation. Regularity and amount.

Vital signs. Temperature, pulse.

Elimination. Bowel and urinary function.

Pain. Cyclical. Backache. Pelvic pain. Pain elsewhere in the body.

ABNORMALITIES OF MENSTRUATION

Menstruation is easily upset by the mental state of the woman or by generalised diseases such as anaemia or disturbance of thyroid function.

Amenorrhoea

The absence of menstruation, either temporarily or permanently, is most commonly caused by pregnancy. However, lack of pituitary or ovarian secretions will also result in primary amenorrhoea in which the girl never starts menstruation and secondary sex characteristics do not develop. An *imperforate hymen* will cause amenorrhoea due to retention of the menstrual flow. In this condition normal secondary sexual characteristics develop but menstruation does not take place, although there may be cyclical discomfort. On examination the hymen is seen to be bulging as a result of the retention of the menstrual blood in the vagina (haematocolpos). It is treated by incision of the hymen and antibiotics to control infection.

Dysmenorrhoea

Pain at the time of menstruation may be primary, when the cause is physiological, or secondary to some other disease. *Primary dysmenorrhoea* may develop in the young girl once she starts to ovulate. At the time of menstruation she may have cramp-like pains, vomiting and faintness; the degree of disturbance varies. Prevention of constipation, plenty of exercise and rest on the first day of menstruation with a hot-water bottle to relieve discomfort may be all that is needed. If the condition is not controlled by these means or by simple analgesia, hormone treatment may be started or, very occasionally, a dilatation and curettage. In those patients in whom the dysmenorrhoea is very distressing, denervation of the uterus may be carried out but this is a major operation and is avoided if possible. *Secondary dysmenorrhoea* is usually the result of pelvic disease such as inflammatory conditions, endometriosis, uterine displacements or tumours. The woman develops dysmenorrhoea after many years of painless menstruation. The cause is treated.

Premenstrual tension

Prior to menstruation there is retention of fluid in the body and in some women oedema of the ankles or abdominal distension may be present. Many women find that they are more irritable or emotional the week before they menstruate.

Menorrhagia

An increased menstrual flow, either in amount or in the number of days, this may arise due to endocrine disturbances or local conditions such as fibroids, displacements or inflammations of the uterus and pelvic organs. An examination is carried out under anaesthetic and the cause treated.

Metrorrhagia or intermenstrual bleeding

This occurs as bleeding unconnected with menstruation. Carcinoma of the body of the uterus, cervix, vagina or urethra may all cause this type of bleeding and therefore it must always be investigated. Ulceration of the vagina, erosion of the cervix and chronic cervicitis or a urethral caruncle may also be more benign causes. The cause is treated.

Postmenopausal bleeding

Bleeding once menstruation has ceased is also a sign of the above conditions and must therefore be fully investigated and the cause treated.

BENIGN TUMOURS OF THE UTERUS

Fibromyomata (fibroids)

The most common tumour of the uterus is the benign myoma. It originates in the muscle as either a tiny single seedling or a number of seedlings and can grow as large as a football. The majority of these myomata remain in the muscle wall (intramuscular or intramural), but occasionally they grow outwards towards the peritoneal cavity (subserous) or in towards the uterine cavity (submucous). Submucous and subserous myomata may develop a peduncle or stalk.

The tumour consists of involuntary muscle and connective tissue and is most common in women between the ages of 35 and 50 who have not had children.

Clinical picture

This will depend on the site of the tumour, its size, whether it is pedunculated, and how many there are. Frequently there are no symptoms. However, as the tumour grows in size the abdomen becomes enlarged, and subserous myomata are associated with heavy menstrual periods (menorrhagia) because of the increased vascularity of the uterus and the presence of a hyperplastic endometrium, possibly due to an imbalance of oestrogen. Anaemia is therefore frequently present as well. Some women complain of spasmodic dysmenorrhoea. As the tumour increases in size it may press on the bladder or bowel, causing frequency of micturition or constipation, and there may be backache.

If the tumour has a pedicle, this may become twisted, so cutting off its blood supply and causing necrosis. A submucous myoma can cause infertility, either by interfering with the implantation of the fertilised ovum or because of distortion of the uterine cavity causing an abortion. The tumour may develop cysts, become calcified or necrotic and, very rarely, it may develop malignant changes.

Treatment

This is only necessary if the tumour has reached the size of a 14-week pregnancy or is causing menorrhagia or pressure symptoms. If the tumour is large or there are many of them and the woman no longer wants to bear children, a hysterectomy will be undertaken. However, if the woman is under 40 and wants further children and there are no other complications, a myomectomy will be carried out.

Polypi

These may occur either in the cervix following chronic cervicitis or from the endometrium in the body of the uterus. Cervical polypi cause bleeding following intercourse and are removed by being twisted on their pedicle (avulsed). Uterine polyps cause menorrhagia or metrorrhagia and are removed by curettage.

MALIGNANT TUMOURS OF THE UTERUS

Carcinoma of the cervix

This is the second most frequent form of cancer in women, carcinoma of the breast being the most common. It is more frequent than carcinoma of the body of the uterus and occurs most commonly in those who have had frequent sexual intercourse when young, although the condition may not be diagnosed until after the age of 40. It is classified as follows.

Stage 0—carcinoma in situ: in which there are abnormal cells on the surface of the cervix but the latter has not been invaded. It is diagnosed by a cervical smear (Fig. 33.1), punch biopsy, cone biopsy or colposcopy. There are no symptoms. Treatment is by cone biopsy, but in a number of cases this can result in haemorrhage or infection. Follow-up of the patients after this procedure is essential, and if there is any recurrence of the abnormal cells, a total hysterectomy and removal of a cuff of the vagina are carried out. Cryotherapy or laser ablative therapy can now be used under a local anaesthetic in out-patients.

Stage I: the disease is confined to the cervix.

Stage II: the disease spreads to the body of the uterus and the upper vagina. There may still be no signs at this stage, although bleeding after intercourse may be present. Treatment at this stage and at stage I is by the insertion of radium or caesium, pelvic irradiation or a Wertheim's hysterectomy.

Stage III: invasion of the lower vagina or pelvic walls.

Stage IV: involvement of the bladder or rectum with metastases to other organs via the lymphatics. There may now be an offensive discharge and pain and the condition is inoperable, although radiotherapy may relieve symptoms.

Carcinoma of the body of the uterus

This condition arises from the endometrial lining of the uterus, usually after the menopause. It is more common in those who have no children. It spreads to the lymph nodes of the pelvis, ovaries,

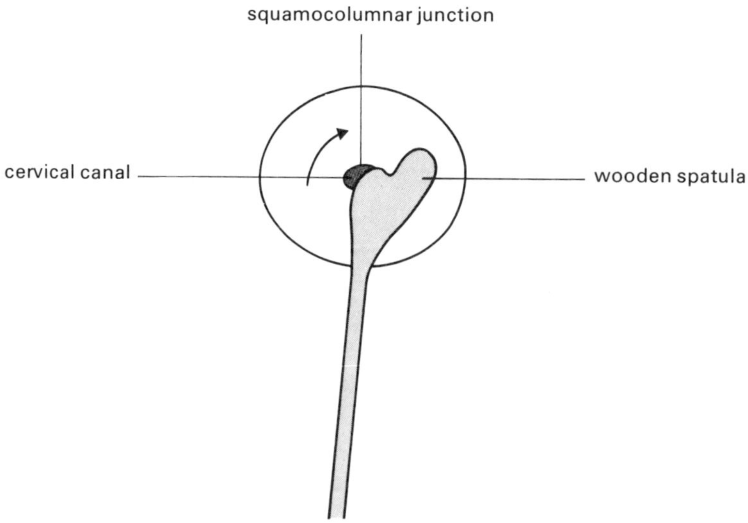

Fig. 33.1 *Taking a cervical smear.*

rectum, bladder, intestines and peritoneal cavity but does not usually metastasise to other parts of the body.

Clinical picture

Bleeding continues after the menopause, the vaginal discharge being profuse, blood-stained and offensive and occurring at a fairly early stage. Pain is a late symptom.

Management

If diagnosed early enough, a total hysterectomy is done with a bilateral oophorectomy and removal of the upper third of the vagina. The lymph glands are checked for any evidence of the spread of the disease and if present radiotherapy will be used on the pelvis. In inoperable cases hormone therapy may be employed.

Sarcoma

This type of cancer is rare but spreads rapidly to the bladder, rectum, ovaries and peritoneum. It sometimes develops from myomata. The prognosis is poor as the symptoms do not appear until late. Treatment will be by means of a Wertheim's hysterectomy if the sarcoma is operable. Cytotoxic drugs may be used.

Chorion epithelioma (malignant trophoblastic tumour)

A small part of the chorion, the outer membrane surrounding the fetus, may persist and continue to invade the uterine tissue. At the same time it will produce the hormone chorionic gonadotrophin. More than half of the tumours occur following a hydatidiform mole (Fig. 33.2), the remainder follow an abortion or pregnancy. A hydatidiform mole (benign trophoblastic tumour) is a benign tumour of the placenta which is full of grape-like vesicles. No fetus is present, and the abdomen is usually larger than the woman's dates would suggest. Vaginal bleeding is present. Ultrasonic echo scanning shows an absence of fetal parts. The urine is strongly positive to the pregnancy test. If the woman wishes to have further children, she will be allowed to expel the mole spontaneously or if necessary be given Pitocin to encourage its expulsion. Five days later a curettage is performed to ensure the uterus is empty. In older women a hysterectomy will be done. For the next year at least the woman is followed up with dilute pregnancy tests to exclude the development of chorion epithelioma. She is also advised not to become pregnant during this time.

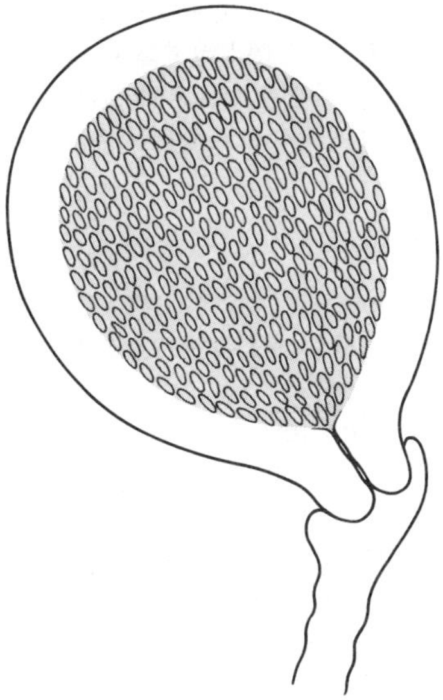

Fig. 33.2 *Hydatidiform mole.*

Chorion epithelioma is highly malignant and will rapidly spread to the lungs, brain, liver, intestines or vagina. The symptoms are the same as those of the benign tumour, although evidence of metastases may also be present. The earlier the tumour is treated and the more radical the treatment, the more likely it is to be effective. In the early stages a hysterectomy and the administration of cytotoxic drugs before and after the operation appear to be the most effective means of control. If the disease has spread, cytotoxic drugs alone will be used unless bleeding from the uterus is a problem in which case a hysterectomy will also be done. The cytotoxic drugs most commonly used are intravenous methotrexate with intramuscular folinic acid to prevent some of the side-effects, or intravenous actinomycin D. The patient is followed up for at least 2 years to check for any recurrence of the growth, and is advised to avoid pregnancy during this period.

DYSFUNCTIONAL UTERINE BLEEDING (METROPATHIA HAEMORRHAGICA)

In this condition there is abnormal uterine bleeding for which no cause can be found. It is associated with an excess production of oestrogen and therefore the administration of progesterone may be effective. It may be necessary in the older woman to do a hysterectomy.

ENDOMETRIOSIS

Small amounts of endometrium are present in abnormal sites such as the ovaries, which undergo the same cyclical changes as the endometrium in the uterus. The patient complains of irregularities of menstruation and dysmenorrhoea, the condition being diagnosed by laparoscopy or laparotomy. Hormone therapy is used to suppress the activity of the ovaries, and is continued for up to 12 months. If it is not effective, surgical treatment may be necessary. In the younger woman who still wishes to have children, as much of the endometrial cyst is removed as possible. However, in older women not responding to hormone treatment, a total hysterectomy will be done and this may also be accompanied by an oophorectomy.

ENDOMETRITIS

Infection of the endometrium may arise following delivery of an infant or an abortion if there is retention of some of the placenta or the products of conception. It may also develop following a uterine operation, gonococcal infection or growths. It is treated by drainage and antibiotics, and the woman is also checked for malignancy.

CERVICITIS

This may arise following damage to the cervix through a pregnancy, a dilatation and curettage, or gonorrhoea. The stratified epithelium which normally covers the cervix is replaced by columnar epithelium and this causes the cervix to appear red and swollen. Although it is frequently seen at the first postnatal examination, spontaneous recovery may occur. However, if the woman is complaining of a profuse discharge which has lasted for several weeks, treatment will be necessary. This consists of destroying the surface cells with diathermy, cauterisation or cryosurgery (freezing). The patient will have a heavy discharge following these procedures as the destroyed tissue is lost. Because of the risk of secondary haemorrhage 1 or 2 weeks after the procedure, the woman is advised not to have sexual intercourse for a month. The condition may become chronic.

CERVICAL ECTROPION

The cervix may develop a split in it following childbirth, and there may also be a discharge. It may be necessary to suture the split edges together, which is called a trachelorrhaphy.

OPERATIONS FOR DISEASES OF THE UTERUS AND CERVIX

The main aim in this type of surgery is to preserve as much function as is possible, particularly in women still in the childbearing age group. Nearer the menopause or after it, it may be preferable to do more radical surgery. However, if malignancy is present, whatever the age of the woman, radical surgery will be inevitable.

Vaginal hysterectomy

A total hysterectomy may be done vaginally and can also include removal of the ovaries and Fallopian tubes. The uterus is removed via the vagina and the vaginal walls are repaired. There is no abdominal wound.

Total hysterectomy

This may be done either abdominally or vaginally and consists of removing the uterus and the cervix. The ovaries and Fallopian tubes may be removed at the same time. It may be done for fibroids or endometriosis.

Wertheim's hysterectomy

The uterus, ovaries and Fallopian tubes plus the upper third of the vagina and pelvic lymphatic glands are removed for carcinoma of the uterine body.

Myomectomy

This operation is carried out to shell out individual fibroids which are removed through an incision.

Dilatation and curettage

The cervical canal is dilated with dilators of increasing size and the lining of the uterus scraped with a curette (Fig. 33.3).

Evulsion of polypi

If the polypi are within the uterine cavity, the cervix is dilated, a polypus is then held in sponge-holding forceps and the pedicle twisted until the polypus separates.

Hysterotomy

The uterine cavity is opened either abdominally or vaginally in order to remove its contents, usually a fetus.

SPECIFIC NURSING CARE OF AN ABDOMINAL HYSTERECTOMY

Preoperatively

The effect of removal of the uterus will be explained, and if the ovaries are to be retained the woman can be reassured that she will not have an early menopause. If a malignant condition is present, investigations will be carried out to exclude spread to other organs. The haemoglobin will be

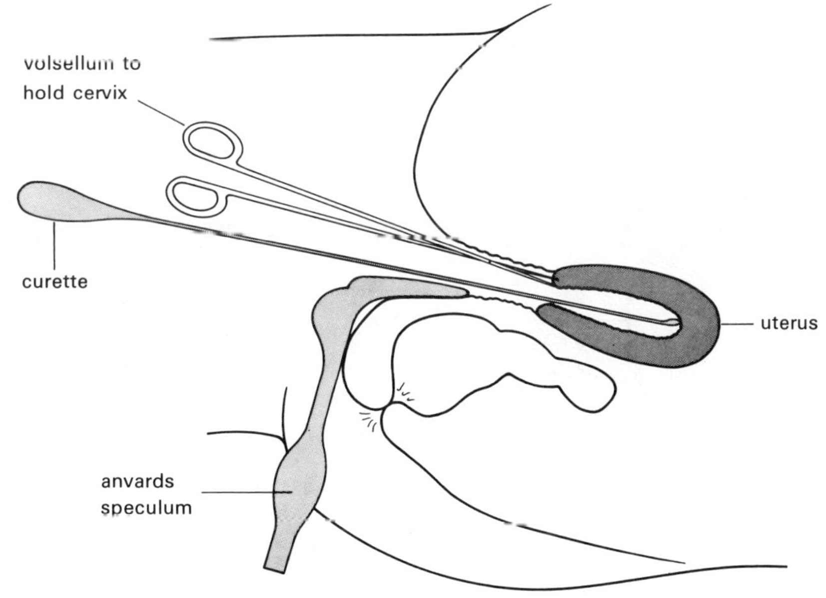

Fig. 33.3 *Dilatation and curettage.*

checked and a midstream specimen of urine sent to the laboratory for culture and sensitivity. Any anaemia or urinary infection is treated. The abdomen and pubic area will be shaved.

Postoperatively

The patient usually returns from theatre with a urinary catheter in position and may also have a vaginal pack. The latter is removed after 24 to 48 hours but the catheter is left in position for at least a week. The patient is cared for in the same way as for any other abdominal operation, fluids being commenced by mouth once the bowel sounds are present. Complications are those of an abdominal operation, although urinary problems and deep vein thrombosis are also common.

DISPLACEMENTS OF THE UTERUS

The uterus in the adult woman is normally in an anteverted and anteflexed position. During development it may not progress from the retroverted position.

Retroversion

This may also occur in the presence of endometriosis, adhesions or tumours. There are usually no symptoms, although it may cause infertility or abortion. If infection is present, the woman may complain of dysmenorrhoea and backache. Treatment is either by means of inserting a Hodge's pessary or by surgery to shorten the round ligaments.

Uterovaginal prolapse

Following childbirth there is some relaxation of the vagina which is normal, but any more descent of the uterus is abnormal. The uterus is always retroverted to some extent before it prolapses. The prolapse may be of various types (Fig. 33.4).

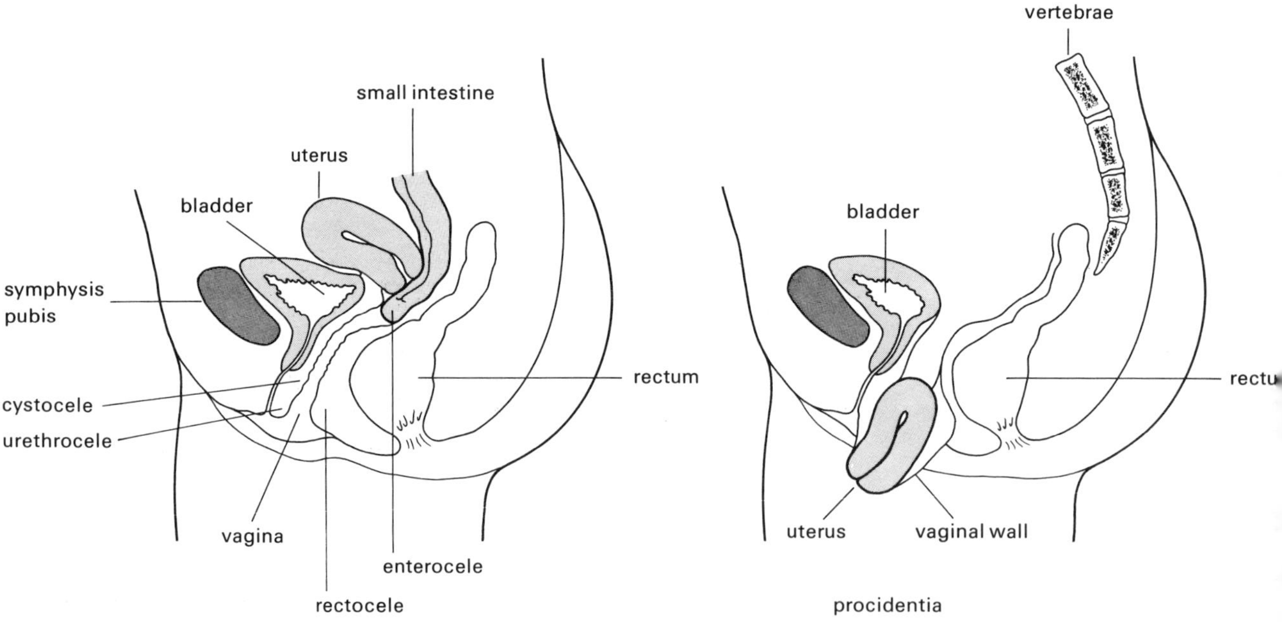

Fig. 33.4 *Types of prolapse.*

Cystocele

The anterior vaginal wall protrudes downwards, the base of the bladder bulging into it. It is frequently associated with an *urethrocele* in which the urethra bulges into the lower part of the vagina.

Rectocele

This involves descent of the posterior vaginal wall, into which the rectum bulges. If the pouch of Douglas herniates into the posterior vaginal wall containing small intestine, it is called an *enterocele*.

Procidentia

The vaginal walls are completely turned inside out and the uterus lies partly or completely outside the vagina. It may also distort the ureters causing an obstruction and back pressure of urine in the kidney.

Clinical features

As the uterus descends it produces a sensation of fulness in the vagina—'something coming down'. Low back pain can occasionally be caused by the traction of the ligaments. If the bladder or urethra is involved, micturition may be affected. The woman may complain of frequency, difficulty in passing urine or *stress* incontinence, incontinence of urine when the intra-abdominal pressure is raised, as in coughing or laughing. If the rectum or small intestine is involved, there may be difficulty with defaecation. The prolapsed vagina may become ulcerated or inflamed, so causing bleeding or discharge. The symptoms are usually worse on standing and relieved by lying down.

Management

If the woman is unable to have an operation, a ring pessary may be used to hold the uterus in position, and this is removed and inspected every 3 to 4 months. Usually the prolapse is treated by a repair operation carried out via the vaginal route; occasionally a hysterectomy is required.

Anterior colporrhaphy

The excess mucous membrane of the anterior vaginal wall is removed. The base of the bladder is then replaced upwards into its normal position and fixed there by sutures.

Posterior colpoperineorrhaphy

The excess mucous membrane of the posterior vaginal wall is removed. The perineum is then restored by stitching together the two levator ani muscles. The vaginal mucous membrane and skin are then sutured, a subcuticular stitch usually being used for the latter. These two operations may be combined, the cervix also being amputated and the transverse cervical ligaments shortened—a *Manchester repair*. In some patients a vaginal hysterectomy may be done and a repair in which the pelvic ligaments are sewn together.

Specific nursing care

Preoperatively

If there is much oedema of the prolapsed organs, the patient will be admitted several days prior to the operation and will remain in bed. A midstream specimen of urine will be taken to check for urinary infection which if present is treated. A high vaginal swab may be taken to rule out vaginal infection and if there is a discharge, a vaginal douche or pessaries given. Adequate preparation of the bowel is essential, especially if a posterior repair is to be done.

Postoperatively

If an anterior repair has been done, a catheter is usually introduced in theatre and is left in for 7 days. It is required because retention frequently occurs. A vaginal pack may be in position if a Manchester repair has been done, and this will be removed after 24 or 48 hours. When it is removed the patient must be observed carefully for haemorrhage, particularly if she has been taking contraceptives or the operation was done immediately prior to menstruation. The perineal wound in a posterior repair should be kept dry but the catgut sutures will dissolve and only require removing if oedema is present. A bowel action is avoided for the first few days postoperatively following a posterior repair, after which a mild aperient will be given, the perineum being cleaned after a bowel action. The patient usually begins taking daily baths 24 to 48 hours after operation, and gets up the day following operation.

Complications

The possible complications include urinary retention, urinary infection, vesicovaginal fistula, pelvic and perineal haematomas, surgical emphysema, deep vein thrombosis and paralytic ileus. The last-mentioned can occur even following a vaginal operation. If the bladder is injured, surgical emphysema may develop in the lower abdomen. A deep vein thrombosis can develop either in the veins of the legs or in the pelvic veins and may lead to a pulmonary embolism.

Advice on discharge

The woman should be advised to avoid heavy lifting for at least 3 months, not to stand for long periods and not to resume sexual relations for 6 weeks. She will be given an out-patient's appointment for 3 months later, at which time she will be checked for dispareunia, continuing stress incontinence and the presence of a fistula.

OVARIAN TUMOURS AND CYSTS

The majority of ovarian tumours are benign and cystic. They may arise from the normal development of the follicle, in which the latter continues to grow in size, or similarly from the corpus luteum after ovulation. These are called *functional cysts*, and only require surgery if they persist for more than 3 months.

Pseudomucinous cysts

These cysts are usually found in one ovary and do not affect the menstrual cycle. They may become very big, consisting of many lobes which contain a dark green fluid or slimy white material (pseudomucin). The lobes may rupture, spilling the contents into the abdominal cavity so that the cells grow on the peritoneum and secrete pseudomucin. This condition is known as pseudomyxoma peritonei. Daughter cysts may also develop. The cysts are removed surgically with as much of the ovary being preserved as possible in the younger woman.

Serous cysts

These are thin-walled cysts with only one lobe which may affect both ovaries but only grow to a moderate size. About one-third of them become malignant. Preservation of the ovary is attempted in the younger woman but removal of both ovaries, Fallopian tubes and a total hysterectomy are usually done in the woman over 40.

Teratomata or dermoid cysts

These cysts contain all the three embryonic layers and may contain hair, bone and teeth. They occur in the younger woman and therefore an ovarian cystectomy is usually done.

Endometriomata (chocolate cysts)

These are not as common as the cysts already mentioned and are described under endometriosis (see p. 244). There are also a very small number of benign growths which are formed of connective tissue and are therefore not cystic.

Malignant tumours of the ovary

These constitute a very small percentage of all ovarian tumours, the majority of them arising due to malignant changes in serous cysts, although other types of cyst may undergo these changes also. A small proportion are metastases from the breast or gastrointestinal tract. These tumours grow rapidly and usually cause the development of ascites. The uterus, ovaries and Fallopian tubes will be removed by surgery and this will be followed by radiotherapy or chemotherapy. If ascites is present, a paracentesis abdominis will be necessary to remove the fluid with a cannula.

There are also two rare tumours, one of which has a masculinising effect and the other a feminising effect; both are treated by removal.

Clinical picture of an ovarian cyst

The abdomen becomes enlarged and symptoms may arise due to pressure on the bladder or bowel, so causing frequency, difficulty in passing urine or constipation. If the cyst is on a pedicle, it may become twisted on itself (torsion), leading to gangrene. If it ruptures, secondary growths may develop on the peritoneum. Both torsion and rupture will lead to peritonitis and shock.

Ovariectomy is the term usually used for removal of a diseased ovary and *oophorectomy* for the removal of a healthy ovary. An *ovarian cystectomy* involves removal of a cyst from an ovary.

ACUTE SALPINGITIS

This condition arises as a result of infection in the Fallopian tubes and usually involves both tubes and the ovaries. It may be the result of infection in the vagina and uterus spreading to the tubes, infection from the adjacent pelvic cavity or via the bloodstream. Therefore gonorrhoea, septic abortion, a retained placenta and appendicitis may all be causes.

Clinical picture

The woman has a high temperature and complains of a severe pain in the iliac fossa and generally feels unwell. She finds a pelvic examination very painful.

Management

Because of the type of infection, barrier nursing is implemented. Rest is necessary while the temperature is raised. A vaginal swab is taken for culture and sensitivity and large doses of the appropriate antibiotic commenced either intravenously or intramuscularly. Analgesics and local application of heat will be necessary to relieve the pain, and fluids are encouraged. Vulval swabbing will be necessary while the woman is in bed. If the condition is not treated early enough, it may lead to a pelvic peritonitis, hydrosalpinx, pyosalpinx, infertility, ectopic pregnancy or chronic salpingitis.

CHRONIC SALPINGITIS

The woman is in a state of general ill-health and complains of dysmenorrhoea, menorrhagia and dyspareunia. She may have episodes of pelvic pain and her temperature may be raised.

Management

The initial treatment involves rest and antibiotics. Once the patient is fit enough, the uterus, Fallopian tubes and as much of the ovaries as is necessary, are removed. Removal of the Fallopian tubes is called a salpingectomy.

PELVIC PERITONITIS

This may follow any infection of the genital tract or the lower gastrointestinal tract. Therefore acute salpingitis, ruptured ectopic pregnancy, ruptured dermoid cysts and conditions such as appendicitis may be causes. If the infection is contained within the pouch of Douglas, a pelvic abscess forms. The patient is extremely ill with a swinging temperature and diarrhoea.

Management

Bedrest is maintained while the temperature remains raised. Large doses of antibiotics are given and an incision is made in the posterior fornix of the vagina to drain the abscess (posterior culdotomy). The patient should sit up to encourage drainage, and strict attention is paid to vulval hygiene with frequent changes of sterile sanitary pads.

CONDITIONS OF THE VULVA

Pruritus vulvae

Itching of the vulval area may arise due to a number of disorders such as: skin diseases or fungal infections; discharge from the vagina, urethra or Bartholin's gland; diabetes mellitus; allergies to soap, douches, spermicidal cream or nylon tights; threadworms, lice or scabies; carcinoma of the vulva; vulval congestion during pregnancy or at the menopause due to the alteration in the levels of hormones; kraurosis vulvae, a degenerative condition in which the tissues shrink causing the vagina to become narrowed; and psychological factors. Leucoplakia also causes pruritus vulvae, the epithelium of the labia, the clitoris and the fourchette becoming thickened and later shiny, cracked and fissured, as if the parts had become covered in white paint. This is considered to be a precancerous condition.

If the irritation has caused eczema of the vulva, groins and inner thighs, it is usually called intertrigo.

Treatment

If possible, the cause is found and treated. Regular washing of the area with plain water after passing urine is encouraged, but soap is avoided. The woman is advised to wear cotton pants and avoid tights. Oestrogens may be given to the post-menopausal patient and a night sedation to ensure a sound sleep. Local applications such as antihistamine or cortisone cream or a dusting powder may be applied. If none of these is effective and there are changes in the cells of the skin, a simple vulvectomy will be done in which the labia majora, minora and clitoris are removed.

Benign tumours

Infective warts or papillomata are treated with an application of 20% podophyllin in tinc. benz. co. to each wart. The application is washed off after 8 hours. If this is ineffective, diathermy is used.

Fibromata and lipomata may also occur and these are usually removed surgically if necessary.

Carcinoma of the vulva

This is a squamous cell carcinoma of the skin and appears as one or more nodules or warts. There may be irritation of the vulva and the skin of the vulva may be altered in appearance. A discharge or slight bleeding may be present. Several biopsies are taken from the affected area to confirm the diagnosis.

Treatment

A radical vulvectomy is done in which the whole of the vulva is removed, the fat of the femoral triangle and the pelvic lymph nodes.

Specific postoperative care

In a simple vulvectomy the skin edges are drawn together, but in the radical operation this is not usually possible and therefore there is a large area of tissue which will have to heal by granulation. A catheter is normally left in position for 5 to 10 days to keep the area clean, and non-adhesive dressings are applied. A bowel action may also be avoided for the first 5 days, and therefore a low-residue diet may be given. As there is a tendency to shock, the patient may come back from theatre with a blood transfusion in progress. Antibiotics may be prescribed to prevent wound infection or urinary tract infection. While the patient remains in bed she will be nursed on her back, and therefore breathing exercises and leg exercises will be necessary to prevent complications. Once up she may start daily baths.

Bartholin's cyst

On each side of the vaginal orifice are two glands and their ducts which may become blocked due to inflammation or infection with *Esch. coli* or gonococcus. The glands become distended and if the infection is not resolved, a Bartholin's abscess may develop.

The patient complains of acute pain in the vulva and a red swelling can be seen. Treatment is by antibiotics. If an abscess develops, *marsupialisation* is necessary. In this procedure the surgeon opens the gland and sews the edges to the vaginal wall to enable it to drain. A pack is left in for 48 hours. If a chronic retention cyst is present, it is completely excised by dissection.

Vesicovaginal fistula

A tract is present between the rectum and vagina, usually as a result of a third-degree tear following a difficult delivery, surgery or radiotherapy. Incontinence of urine or faeces is present. Small fistulae may not be visible on examination with a speculum and it may be necessary to introduce a dye into the bladder after inserting three swabs into the vagina. The level at which the swabs are stained will then give an indication of the fistula's position. A vesicovaginal fistula requires a catheter to be inserted and to remain draining for 2 to 3 weeks. Postoperatively it is particularly important to ensure that the catheter is draining adequately. Prior to an operation to repair a vesicovaginal fistula, the patient should be prepared in the same way as for any operation on the gastrointestinal tract. Following the operation a low-residue diet is given to prevent the bowels being open for 5 days, thus allowing healing to take place, after which liquid paraffin or a similar aperient is given.

INFERTILITY AND DISORDERS OF EARLY PREGNANCY

The ova are formed in the Graafian follicles of the ovaries, and when a follicle ruptures the ovum is released into the fimbriated end of the Fallopian tube. As it travels along the Fallopian tube it will come into contact with any spermatozoa which have reached this point from the vagina where they have been deposited by the male. One of these spermatozoa enters the ovum and fertilises it.

The fertilised ovum starts dividing into a ball of cells (morula) and at the same time is propelled along the Fallopian tube by peristalsis and the action of the cilia. About 7 days after fertilisation the morula reaches the uterine cavity. At this point it consists of an amniotic cavity containing amniotic fluid and the developing embryo. The outer layer of cells (the trophoblast) burrows into the endometrium, penetrating to the blood capillaries from which nourishment for the developing fetus is gained.

These processes are under the influence of progesterone from the corpus luteum in the ovary which also causes the endometrium to become thicker and more vascular. The trophoblast undergoes changes, eventually, after the twelfth week, becoming the placenta which is attached to the fetus by the umbilical cord. The latter contains two arteries, through which the fetus receives its nourishment from the mother's circulatory system, and one vein. The fetus, which is recognisable by 6 to 8 weeks after fertilisation, is surrounded by fluid and enclosed in two membranes, the amnion and the outer chorion.

Infertility

Nearly a third of all cases of infertility are due to some problem in the male partner and therefore a seminal fluid analysis is done, after which, if it is satisfactory, the female is investigated.

Infertility may arise due to infrequent ovulation by the ovaries, blockage of the Fallopian tubes following salpingitis, fibromyomata (fibroids), widespread endometriosis or more general diseases such as myxoedema or diabetes.

Investigations

The woman is asked to take and record her temperature each day before getting up. If ovulation has taken place, there should be a rise of 0.5°C in the last 14 days of the cycle. An examination of the cervical mucus will also show changes during ovulation. The blood progesterone level is also recorded. A full general medical examination is done to rule out endocrine and other diseases.

Laparoscopy This examination is carried out prior to the menstrual period. Following a general anaesthetic, the abdominal cavity is inflated with carbon dioxide or nitrous oxide gas to allow the intestines to rise out of the pelvic cavity. The laparoscope is then introduced through a small incision in the abdominal wall, so enabling the surgeon to see the pelvic organs.

Hysterosalpingography A radio-opaque dye is injected through the cervix, and its passage observed under x-ray. The process is carried out during the first 10 days of the cycle, and if necessary a general anaesthetic can be given.

Postcoital test This test is done to see if the cervix is producing antibodies against the sperm. A specimen of the cervical mucus is taken at the time of ovulation and up to 12 hours after intercourse, and is examined under a microscope to see the number of motile sperm. The test is repeated on further cycles and, if negative on three occasions, the semen is tested against the cervical mucus. Blood prolactin levels are also recorded as a high level of prolactin in the blood will cause infertility.

Treatment

If reduced ovulation is the cause, clomiphene or human gonadotrophins may be prescribed. The former may give rise to twin pregnancies and the latter, if not carefully controlled, to multiple pregnancies. A high serum prolactin may be reduced with bromocriptine. Tubal blockage may be treated surgically but at present this is not very successful. If there are adhesions around the tubes, these can be removed (salpinolysis). An opening can be made at the end of the tube (salpingostomy), the blockage may be removed and the two ends of the tube joined together (tubal anastomosis and reimplantation). Other means of overcoming infertility are in-vitro fertilisation and artificial insemination. The former is done when the Fallopian tubes are blocked or have been removed and the latter for impotence or hypospadia in the male.

Abortion

The expulsion of the fetus before the twenty-eighth week of pregnancy is termed an abortion. Premature labour is the term used if labour commences between the twenty-eighth week and term. However, a fetus of less than 32 weeks is unlikely to survive.

Spontaneous abortion

This is the most common complication of pregnancy and is known to be nature's way of getting rid of abnormal fertilised ova, although there may be other causes. Any abnormality in the balance of oestrogen and progesterone will prevent the fertilised ovum from embedding in the uterus. Maternal disease and infection or damage to the cervix are other causes. Tumours and congenital abnormalities of the female tract may also cause an abortion, and trauma or severe fright or shock may precipitate labour.

Threatened abortion

In this there is uterine bleeding which may be quite heavy but there are no uterine contractions, or very weak ones. On examination the cervix is closed. The treatment is rest and in some cases progesterone is given.

Inevitable abortion

Uterine bleeding is heavy and there are painful uterine contractions. On examination the cervix is found to be dilated. The membranes may rupture. This will either go on to a *complete abortion* in which all the products of conception are expelled, or an *incomplete abortion* in which the membranes and placenta are partly or completely retained but the fetus is expelled.

In the latter case the uterus is evacuated under a general anaesthetic. A blood transfusion may be necessary to replace the blood lost, and intramuscular ergometrine is given to control bleeding.

Habitual abortion

Some women appear unable to carry a pregnancy to full term and suffer from repeated abortion. This may be due to the incompetence of the cervix, and is treated by the insertion of a Shirodkhar suture around the cervix to hold it closed. The suture has to be removed before the birth of the baby.

Induced abortion

Illegal termination of an unwanted pregnancy by an individual not abiding by the terms of the law is called a criminal abortion. The introduction of instruments or very strong douches may provide a very serious risk of septic abortion, profound shock, acute renal failure or death. A therapeutic abortion is done if two registered medical practitioners are agreed that it is necessary on the grounds of medical, psychological or social reasons. The later this is performed in the pregnancy the more hazardous it is. The Department of Health must be notified of the details. The products of conception may be removed by curettage or suction if early enough, otherwise a hysterotomy will be necessary. A septic abortion will require treatment with antibiotics and a blood transfusion as well as evacuation of the uterus.

Extrauterine pregnancy (ectopic gestation)

An extrauterine pregnancy is one in which the fertilised ovum is not embedded in the uterus but at another site (Fig. 33.5). In the majority of cases this is in the Fallopian tubes, but on rare occasions it can also occur in the abdominal cavity, the broad ligament, cervix or ovary.

Those that occur in the Fallopian tubes usually do so because the tubes have some abnormality which prevents the fertilised ovum passing along them. This may be due to chronic inflammation from gonorrhoea or other pelvic infection, kinking or spasm of the tubes. If the fertilised ovum continues to develop within the Fallopian tube, the tube will rupture, causing the woman severe loss of blood and shock. Sometimes the fertilised ovum is expelled into the peritoneal cavity through the fimbriated end of the tube. Again haemorrhage and shock may occur. Should an abdominal pregnancy occur, it is unlikely to result in a normal fully developed baby because the fetus is not protected by the uterus. It is also a serious risk to the mother, leading to abdominal haemorrhage, and the fetus is therefore removed surgically.

Clinical picture

The patient may have recognised the symptoms of pregnancy such as amenorrhoea, nausea, vomiting and discomfort in the breasts. There may also be a small amount of vaginal bleeding. Occasionally patients may complain of fainting attacks or pain in the shoulder from the effects of the blood in the abdominal cavity on the phrenic nerve. In a ruptured ectopic pregnancy the patient is severely shocked, white and has a rigid, tender abdomen.

Management

If a tubal pregnancy is suspected, a laparoscopy or laparotomy is done to confirm the diagnosis, and if present the whole of the tube is removed. A ruptured tubal pregnancy is a surgical emergency, the tube being removed and a blood transfusion given to replace lost blood and restore the blood pressure. Postoperatively urinary output must be

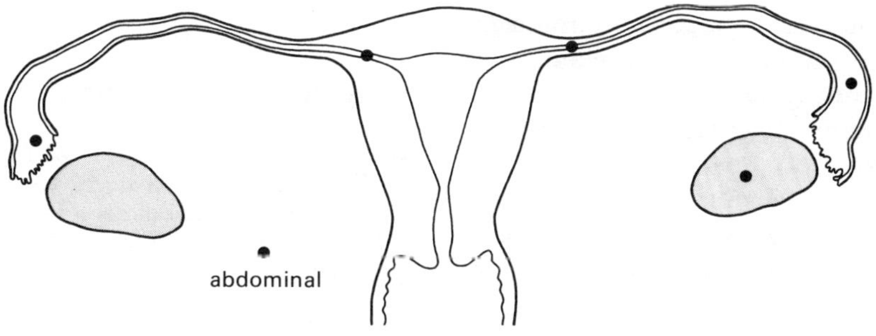

Fig. 33.5 *Sites where an ectopic pregnancy may develop.*

monitored carefully as the severe shock may cause renal failure.

Advice on discharge

The woman must be told that her chances of conceiving are reduced and there is the possibility of another ectopic pregnancy in the other tube and therefore she should seek medical advice early if she does become pregnant.

Caesarean section

Caesarean section is the removal of the baby, placenta and membranes through the abdominal wall. It is carried out if a vaginal delivery is dangerous for the mother or baby. Therefore, if there is disproportion between the size of the baby and the size of the mother's pelvis, signs of fetal distress or the baby is lying in a difficult presentation, a caesarean section will be carried out. It will also be necessary if the mother has diabetes, severe toxaemia, tumours in the uterus or pelvis or placenta praevia, in which the placenta is over the exit of the uterus.

The patient is prepared for abdominal surgery under a general anaesthetic, although local or spinal anaesthesia may be used. The bladder must be emptied. An incision is made transversely into the lower abdomen and another in the peritoneum, after which the lower part of the uterus is incised. The baby is delivered through this opening, the cord is clamped and cut and the baby handed to the midwife for resuscitation. Ergometrine is given intravenously to stimulate contractions and the placenta and membranes are removed. The cervix is dilated with the surgeon's finger to aid drainage postoperatively, and the uterus, peritoneum and abdominal wound are sutured.

The specific postoperative care is that for an abdominal gynaecological operation. The most common complication is haemorrhage; sepsis may also develop if the membranes are not completely removed from the uterine cavity. Paralytic ileus is another hazard due to the spillage of liquor amnii and blood into the peritoneal cavity and deep vein thrombosis and infection of the wound are other complications.

The woman may be able to have her next baby by vaginal delivery, depending on the reason for the caesarean section, but the delivery must take place in hospital because (very rarely) the uterus may rupture, in which case a hysterectomy is necessary.

STERILISATION

In some patients further pregnancies are contraindicated due to some medical condition. Although contraceptives such as the pill, intrauterine devices or occlusive diaphragms may be used, none is 100% effective. Therefore it may be considered preferable for the woman to be permanently sterilised, either by means of a laparoscope or by laparotomy. The Fallopian tubes can be cut or sealed by ligatures or diathermy. All of the implications of sterilisation must be fully discussed with the woman and her partner before the operation, as it can only rarely be reversed.

SUGGESTED WORK

1. Find out which are the most common gynaecological conditions treated in your hospital. Why is this so? Are there any other preventative measures that could be taken?

2. How well do the patients in your ward understand the function of their bodies? Are there any old wives' tales which are commonly believed?

SUGGESTED READING

Bailey R. E., Grayshon J. (1982). *Obstetric and Gynaecological Nursing*, 3rd edn. Nurses' Aids Series. London: Baillière Tindall.

Trevor W. (1973). *Elizabeth Alone*. London: Bodley Head.

34

Burns and Plastic Surgery

Extensive burns remove the protective covering of the body allowing large amounts of fluid to escape. They therefore very rapidly lead to shock and electrolyte imbalance and can lead to infection. They can also be very disfiguring. The nurse will therefore have to take strict precautions to prevent infection and will be involved in the accurate monitoring of fluid intake and output. She will also need to give psychological support and reassurance if disfigurement is present.

Specific emphasis in the nursing history

Skin. Extent of burns and other injuries.

Vital signs. TPR blood pressure.

Breathing. Note any difficulty, especially if burns of face.

Excretion. Note urinary output.

Mobility. Any joints affected? Need for being bedfast.

Social. Distance of relatives from hospital. Are there any difficulties in visiting?

Leisure pursuits. Look for a suitable pastime for the recovery phase.

BURNS

Burns are caused by dry heat from flames or the flash of exploding gas, corrosive chemicals, electricity, radioactivity, x-rays, friction and sunburn. Liquids and steam at a high temperature cause scalds which are usually more superficial, unless there is prolonged contact.

Burns are classified according to the extent of the surface skin involved and the depth or thickness of skin destroyed. The extent of the surface skin area affected is estimated by the 'rule of nines', (Fig. 34.1). Burns involving more than 15% of the surface area in an adult and 10% in a child will cause shock unless adequate preventative measures have been taken.

The depth or thickness of skin destroyed will affect the ability of the skin to regenerate and will also add to the degree of shock. A superficial or partial thickness burn will at the most affect the epidermis and part of the dermis. It will therefore heal without skin grafting unless infection occurs. A deep, or full thickness, burn includes the whole of the dermis and may also involve the underlying structures (Fig. 34.2).

The destruction of large areas of skin has two main effects. The first is that the natural barrier to infection has been removed and the presence of dead moist tissue enables bacteria to enter. The other effect is that the blood supply to the area increases and the capillaries become more permeable, allowing fluid and protein to leak from the circulation into the tissues causing oedema. Added to this the destruction of skin allows fluid and protein to escape from the surface of the body. The amount of fluid in the circulation is therefore reduced and the patient suffers from shock. Exposure of the nerve endings will cause pain and add to the shock. If the shock is severe and prolonged, acute renal failure will follow.

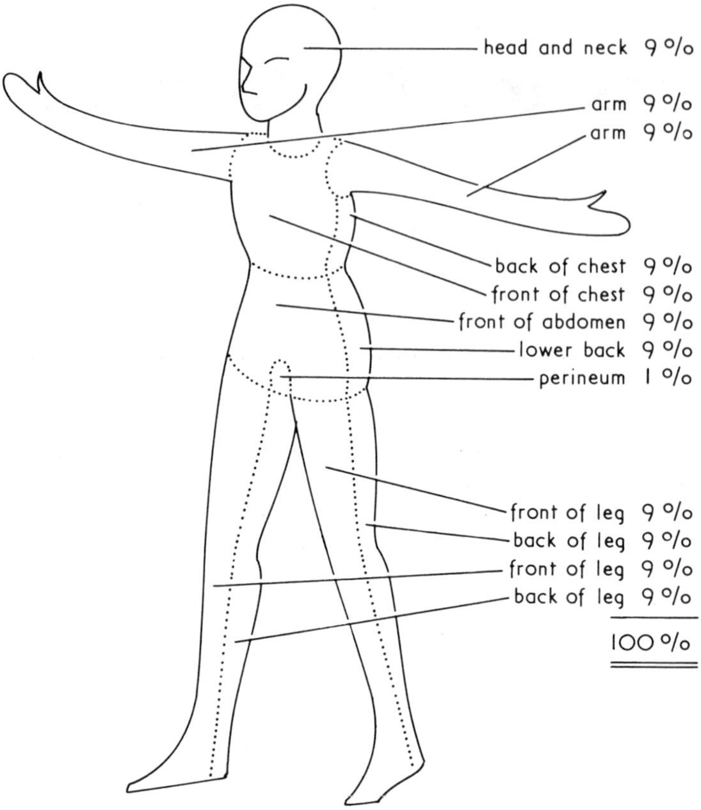

Fig. 34.1 *'Rule of nines'.*

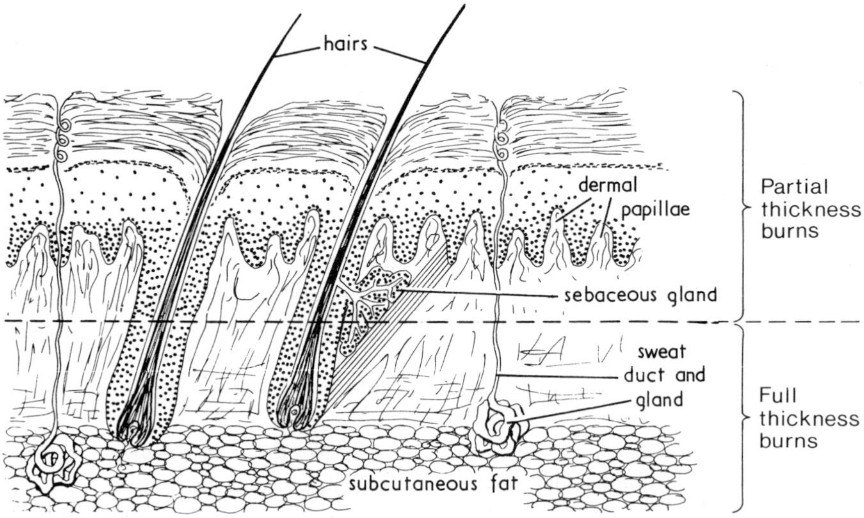

Fig. 34.2 *The extent of partial and full thickness burns.*

Treatment

The aim is to control shock, prevent infection and treat the burn. In order to control the shock an intravenous infusion of plasma or dextran—substances which do not leak from the circulation because of their large molecular size—is given. Sodium chloride 0.9% may also be used in conjunction with either of these. For each 9% of estimated loss, 1200 ml of fluid may be required. In serious burns 1500 ml are given in the first 8 hours, after which the patient's condition is assessed and, if required, a further 1500 ml are given in the following 12 hours. If after this period the patient has still not fully responded, a further 1500 ml will be given over the next 16 hours. Haematocrit readings, that is the proportion of cells to plasma, indicate the progress of the patient. Oral fluids with added dextrose are given in small amounts at half-hourly or hourly intervals, the patient being discouraged from drinking large amounts which may cause vomiting.

A strict fluid balance chart will be maintained and the insertion of a catheter may be required if the burns are extensive. A urinary output of more than 50 ml an hour in an adult is considered satisfactory. Analgesics must be given as required to control the pain or this will increase the shock. The pulse and blood pressure are monitored half-hourly until satisfactory. Observations of the temperature and respirations will also be necessary.

The wound is cleaned gently, blisters being snipped and loose tissue removed. If necessary, removal of dead tissue (debridement) may have to be done in theatre. The wound may then be covered with sterile Vaseline gauze and a firm crepe bandage. Dressings should be left undisturbed for as long as possible, but if they become soaked they should be changed or bacteria will enter. Many burns are treated by exposure and therefore if they are extensive, the patient will need to be nursed in a 'sterile' room, in which the room temperature is kept constant. Antibiotics may be given to prevent infection. If limbs are affected, they are elevated to reduce the oedema, and splints are applied to prevent contractures (Fig. 34.3).

If the patient's condition allows it, daily saline baths may be commenced. If full thickness burns are present, plastic surgery will be required and any contractures will need to be released. Once the patient is able to eat, a diet high in calories and protein will be encouraged, and if necessary a nasogastric tube passed. Subclavian feeding is occasionally necessary.

Complications

Contracture of joints.
Renal failure.
Septicaemia.
Electrolyte imbalance.
Pressure sores.
Respiratory involvement, particularly following burns of the face and chest.
Duodenal ulceration.
Gastric dilatation.
Intestinal ileus.
Anaemia.
Osteoporosis if bedrest is prolonged.

PLASTIC SURGERY

In this form of surgery the aim is to improve not only the function of a part but also the appearance. Sometimes it may be done purely for the cosmetic effects. It may be used to correct congenital abnormalities such as a cleft lip and palate, following extensive surgery for cancer of the jaw or larynx, after major burns, or on wounds or ulcers which fail to heal. The treatment may take some time and involve several operations, therefore the psychological support of the patient is very important.

There are various types of skin grafting which may be used depending on the extent of skin required and the need for a good cosmetic effect.

Free skin grafts

In these grafts the skin is completely detached from its donor area and transferred to the recipient area. These are divided according to the depth of skin

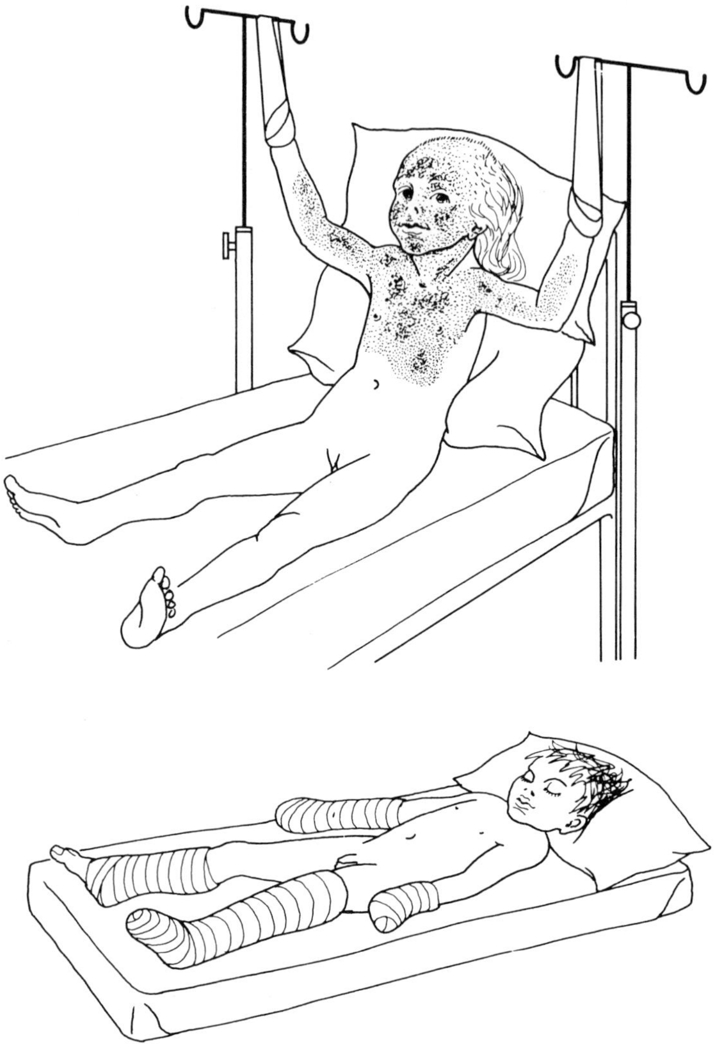

Fig. 34.3 *Care of burns.*

removed. A *Thiersch* (*split skin graft*) consists of the full thickness of epidermis and the top layer of the dermis; it is a commonly used type. *Patch* (*postage stamp*) *grafts* are an adaptation used for large areas, where the cosmetic effect is not of prime importance. The donor skin is divided into small rectangles or strips and laid on the recipient area with spaces between.

A *partial thickness graft* is one in which the full thickness of the epidermis and up to two-thirds of the dermis are removed.

A *Wolfe graft* is a full thickness skin graft including the full thickness of the epidermis and the dermis but not the underlying subcutaneous tissue.

Pedicles and flaps

These are a type of full thickness graft in which one end is left attached to its original site, so maintaining its blood supply. A flap may be rotated so that the free edge covers a neighbouring raw area, it is then called a rotational or sliding graft. The *pedicle* or *tubular graft* also includes some of the subcutaneous layer and is used where reconstructive surgery is required. The skin is taken from a distant part of the body by means of an intermediate attachment. The donor skin is first formed into a tube by raising the skin and stitching the two edges together. After 3 weeks one end is released and attached to a wound made in the intermediate site such as the arm. Once this has taken, the other end of the graft is freed from its intermediate site, unrolled and sutured in place. The donor area may be covered with a Thiersch graft or sutured.

Skin grafts may be removed from the donor area with a special knife or dermatome (Fig. 34.4). Mixed plasma and leucocyte extract or Thrombin Topical may be used to fix the flap in position. Where possible the skin graft is taken from the patient himself (autograft) as these are the only ones which take permanently. However, if temporary skin covering is required to prevent skin infection, skin will be taken from another person (homograft), but these grafts are rejected after 3 to 4 weeks. By this time the patient's condition will

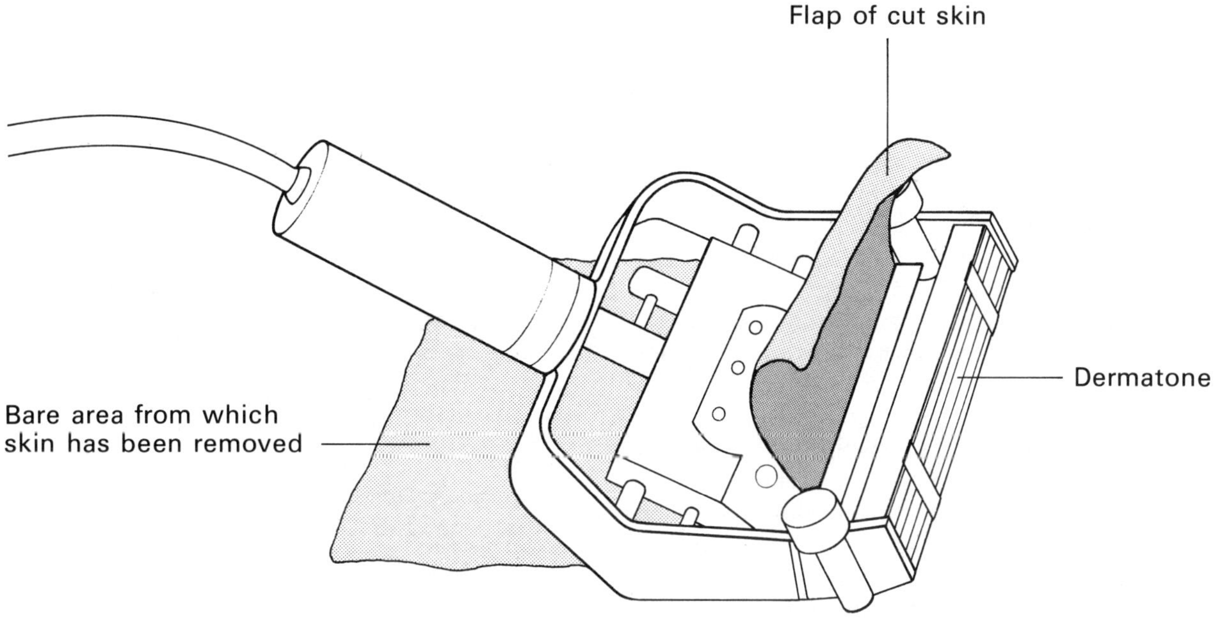

Fig. 34.4 *Dermatome.*

probably have improved and he may be able to provide his own donor sites. Homografts are stored in a skin bank.

The sites used vary according to availability of skin and the purpose for which the skin is required. The inner aspects of the thigh, arms or lower legs are the most common sites, but where severe burns are present it may be necessary to take skin from the abdomen or buttock.

It has now become possible to grow the patient's skin cells in the laboratory and so produce larger grafts.

Specific care of a patient following skin grafting

Prevention of infection of the site and maintenance of the patient's general condition in the optimum state are the main aims of care. On return from theatre the graft has usually been covered by Vaseline gauze, on top of which a pad has been placed, a firm crepe bandage maintaining its position. This is to prevent serous fluid from lifting the graft and so interfering with healing. If the graft is on a limb, this is elevated to encourage drainage. The wound is checked daily but the dressing is not removed for 7 to 10 days. If there is much oozing postoperatively, the top dressing is replaced but the Vaseline gauze is left in position. After the first dressing, which may have to be soaked off, it is redressed daily until complete healing has taken place. If blisters are present, these will be snipped to allow the serous fluid to drain away. The presence of a raised temperature, a discharging or smelly wound or persistent pain suggests that infection is present, in which case the dressing will have to be removed and a swab taken so that the appropriate antibiotic can be given. The area may be washed normally once it is fully healed and lanolin massaged in to restore the skin's suppleness. Full thickness grafts will also require the sutures to be removed; if a good cosmetic effect is required, this will be after 3 or 4 days. If the legs have received grafts, the patient will wear elastic stockings to prevent fluid accumulating.

The donor site is also left to heal for 7 to 10 days. These sites are usually more painful than the recipient site, the patient requiring analgesics. The dressing is soaked off and the wound redressed until complete healing has taken place.

SUGGESTED WORK

1. Do a survey on patients admitted to hospital with burns to find out the most common causes and the age group most frequently affected.
2. Discuss with a patient who has had plastic surgery what he felt were the greatest problems and whether these were dealt with adequately.

SUGGESTED READING

Danis D. M. (1982). Burn care. After-care instructions. *Journal of Emergency Nursing:* **8**(5): 257.

* * *

JEAN COX (aged 12) is the oldest of four children. On Guy Fawkes night a firework was thrown into a group and exploded, setting fire to her clothing and causing full thickness burns of her upper chest and arms. She is shocked and her parents are also very distressed.

Medical plan
Intravenous infusion of plasma. Exposure of burns. Skin graft.

Identification of the patient's needs and problems on admission and action arising from these

Shock
Raise the foot of the bed and maintain an even, warm temperature in the room. Control and monitor the intravenous infusion according to the instructions. Monitor and record her blood pressure and pulse half-hourly until stable.

Pain
This may not be as much as might be expected because the burns are full thickness. Administer prescribed analgesics as required.

Protection from infection
Nurse in strict isolation, explaining to Jean and her parents why this is necessary, and exclude visitors with any infection. Administer antibiotics as prescribed. Maintain a 4-hourly temperature chart.

Wound
Expose the wound and keep it as clean and dry as possible by regular wound toilet.

Nutrition
Initially limit oral fluids to 30 ml hourly and maintain a fluid balance chart. When she is able to eat, find out her likes and encourage a diet high in calories and protein. Give Hycal drinks. Keep the doctor informed of the blood electrolyte results. Administer any deficiencies orally or via the intravenous infusion as prescribed.

Excretion
Monitor urinary output carefully and report it if this becomes less than 50 ml/hour. Report any vomiting.

Pressure areas
Check sacrum, heels and elbows in particular. Take care when moving her not to drag her up the bed. She will need to be moved frequently.

Prevention of joint contractures
Check movement of the arms, which will rest in the optimum position.

Hygiene
When bedbathing Jean it is particularly important to respect her privacy. She may prefer plain water rather than mouthwash to clean her teeth.

Prevention of respiratory complications
Encourage Jean to breathe deeply. Once the shock has been controlled she should gradually be sat up in bed.

Psychological
Even at this early stage she may be worried about the long-term effects of the burns. Explain that the scar will become less unsightly in time and she will be able to find ways of concealing it. Arrange for the plastic surgeon to come and discuss what can be done.

Initially boredom will not be a problem, but as she recovers she will need to be provided with a variety of suitable interests, and a television. Suggest to her parents that friends could be encouraged to write or telephone her. Check whether she should be doing some school work as this may take some time to arrange.

35

Conditions Affecting Structures in the Neck

The most common condition requiring surgery of the neck is an abnormality of the thyroid. The nurse not only has to be aware of the effects of surgery within the limited space of the neck and the potential hazard of asphyxia, but she must also be able to recognise the effects of abnormal secretion by the thyroid gland at an early stage in its development and report them promptly.

Specific emphasis in the nursing history

General appearance. Does the patient appear to be hotter than the weather warrants? Is the patient flushed? Is there any loss of weight? Notice any protrusion of the eyes or any soreness.

Vital signs. Note the pulse particularly.

Breathing. Is there any increase in the respiratory rate?

Mobility. Is the patient overactive?

Nutrition. What is the patient's appetite like?

Attitude. Is the patient overexcited, irritable or easily upset?

Social. Have the family found it difficult to get on with the patient?

THE THYROID GLAND

The thyroid is an endocrine gland situated in the lower part of the neck in front of the trachea and larynx (Figs. 35.1 and 35.2). It has a rich blood supply from the four thyroid arteries, and on either side and in close proximity to it lie the recurrent laryngeal nerves. The gland is composed of follicles lined by cubical epithelium which takes up the circulating iodine and converts it to thyroxine, storing it in the follicles. This thyroxine stimulates metabolism and controls growth. The control of the production of thyroxine is under the influence of the pituitary gland which produces the thyroid-stimulating hormone. Lack of thyroxine in the blood stimulates the pituitary to produce more thyroid-stimulating hormone and as a result of this more thyroxine is produced by the thyroid gland.

Simple goitre

Lack of available iodine in the blood prevents the thyroid from producing sufficient thyroxine and this stimulates the pituitary to produce more thyroid-stimulating hormone. In response the thyroid enlarges in an effort to produce more thyroxine, but as it lacks the essential iodine it is unable to do this. Gradually the thyroid becomes larger, forming a goitre, and may press on other structures in the neck. It may cease to produce an adequate amount of thyroxine, causing myxoedema. The goitre may be parenchymatous, with proliferation of the epithelial cells, colloid, with large vesicles filled with an excess of colloid, or nodular, with encapsulated nodules of glandular or colloid tissue.

The administration of iodine and thyroxine may be sufficient to cause the gland to shrink, but if dyspnoea is present, part of the gland will have to be removed.

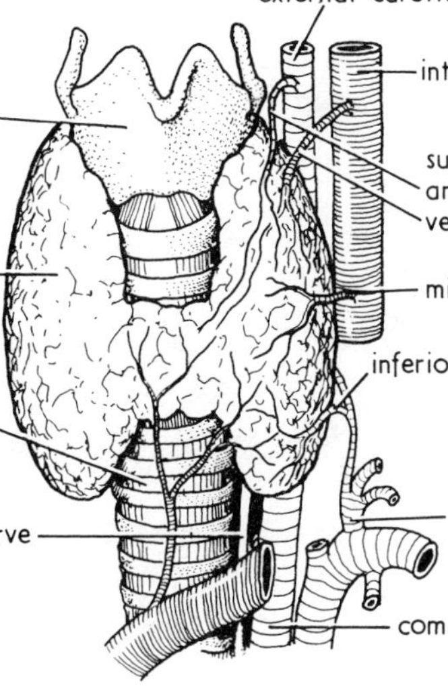

Fig 35.1 *The thyroid gland and its neighbouring structures.*

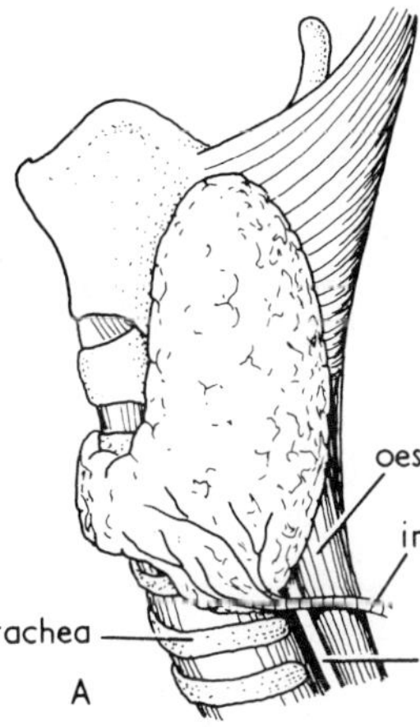

Fig. 35.2 *Side view of the thyroid gland.*

Thyrotoxicosis (toxic goitre)

This condition much more commonly affects women between the ages of 15 and 30 than men. The overactive thyroid causes metabolism to be speeded up abnormally. This results in an enlarged thyroid gland; an increased pulse rate, even in sleep, due to atrial fibrillation; increased respiratory rate with an increase of oxygen consumption; exophthalmos, prominent staring eyes and lid retraction; increased heat production causing a warm, moist skin; fine tremor of the fingers when the hands are held out; increased appetite, but a loss of weight, the body's stores being used up; and excessive nervousness and irritability.

Treatment

Medical treatment is with antithyroid drugs such as carbimazole 5–10 mg 8-hourly. If there is any reaction to this, propylthiouracil may be prescribed. The treatment is usually continued for 18 months to 2 years. However, a large proportion of cases relapse and require surgery and there is the possibility of the patient developing agranulocytosis, aplastic anaemia or skin rashes. Prior to surgery the drug is important in reducing the toxicity of the patient.

Subtotal thyroidectomy (Figs. 35.3 and 35.4) An incision is made about 2.5 cm above the sternal notch, following the natural skin crease. The

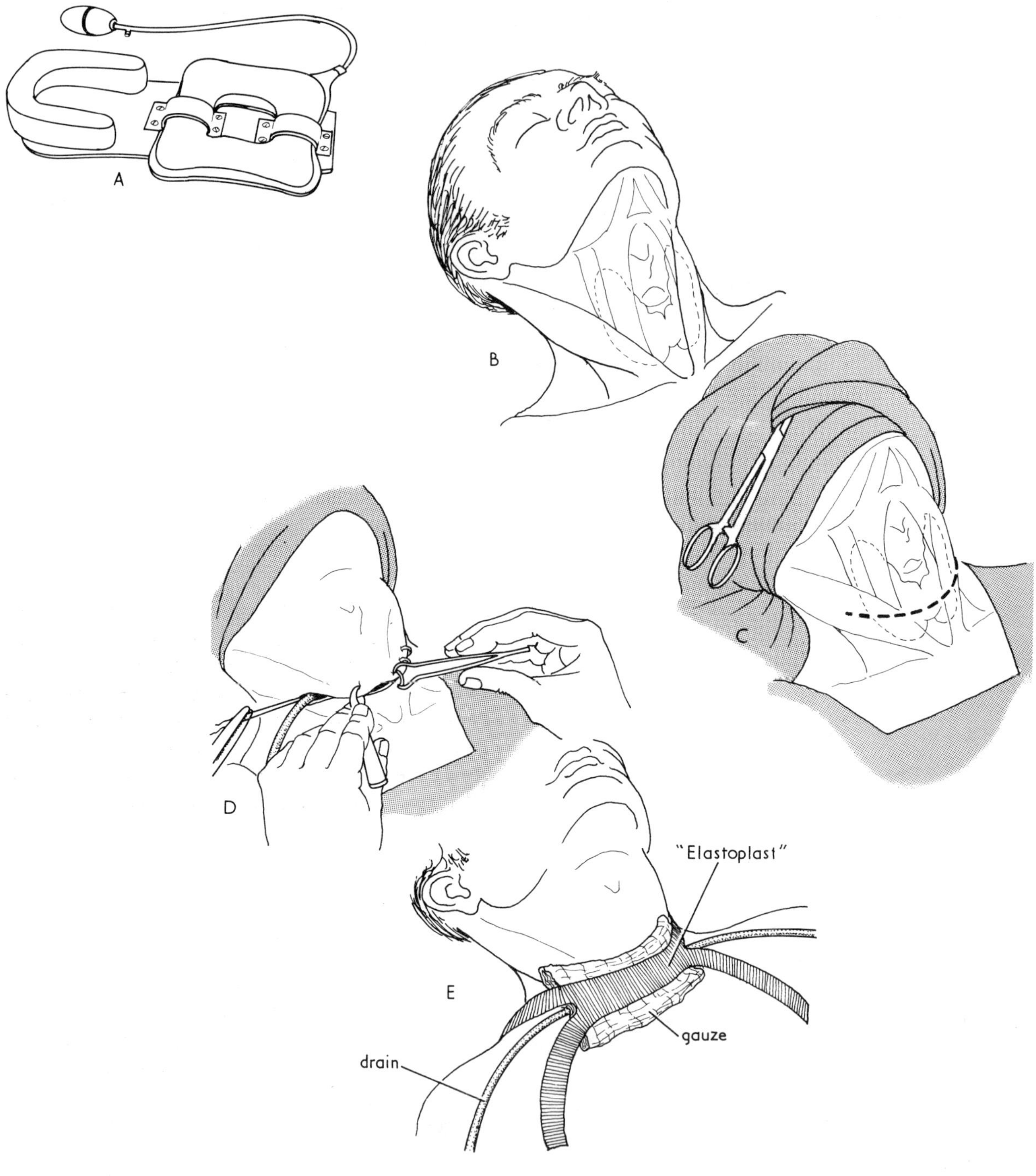

Fig. 35.3 *Thyroidectomy. (a) The support for the neck during the operation. (b) The position of the thyroid gland. (c) The incision. (d) Insertion of clips. (e) The final dressing.*

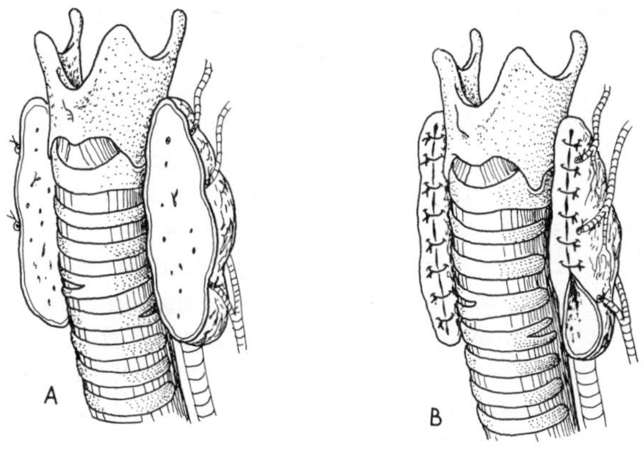

Fig. 35.4 *The extent of excision in a thyroidectomy.*

thyroid is freed from the surrounding structures and, after ligation and division of the blood vessels, almost all of the thyroid gland is removed leaving only a small part of each lobe. A total thyroidectomy would be done for carcinoma of the thyroid.

Specific preoperative preparation

Radioactive iodine is given by mouth to the patient and the amount taken up by the thyroid measured with a scintillation counter placed near the gland. The amount excreted in the urine is also measured. The greater the activity of the thyroid, the more radioactive iodine it takes up, and therefore there is less in the urine. Blood tests are carried out to measure the protein-bound iodine, the levels of which are raised in thyrotoxicosis (whereas in a goitre they are reduced). A sleeping pulse rate will also be recorded. The neck is x-rayed for the position of the trachea.

The patient tends to be easily upset and will therefore require careful handling from the time of admission, sedatives being prescribed if necessary. The patient will need to be in a cool, airy part of the ward away from distressing sights. If exophthalmus is present, the eyes will require special care, with lubricant drops at night and dark glasses in the day. The carbimazole will have been discontinued 10 to 14 days prior to the operation, and Lugol's iodine 0.1–0.3 ml three times a day will be given in milk, to reduce the vascularity of the gland. The patient may require to be digitalised or given propranolol. The physiotherapist will encourage deep breathing and coughing. The axillae, chest and upper arms will be shaved.

Specific postoperative care

As soon as the patient has recovered from the anaesthetic and has satisfactory blood pressure, he is sat up with the neck well supported. There may be two Redivac drains, which are removed after 24 and 48 hours. The sutures are removed after 2 to 3 days to produce a good cosmetic effect. On the evening of the operation the patient is encouraged to take sips of water, and by the first postoperative day can eat a light diet. Mobilisation is straightforward.

The patient is observed carefully during the first 4 to 6 hours for haemorrhage which may escape and drain behind the neck or be trapped in the tissues of the neck causing pressure on the trachea. It is therefore important when checking the patient for the nurse to slide her hand behind the neck to check for any bleeding. If the patient is becoming dyspnoeic due to the pressure from a haematoma or oedema, the clips or sutures must be removed immediately to relieve the pressure. The patient will have to return to theatre to have the bleeding points religatured.

Dyspnoea and cyanosis, particularly if stridor is present, may indicate that damage has been done to both the recurrent laryngeal nerves, and the patient will require a tracheostomy. If the nerves do not recover, a permanent tracheostomy will be necessary. Damage to one of the nerves causes hoarseness of the voice, but this is usually temporary.

The patient may develop a dry cough with pain on swallowing and coughing, and occasionally respiratory distress as a result of tracheitis is a complication. Steam inhalations help to relieve it.

If the patient was operated on while still toxic, a thyroid crisis may develop, usually in the first 24 hours, although it is uncommon. The patient develops a very high temperature, rapid pulse, dyspnoea and extreme restlessness. Rapid and effective treatment is essential to prevent death from exhaustion. Neo-Mercazole is given to diminish the activity of the glandular tissue and propranolol or digoxin to control the heart rate. Sedatives, oxygen, an intravenous infusion would also be required and measures taken to relieve the temperature.

Accidental removal or damage to the parathyroids will cause tingling and numbness of the face and hands, painful spasms of the hands and feet (carpal pedal spasms), leading to cramp and convulsions (tetany). At the first indication of this the patient will be given calcium gluconate 10 ml of a 10% solution intravenously, followed by oral calcium. In mild cases oral calcium may be sufficient.

If too much of the thyroid gland has been removed, myxoedema will develop but this will not be evident until the patient returns to out-patients. All the metabolic processes slow down and the patient becomes mentally and physically slow, putting on weight and losing some hair, which is dry and brittle. The pulse is slow and the temperature subnormal.

Radioactive iodine This may be used in larger amounts than in diagnosis to destroy the thyroid cells. It eventually causes myxoedema and it is thought that there may be some risk of carcinoma or leukaemia in the young. It is therefore reserved for the older patient who is unsuitable for surgery or those patients who have had more than one thyroidectomy and are still not controlled.

Malignant tumours

These are rare, mainly affecting women over the age of 40. The patient complains of dyspnoea, dysphagia and pain in the neck and there may be hoarseness. Treatment is by a total thyroidectomy and thyroxine must be taken indefinitely.

THE PARATHYROID GLANDS

These are four small glands the size of a pea, situated on the posterior surface of the thyroid gland. There is one at each of the four poles of the thyroid lobes. They secrete parathormone which controls the amount of calcium and phosphorus in the blood. The amount of parathormone produced is regulated by the amount of calcium in the blood.

Hypoparathyroidism leading to tetany arises from atrophy or surgical removal and has been dealt with under the complications of a thyroidectomy (see above).

Hyperparathyroidism (osteitis fibrosa cystica) may arise due to an increase in the amount of secreting tissue or due to a tumour of the parathyroid. There is an increase in the parathormone which leads to a high blood calcium level. Calcium is removed from the bone and excreted in the urine, with the result of cyst formation in the bones leading to pathological fractures and calculi forming in the renal tract. There are also gastric disturbances and mental changes such as lethargy and confusion. The diagnosis is based on the blood calcium level and an x-ray of the bones.

Parathyroidectomy

The whole tumour may be excised surgically or, in the case of hypertrophy, a subtotal resection of the gland may be done. If the whole gland has been removed, calcium and vitamin D will have to be given. Otherwise these medicines are given until the skeleton has recalcified. Signs of tetany must be watched for.

TUMOURS AND CYSTS OF THE NECK

The most common tumours of the neck are the benign *lipomas*, tumours of adipose tissue. However, *secondary carcinoma* may also develop in this region and, less commonly, *lymphosarcoma* in the lymph nodes. If carcinoma develops, the lymph nodes become hard and matted together and may eventually ulcerate through the skin. These tumours are excised and if malignant may require a complete removal of the lymph glands in the neck—block dissection. In some cases radiotherapy is used.

Carotid body tumours are small tumours in the beginning of the carotid artery which may be excised with difficulty or be treated by radiotherapy.

Congenital tumours, cysts and fistulae of the neck

The neck and pharynx are formed from five bars of tissue called branchial arches, between which are depressions or clefts. The second arch develops rapidly and a lateral downgrowth from it eventually reaches and joins with the fifth arch producing an enclosed cavity, the cervical sinus.

Branchial (lateral cervical) cysts

These are embryonic dermoid cysts which arise by distension with fluid of the cervical sinus and unobliterated portions of the second branchial cleft. They are found in front of the upper part of the sternomastoid muscle and often do not arise until adulthood.

Branchial fistula

This is a tiny opening in the front of the lower part of the neck, slightly to one side. The track of the fistula passes up into the neck and may become infected in which case it will be excised.

Thyroglossal (median cervical) cysts

Another fairly common form of embryonic maldevelopment of the neck is a thyroglossal cyst (Fig. 35.5). Towards the back of the tongue in the centre is a depression called the foramen caecum, and it was at this point that the thyroid gland developed in the fetus and where the opening of the thyroglossal duct, now obliterated, was. As the fetus developed the thyroid gland gradually descended to the lower part of the neck, its duct and the passage produced by its descent being obliterated before birth. If the thyroglossal duct does not disappear, cysts may develop anywhere along the track and these frequently become infected. The cysts may then track through to the surface of the skin forming a thyroglossal fistula. The treatment for both cysts and fistulae is excision.

WOUNDS OF THE NECK

The most common type of injury to the neck occurs as a result of attempted suicide. Damage to the

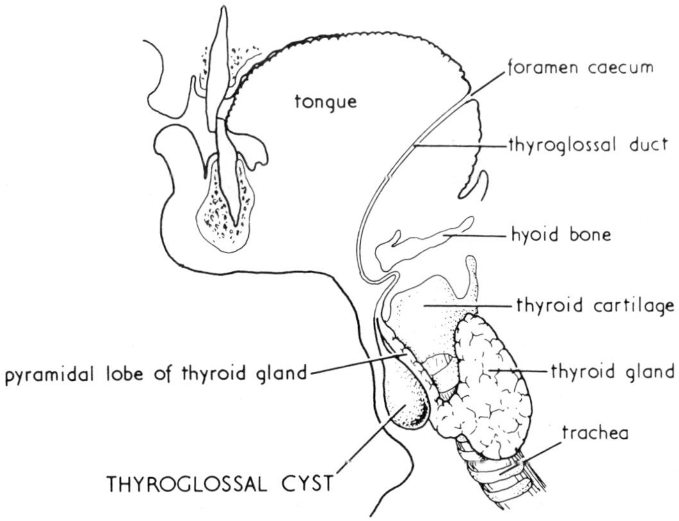

Fig. 35.5 *Thyroglossal cyst.*

large blood vessels in the neck will quickly lead to death but if these are spared, the trachea may be damaged, interfering with the ability to breathe. In this case a tracheostomy will be necessary. Infection frequently occurs and therefore antibiotics are given; if it is not adequately treated, it may spread down into the chest.

ACUTE CERVICAL ADENITIS

The lymph nodes of the neck drain the face, mouth, nose, ear, scalp and tonsils. Infection may spread from any one of these sources, although the tonsils are the most likely. The glands in the neck become enlarged and tender. In the majority of cases they respond to antibiotic treatment, but if abscesses develop, they may require drainage.

TUBERCULOUS ADENITIS

The glands which may already be infected by other bacteria are invaded by the tubercle bacillus. The infection may be localised to a few glands or be diffuse, and cold abscesses may develop. Diagnosis is made by doing a Heaf or Mantoux test which, if positive, indicates the presence of a tuberculous infection. Evidence of tuberculosis in other parts of the body such as the lungs will help diagnosis. If the glands are localised, they may be excised. Whether they are excised or not, antituberculous drugs such as streptomycin, para-amino salicylic acid and isoniazid will be given. Other antibiotics will be necessary to deal with any superimposed bacterial infection. If the tonsils and adenoids are infected, they will be removed and the general health of the patient built up with extra vitamin D. Splinting of the neck may be required and this will be done with some form of stiff collar.

SUGGESTED WORK

1. Compare the care of a patient following subtotal thyroidectomy in your hospital with that described in the text. Note any variations and find out the reason why these occur.

2. Discuss with a patient who has thyrotoxicosis the effects her condition has had on her and her family.

* * *

Mrs ANNE BLAKE (aged 28) is married with two children aged 5 and 7 years. She was diagnosed as having thyrotoxicosis 2 years ago when she commenced medical treatment with Neomercazole. However, when the treatment was reduced she had a return of the symptoms and it was decided that she should have surgery. She has a slight exophthalmus.

Medical plan
Subtotal thyroidectomy.

Identification of the patient's needs and problems in the immediate postoperative period and action arising from these

Recognition of haemorrhage and shock
Monitor the blood pressure, pulse and respirations quarter-hourly until stable and the temperature 4-hourly. Report any abnormality. Observe for restlessness or pallor.

Recognition of respiratory complications
Note any difficulty in breathing, noisy breathing or cyanosis. If this occurs, check the wound for distension due to oedema or haematoma. If present, the sutures will have to be removed, so check that the stitch cutter is near the patient.

Wound
Observe for haemorrhage by feeling behind the neck as well as checking the wound. Sit the patient up with the wound supported once the blood pressure is satisfactory. Check that the vacuum drains are functioning.

Nutrition
Encourage sips of water in the evening following the operation.

Recognition of a thyroid crisis
Note any sudden rise in pulse and temperature or the patient becoming restless. Report to the doctor immediately.

Recognition of damage to the laryngeal nerve
Check that the patient's voice is normal and report any undue huskiness. Also note any cough or pain associated with swallowing or coughing, and report.

Recognition of tetany
Report any tingling in the fingers or cramps.

Pain
Administer prescribed analgesics as required. Aspirin mucilage may help a sore throat.

Mobilisation
Encourage movement in bed to prevent a deep vein thrombosis and respiratory complications.

Psychological
Reassure Mrs Blake that she may move her head without damaging the wound. Explain that the scar will be hidden in the lines of her neck once it has fully healed.

Hygiene
Wash the patient on recovery from the anaesthetic and put her own nightdress on. Give her a mouthwash.

Social
Make sure that Mrs Blake's husband reassures her regarding the arrangements made for the children.

SUGGESTED READING

Taylor S. *et al.* (1984). *Surgical Management.* Ch. 34, p. 269. London: Heinemann Medical.

36

Conditions of the Face and Mouth

The person who is to undergo surgery on the face or mouth is acutely conscious of the effects his appearance may have on other people. The baby and young child are spared the mental distress that this type of surgery can produce. The nurse must be fully informed of the surgery which is to be done and its effects both immediately after the operation and in the longer term. She must be aware of what the patient has been told so that she does not give him conflicting information. The patient will require a lot of reassurance that his appearance will improve, but if he has been adequately prepared for the immediate postoperative effects of the surgery, this will be easier. The emphasis in the physical care will be on oral hygiene.

Specific emphasis in the nursing history

General appearance. Note the presence of asymmetry of the face, loss of weight, excess salivation, dribbling, bad breath or weakness.

Pain. Note the degree of pain and the rate it has progressed since its commencement. Is there any pain elsewhere, such as in the ear?

Nutrition. Is there any difficulty in eating or swallowing or any evidence of bleeding in the mouth? What is the state of oral hygiene?

Breathing. Note any difficulty in breathing or noisy chest sounds. Is the patient a smoker?

Vital signs. Is there any evidence of infections such as a raised temperature?

Social. Has the patient any children as relatives that he may want to keep in contact with but not be seen by. In the case of a child, have the parents other children or commitments? Can one of them stay with the child?

Surgery on the mouth may involve surgeons from different specialties, such as the plastic or orthopaedic surgeon, but the nursing care remains the same.

CLEFT LIP AND CLEFT PALATE

Between the fifth and tenth week of fetal life the parts of the lip and palate fuse together. If some genetic or environmental factor interrupts growth during this time, fusion may not occur, resulting in a cleft lip if the interruption is early on, and a cleft palate if the inhibiting factor continues into the tenth week (Fig. 36.1). Because of the continuing growth of the fetus there will be further facial deformity.

The defect may therefore vary from just a slight deformity on one side of the lip to a complete lack of fusion of the lip and palate. Occasionally there may be a bilateral defect. More than 25% of these children will also have other congenital deformities.

Treatment

A cleft lip is surgically repaired when the baby is 2 to 3 months old. The care of a cleft palate will start with presurgical orthopaedic correction to control the unrestricted growth of the cartilage in the nasal septum and to reposition the maxillary bones.

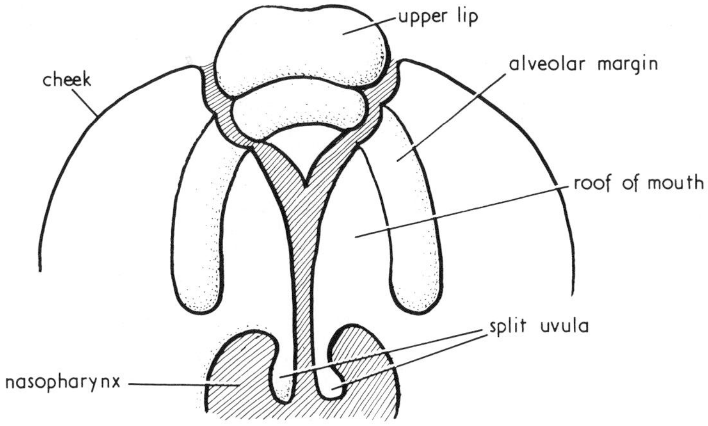

Fig. 36.1 *A cleft palate and cleft lip.*

Within the first 24 hours after birth the baby is fitted with an acrylic feeding plate to occlude the cleft in the palate, thus enabling him to be fed with a teat. A series of appliances is also made to correct the position of the maxilla gradually.

Particular care is taken in feeding the baby at this time. He must not be hurried, and should be winded frequently or he may inhale the feed. The mouth and nose are kept very clean, particularly after feeding. Once winded the baby is placed on his side to prevent inhalation of vomit.

The maxillary correction appliance is worn continuously except when feeding and must be checked frequently to see that it is in the correct position. Extra-oral traction may be applied to speed up the process. Initially the baby will have to remain in hospital, but once the mother is able to manage she may take him home.

When the presurgical orthopaedic correction has produced its maximum effect and no further correction is possible, the baby will be considered for closure of the palate and insertion of a bone graft to stabilise the maxilla (Fig. 36.2). Prior to operation, care is taken to ensure that the infant has had adequate nutrition, that he weighs at least 4.5 kg and that there is no anaemia, chest infection or otitis media. If these are present, they are corrected first. Antibiotic cover is usually given.

Specific postoperative care

A very careful watch is kept on the airway and if suction has to be used, it is done very gently. Tension on the suture line must be avoided and therefore the baby is kept contented to prevent crying, and a metal appliance (Logan's bow, Fig. 36.3) may be placed over the upper lip. The colour of the lips must be observed for any blueness. It is also important to prevent infection of the suture line as this will spoil the cosmetic effect. Cardboard elbow splints are therefore used to prevent the baby from touching the suture line. Feeds are given by a special spoon and the mouth and suture line cleaned afterwards. Sutures are removed on the sixth day.

Secondary plastic surgery may be necessary when the child is older to correct any other defects. Speech therapy will be required to help the child acquire proper speech development.

ACUTE GLOSSITIS

Acute inflammation of the tongue may be due to infection such as thrush which may occur with steroid or antibiotic treatment, wounds or burns. The tongue becomes swollen and painful. Careful oral toilet in patients at risk may help to prevent it.

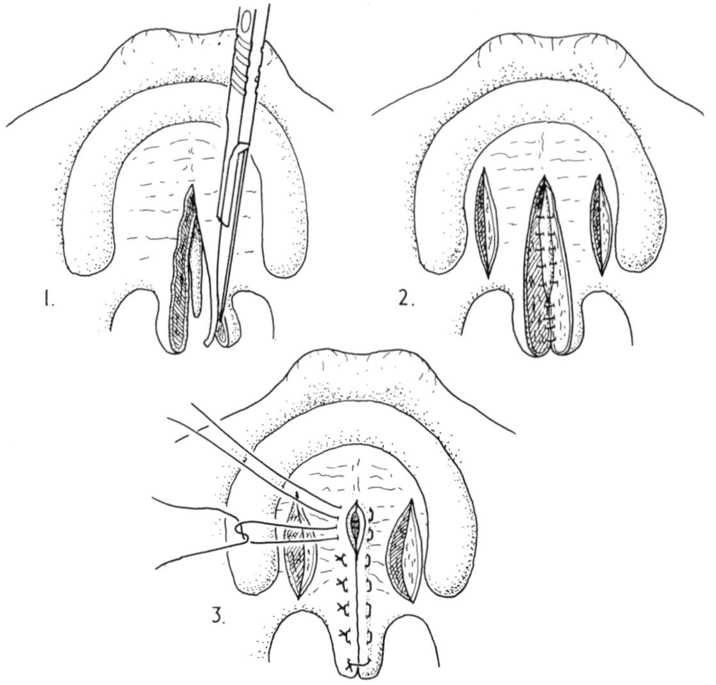

Fig. 36.2 *Repair of a cleft palate.*

Treatment

Chemotherapy, oral toilet and antibiotic pastilles are given as appropriate. Extra vitamin B is given to patients on antibiotics. If an abscess forms, an incision will be necessary. Should the tongue swell excessively and threaten breathing, a tracheostomy may be required.

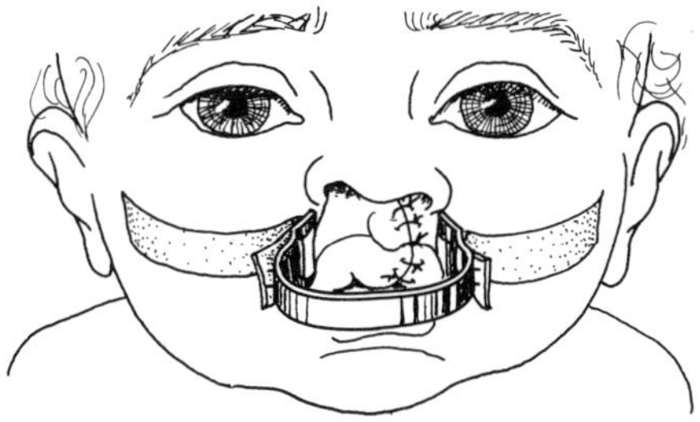

Fig. 36.3 *A Logan's bow.*

CHRONIC SUPERFICIAL GLOSSITIS (LEUCOPLAKIA)

This condition is occasionally due to syphilis but any irritant such as smoking or ill-fitting dentures can cause it. It is a precancerous condition. The tongue looks as if it is covered with cracked white paint, other areas of it being smooth, red and glazed. Later, cracks and fissures appear. The occurrence of pain on smoking or drinking indicates the onset of malignancy. Eventually the pain will be spontaneous.

Treatment

The underlying cause must be treated. If this fails, the affected areas may be excised.

TUMOURS OF THE TONGUE

Benign tumours of the tongue are rare, malignant tumours being much more common. Epithelioma (cancer) of the tongue usually occurs in the middle-aged or elderly man. It starts as a lump or small ulcer with a markedly indurated base which often causes discomfort from the onset. It is usually found at the side of the tongue in the anterior two-thirds, although it may be at the back of the tongue or on the tip. It is sometimes wart-like in appearance and its growth is accompanied by a gradual increase in pain. Referred pain in the ear is characteristic of this condition. The tongue becomes rotated to one side, and eventually fixed to the floor of the mouth, so interfering with speech and swallowing. Secondary infection (stomatitis) causes excessive salivation and dribbling of saliva which may be blood-stained. The infection also causes the breath to smell, and the cervical lymph nodes to enlarge. These lymph nodes become matted together, eventually ulcerating through the skin of the neck. If blood vessels become involved, there may be severe haemorrhages from the tongue or neck. The tongue and the glottis may also become oedematous, so interfering with breathing and leading to asphyxia if nothing is done.

Unless radical treatment is adopted, death occurs usually within 18 months from wasting and exhaustion, bronchopneumonia, haemorrhages or asphyxia.

Treatment

A biopsy is taken to confirm the diagnosis. The growth may be treated by the insertion of radium needles into the tongue, by the use of the cobalt bomb or deep x-ray therapy or surgery. Surgery involves the excision of a large part of the tongue and may require a temporary tracheostomy. There will also be treatment of the lymphatic glands in the neck which drain the mouth, either with radiotherapy or excision (block dissection). If the mandible is also involved, a much more extensive and mutilating operation may be required with bone grafts and plastic surgery.

Prior to operation on the mouth any infection is treated with antibiotics and dental caries are removed.

Specific postoperative care

Because of the inflammation, the tongue will be swollen and this could interfere with breathing, therefore the surgeon will insert a suture in it so that it can be pulled forward. In some patients it may be necessary to carry out a tracheostomy.

Oral hygiene is very important because the mouth is dry and infection may easily enter and spread to the lungs causing respiratory complications. The oral hygienist can provide advice on the best care. Antibiotic cover is continued.

Suction and oxygen must be readily available as they may be required urgently. Frequent swallowing by the patient may indicate that there is bleeding. If the patient is unable to take sufficient nutrients by mouth, a nasogastric tube will be required and in some patients parenteral feeding is the best way of ensuring adequate nutrition. The sutures are removed on the fourth to fifth day.

ULCERS OF THE TONGUE

These may arise as a result of trauma from dentures or broken teeth, general ill-health, tuberculosis or syphilis, and require treatment of the cause.

FRACTURES OF THE JAW

Lower jaw (mandible)

These may arise due to road traffic accidents, fights or falls, and are more common than those of the face. The powerful muscles used in mastication are attached to the mandible and include muscles which close the jaws balanced by those which open the jaws. After a fracture of the jaw one group of muscles may be stronger than those opposing them on one segment of the jaw, whereas in another segment it may be the opposite group which is strongest. This will cause displacement, especially if the patient moves the jaw. If there is a double fracture of the mandible in the canine region, the muscles will pull the section back, so allowing the tongue which is attached to it to fall backwards and cause an airway obstruction.

Management

The airway requires particular attention as loose teeth, blood clots, debris or secretions may cause an obstruction. Therefore the debris should be removed from the mouth and a check made for any damaged or lost teeth. Aspiration may be used to remove secretions and any false teeth should be taken out and kept, even if broken, as they may be used later for splints. If the tongue falls back and blocks the airway, it may be held forward with a suture, or an endotracheal tube or tracheostomy may be necessary.

Although there may be some degree of bleeding initially, this usually stops quickly. If it requires attention, a pack and pressure are in most cases sufficient.

Trauma in the region of the head suggests that there might be some degree of brain damage and therefore neurological observations will be required.

Swelling and bruising will appear in the tissues over the fracture site, reaching their maximum in 48 hours. This will upset the relatives and the patient if he sees it but they can be reassured that it will subside.

The patient will complain of pain if he tries to move his jaws, and will be unable to chew and this will require analgesics.

The fracture is reduced, restoring the bones to their correct position, after which they are immobilised for up to 6 weeks. If the patient has his own teeth, the upper and lower sets of teeth are wired together. The patient has to remain in the recovery room until fully conscious because of the difficulty in gaining access to the airway. When the patient returns to the ward, wire cutters must be by the bedside ready to cut the linking wires immediately if the patient obstructs.

If the patient only has a few of his own teeth, a metal bar may be attached to the base of the teeth of each jaw and then wired together. Those patients who have no teeth have an upper and lower dental plate made without any teeth which is fixed to the jaws with wiring, the two plates then being fixed to each other.

Antitetanus serum and antibiotics are necessary to prevent infection, and the patient will be given a nutritious fluid diet which he may be able to swallow through his teeth. Alternatively a nasogastric tube may be preferred. Care must be taken when giving fluids that they are not given too fast, so causing choking or vomiting. Oral hygiene is essential and either a Higginson's syringe or soft plastic tubing attached to an ordinary syringe may be used to rinse the mouth—again great care must be taken. Once the patient is fit enough, he can be taught to deal with this himself.

Upper jaw (maxilla) and associated facial bones

These fractures are characterised by marked facial swelling, bruising and bleeding from the nose. The face appears lengthened, the middle third of it being flattened. There is extensive bruising around both eyes. If the fracture is in the upper third of the face, there will be leakage of cerebrospinal fluid from the nose. This type of injury is frequently associated with other injuries of the head or body.

Management

The patient will have suffered a head injury and therefore will require neurological observations. He will be checked thoroughly by the doctor for other injuries and treated for shock which will undoubtedly be present. The bones are reduced and immobilised, but unfortunately the mandible is no use for this as it is a movable bone. A plaster of Paris headcap is made which fits firmly on the head, not moving. Into this are fitted wires or metal bars which are used to immobilise the fractures.

The oral splints in the mouth will require brushing with a toothbrush and the mouth is kept clean as described above. A fluid diet is given. Antibiotics will be required to prevent infection.

Dislocation of the mandible

Dislocation may be caused during the extraction of teeth, in yawning or as a result of a blow on the chin if the mouth is open. The surgeon will reduce the dislocation as soon as possible.

CYSTS

Retention cysts

These are cysts in the small mucous glands of the lips and cheeks, arising as a result of the ducts to these glands becoming blocked. They are small, painless, blue or yellow swellings which may gradually become bigger, eventually bursting. Although they heal easily they do tend to recur and are therefore excised.

Dermoid cysts

These cysts result from the inclusion of ectoderm in the lines of fusion in the face and neck during development. They are therefore found in the midline of the palate, tongue or floor of the mouth under the tongue. They form a large painless swelling which contains sebaceous material and sometimes teeth and hair. Treatment is by excision through the floor of the mouth or neck.

Dentigerous cysts

These develop in the follicle around unerupted teeth. They cause the bone to expand and may become infected.

Dental cysts

These are associated with dead teeth or roots. They cause painless swellings which lead to expansion of the bone of the jaw. Treatment of dentigerous and dental cysts is by excision or marsupialisation. In the latter the cyst is incised and packed to enable it to heal slowly. The packing is renewed weekly until healing has taken place.

TUMOURS OF THE JAWS AND LIPS

Epulis is a slow-growing tumour of fibrous tissue developing on the edge of the gum as a result of chronic irritation. Treatment is by excision, which may also require the adjacent teeth to be removed.

Adamantinoma or multilocular cyst is a slow-growing locally malignant tumour which may contain a large number of small cysts. It gradually invades the bone and may destroy large sections of it. It is found in younger people. Treatment consists of radical excision which may require bone grafting.

Malignant tumours of the jaw

Carcinoma or, less commonly, sarcoma may affect the sinuses or the jaws, particularly the maxillary antrum. The patient presents with loose teeth which may fall out, a purulent discharge from the nose, and bleeding. Aching pain develops at a later stage when there may also be bulging of the cheek, displacement of the eyeball, nasal obstruction and deformity of the palate. Eventually the tumour will ulcerate into the mouth, nose, orbit or pharynx. It may spread into the lymph glands of the neck. Diagnosis is by x-ray and biopsy.

Treatment

Treatment involves a combination of surgery and radiotherapy, although in a small tumour surgery alone may be sufficient. As much of the tumour as possible is excised including the hard palate, alveolus and teeth on the affected side. Sometimes the surgery has to be even more radical than this. The remainder of the tumour is frequently irradiated with radium needles which are held in position by a vulcanite and lead denture which protects the mouth and tongue from the action of the radium. Cytotoxic therapy may be used before commencing other treatment or in those patients who cannot be operated on.

Carcinomata of the mouth, gums, cheek, palate and tonsil

These tumours spread to the cervical lymph nodes and are dealt with in the same way as carcinoma of the tongue.

Carcinoma of the lip

An indurated ulcer or warty growth develops on the lower lip, most frequently in men. In its later stages it ulcerates. The growth is treated by radiotherapy and excision of the lymph nodes which drain the area. Occasionally the growth is excised.

Benign tumours of the lips

The commonest of these is the naevis or haemangioma. Papillomata and mucous cysts are also not uncommon.

Rodent ulcer of the face

This is a slowly growing malignant ulcer found on the face. If it is not treated, it will relentlessly erode the tissues of the face, but it rarely metastasises. Treatment is by radiotherapy or excision.

THE SALIVARY GLANDS

Calculi most commonly develop in the submandibular glands or their ducts causing an obstruction and subsequent infection. The gland is swollen and painful, especially after meals. The calculi can often be felt in the floor of the mouth, and can usually be seen on x-ray. Treatment is by excision of the calculi if accessible, or of the whole gland through an incision below the mandible.

Ranula

A small, round, bluish, translucent cyst which develops under the tongue near the frenum, this is treated by excision.

Tumours of the salivary glands

Tumours most commonly occur in the parotid gland, although occasionally they develop in the submandibular gland. A mixed parotid tumour is a firm, round or lobulated, slow-growing tumour, which may become malignant. The indications of this are a more rapid growth, pain, facial paralysis and spread to the lymph nodes. Both benign and malignant growths are removed by surgery, but great care has to be taken to avoid injuring the facial nerve if only part of the gland requires removal. If a total parotidectomy has to be done for carcinoma, there will inevitably be damage to the facial nerve because it enters into the gland near to the ear. This will then require further operations to protect the cornea from injury, such as a tarsorrhaphy in which the lid margins are fused at both the inner and outer canthus, leaving only a small gap opposite the pupil. Removal of the parotid gland is followed by radiotherapy to prevent recurrence. If the tumour is malignant, a block dissection of the cervical glands will also be done.

SUGGESTED WORK

1. Find out what care is provided after discharge from the hospital for the patient who has had radical surgery to the face.
2. Find out through out-patients the progress of a child who has had a repair of a cleft palate some years ago. How good is the cosmetic effect of the operation and how well does the child talk?

SUGGESTED READING

Daly K. M. (1979). Oral cancer: everyday concern. *American Journal of Nursing*; **79**(8): 1415–17.
Dropkin M. J. (1981). Development of self care teaching program for postoperative head and neck patients. *Cancer Nursing*; **4**(2): 103–06.

* * *

Mr JAMES SIMPSON (aged 63) is married with two daughters, both of whom have school-age children and live nearby. He was admitted with a malignant growth of the tongue which had extended to the jaw. The malignancy was confirmed by biopsy.

Medical plan
Excision of tongue and jaw followed by plastic surgery.

Evaluation and adaptation of the continuing postoperative care of the patient

Psychological
Mr Simpson has refused to allow any other member of his family to visit him than his wife.

Even with her he is uncommunicative. The only person he has said anything to is the hospital chaplain. He has said 'What is the purpose of living? No one would want to see me now.'

Action
A case conference will need to be called including his surgeon, the plastic surgeon (if different), the nurse responsible for his care, the chaplain, Mr Simpson's wife, and a psychiatrist. They will need to discuss what the root of his problem is, e.g. not being fit to be seen by his grandchildren, and how he can be convinced that the disfigurement is temporary.

The plastic surgeon may introduce him to a patient who has had the operation to show him what can be done. The chaplain can continue to be the person he can say what he likes to without fear of hurting or shocking him. Encourage Mr Simpson's wife to continue visiting, even if he does not talk, and to maintain his links with his family by letter. The nurse can show him ways of hiding his disfigurement, particularly when his wife visits.

Relatives
Just when he needs them most and they would willingly give the support he requires, he appears to have rejected them.

Action
Explain that it is because he cares so much for them he is frightened they will reject him and he would be unable to cope with his feelings. Ask them to be patient, keeping them informed and particularly maintaining the links with the grandchildren. This may be done by letters, news bulletins and telephone calls.

Respiratory function
The care of the tracheostomy has been continued with no complications. Less suction is required. The tracheostomy wound is clean.

Nutrition
The intravenous infusion is still in progress; however, the electrolytes appear satisfactory. Nasogastric feeding continues with vitamin supplements but Mr Simpson has developed diarrhoea.

Action
Inform the doctor of the electrolyte results and check whether he wishes the intravenous infusion to be continued. Inform him of the diarrhoea so that he may prescribe a suitable bulking agent.

Pain
This does not appear to be severe and it would seem that the analgesics prescribed do not need to be as strong.

Action
Ask the doctor to prescribe a milder analgesic.

Hygiene
The patient is still being bedbathed because of his generally weak condition.

Action
Continue with bedbaths.

Mobility
Mr Simpson has sat out of bed for short periods with no ill-effects.

Action
Gradually increase the amount of time up, walking him to the bathroom when he is fit enough. Until then he can be taken out in the Sani-chair.

37

The Ear, Nose and Throat

Patients with minor conditions affecting their ears, nose, sinuses or throat are treated by their general practitioner or in the hospital out-patient department. In the ENT wards throughput of patients is, on the whole, more rapid than on general wards. Many patients have special communication needs, owing to hearing or speech difficulties, or to the brevity of their stay in hospital. Therefore, it is the role of the nurse to ensure that each patient's individual needs are identified and met.

Specific emphasis in the nursing history

General appearance. Does the patient look healthy or run down? Is there evidence of mouth breathing? Vertigo?

Excretion. Test urine for sugar.

Vital signs. Raised temperature.

Pain. Child holding or rubbing ear. Pain in ear. Headaches aggravated by stooping.

Special senses—ears. Loss of hearing in one or both sides. Tinnitus. Nausea or vomiting.

EXAMINATION OF THE EAR (Fig. 37.1)

The pinna is inspected with the naked eye, and an aural speculum is used to inspect the external auditory canal and the tympanum. The canal is straightened by gentle traction of the pinna in a backward direction. An auriscope, which has its own light source, can be used or, alternatively, a

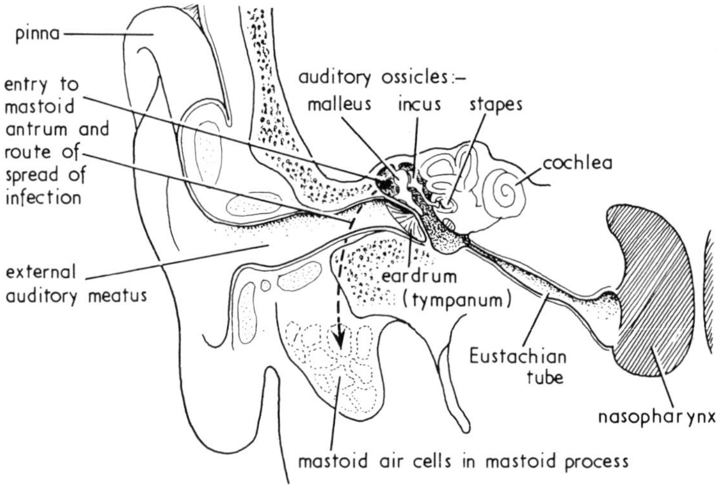

Fig. 37.1 *The ear.*

lamp can be directed from behind the patient and reflected by means of a head mirror. Both ears are examined—the 'good' side before the 'bad'. Vibrating tuning forks are used to test air and bone conduction of sound waves, air conduction being better than bone conduction in normal hearing. Hearing is tested in various ways, according to the subject's age, though the most accurate method is audiometry carried out under carefully controlled conditions in a soundproof room.

PROBLEMS ASSOCIATED WITH THE EAR

Wax

Wax (or cerumen) is produced by modified glands in the external meatus of the ear, normally it is carried outwards by the cilia. However, occasionally it forms a plug which hardens, causing deafness and even discharge, tinnitus or vertigo. Before ear syringing is carried out the patient must be examined by a doctor, the procedure only being undertaken by qualified nurses after appropriate training. The wax is previously softened by a 3-day course of cerumen ear-drops. Tap water, 1% sodium bicarbonate solution or 0.9% saline is warmed to 37°C to prevent dizziness. The patient is sat up with a kidney dish held firmly against the face. The lotion is introduced using an aural syringe and maintaining a steady flow of fluid along the upper wall of the meatus (Fig. 37.2). The ear is then dried and inspected. Complications which may arise following this procedure are giddiness, nausea and perforation of the tympanic membrane.

Foreign bodies

Children often put small objects such as beads or paper into the external auditory meatus. These are generally removed with a ring probe (Fig. 37.3) or by syringing. If the child becomes distressed, a light anaesthetic may be required.

Otitis externa, localised

This condition often occurs in 'run down' people or in those who are prone to infection, such as diabetics. A hair follicle in the external meatus becomes infected, often by a *Staphylococcus*, and

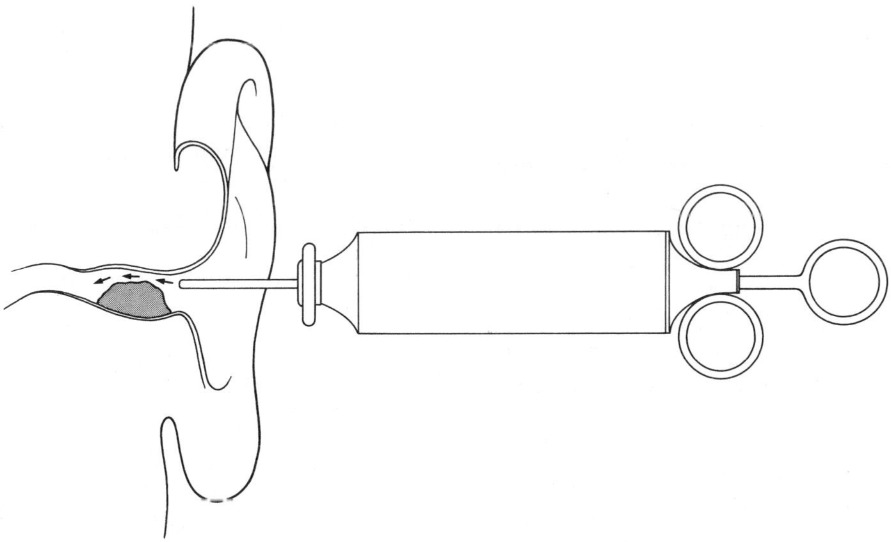

Fig. 37.2 *Ear syringing. The tip of the syringe is directed at the posterior wall.*

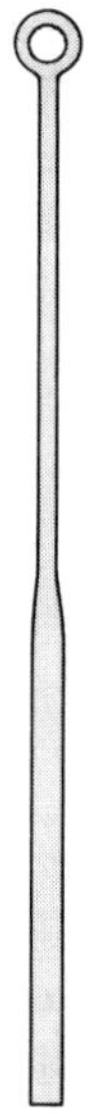

Fig. 37.3 *A Jobson Horne probe.*

this is known as furunculosis. Symptoms include inflammation, swelling and pain, which is worse on examination. The treatment is meticulous ear toilet and renewal of a 10% glycerine and ichthammol wick once or twice a day. Antibiotics and analgesia are prescribed by the doctor.

Otitis externa, diffuse

This condition is caused by a mixture of organisms such as *Staphylococcus pyogenes*, *Pseudomonas pyocyanea*, diptheroids, *Proteus vulgaris*, *Escherichia coli*, *Streptococcus faecalis*, *Aspergillus niger* and *Candida albicans*. It often coexists with other dermatological conditions of the scalp, such as dandruff and seborrhoeic dermatitis. There are diffuse inflammatory changes which cause the patient to scratch and probe the external canal. There may be some discharge. The condition may result from swimming in public baths, trauma during drying, or water remaining in the ears after washing. Europeans in tropical climates may also develop this condition. The treatment is careful aural toilet once or twice a day, and the insertion of a 10% glycerine and ichthammol wick.

Acute otitis media

This is common in young children and may be caused by infection arising from the upper respiratory tract which enters the ear via the eustachian tube, or by trauma to the tympanic membrane. Prompt treatment is essential. The patient experiences severe, throbbing pain and may be pyrexial. Often he suffers some degree of hearing loss, and sometimes tinnitus. A child may be fretful, rubbing his hand over the affected ear. If untreated, the tympanic membrane may rupture spontaneously, giving instant pain relief. However, the perforation will be jagged, and scar tissue formed in the healing process may cause impaired healing.

Treatment comprises rest and antibiotics. A local decongestant may be prescribed to assist drainage of the eustachian tube. If spontaneous rupture seems imminent, a small surgical incision may be made to avoid unnecessary damage to the tympanum (Fig. 37.4). This procedure may be carried out under local or, more usually, general anaesthetic. Gentle suction can be used to remove debris from the middle ear cavity. A Teflon grommet may be inserted following myringotomy (Fig. 37.5) to facilitate drainage. This is usually expelled spontaneously within a month.

The nurse must be aware of the importance of educating the public about completing a prescribed course of antibiotics, as failure to do so may allow a resistant strain of organisms to develop, leading to a chronic infection.

Chronic otitis media

Antibiotic therapy has considerably reduced the

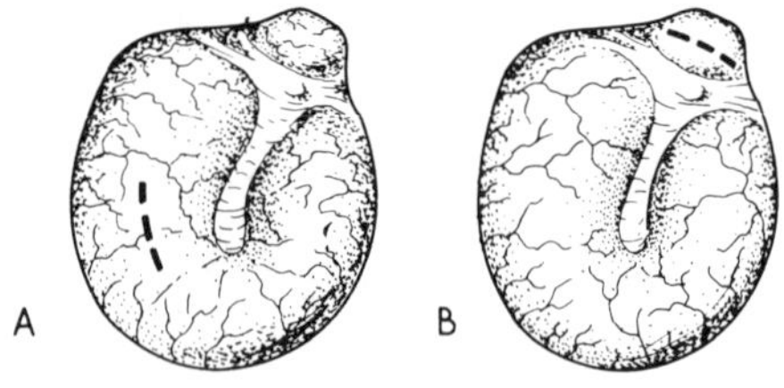

Fig. 37.4 *Incisions for otitis media.*

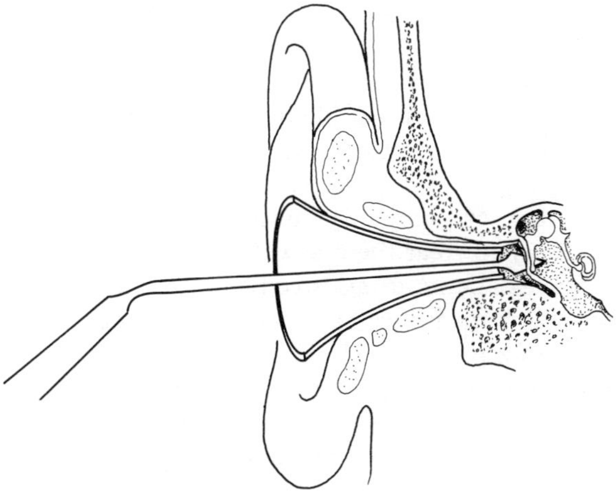

Fig. 37.5 *Myringotomy.*

incidence of acute otitis media, and therefore of the chronic form as well. Eventually infection will erode the ossicles of the middle ear and invade the air cells of the mastoid bone, and patients suffer considerable pain and deafness. Conservative treatment aims at eradicating any focus of infection, such as tonsillitis or sinusitis. Aural toilet is helpful, and efforts must be directed at improving the patient's generally poor state of health.

Acute mastoiditis

This rare condition arises as a result of neglected or inadequately treated acute otitis media. The thin bony partitions between the mastoid air cells break down and there is an increased production of pus through the perforated eardrum. The patient feels generally unwell. If diagnosed early enough, the condition may be treated with antibiotics; otherwise it will require mastoid surgery.

Mastoid surgery

The preoperative preparation specifically includes hairwashing, and shaving the hair in the postaural area, according to the surgeon's preference. The operative area is gently cleansed, though care must be taken to ensure that no fluid enters the ear.

The invention of the operating microscope has meant that in most cases the surgeon can aim to preserve the patient's hearing. There are various degrees of mastoidectomy which can be carried out: cortical, modified radical, and radical mastoidectomy. Reconstruction of the ossicle chain and tympanoplasty are also undertaken. Postoperative care includes the management of the meatal wick, wound drain and postaural pack. The patient rests in bed for 24 hours postoperatively. Labyrinthine disturbance may cause nausea and vomiting, and rest and antiemetic drugs are employed to minimise these problems. The nurse must observe for signs of facial palsy, which is indicated if the patient grins asymmetrically. The patient must avoid getting his ear wet until healing has taken place.

Otosclerosis

Otosclerosis is a progressive ossification and immobilisation of the foramen ovale and stapes which causes conductive deafness. Onset is usually between the ages of 15 and 30 years, and there is often a familial tendency to develop this condition. According to current thinking, males and females are about equally affected, though pregnancy may cause increasing deafness. Tinnitus may also be reported, and the patient can often hear better in noisy surroundings (paracusis). Deafness is unilateral and then bilateral. Stapedectomy is the operation of choice and involves the insertion of a prosthesis after the removal of the stapes (Fig. 37.6).

Postoperatively the patient is nursed lying flat for 24 hours to minimise the symptoms of nausea and vomiting. He must not blow his nose until healing has taken place.

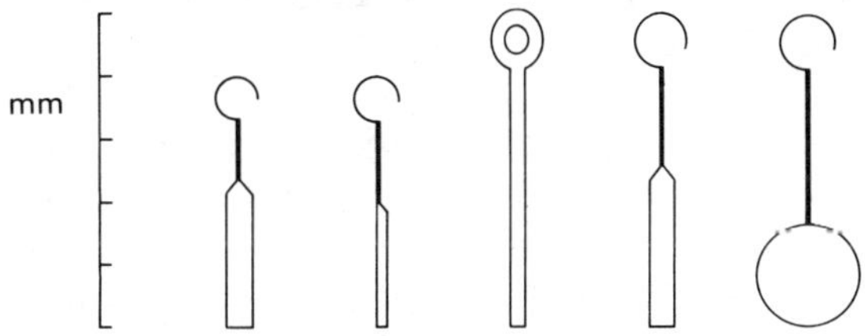

Fig. 37.6 *Types of stapedectomy prostheses.*

Electrical stimulation of the inner ear

This is being developed for the profoundly deaf.

Menière's disease

Menière's disease is thought to be caused by distension of the membranous labyrinth due to increased pressure of the endolymph. This phenomenon is associated with an electrolyte abnormality of the labyrinthine fluids. Onset is usually between 40 and 60 years of age. The patient experiences repeated episodes of tinnitus, vertigo, nausea and vomiting, accompanied by increasing deafness. At first deafness is unilateral, but in about 25 % of patients the other ear may become affected. Eventually surgery may be required, either to decompress the saccule or to destroy the labyrinth, and consequently the hearing on the affected side. The nurse's role is the support and careful observation of the patient.

Deafness in children

Deafness in children must always be investigated promptly. Tests to screen for hearing difficulties should be performed at 6 to 8 months of age, and repeated if the mother or health visitor has any anxieties about the child's hearing. Deaf children require early training to enable them to develop speech and to reach their educational and social potentials. Immunisation of pubescent girls helps to prevent rubella infection of fetuses in the first trimester which leads to consequent birth defects, including deafness.

CARE OF THE DEAF PATIENT IN HOSPITAL

The patient without hearing suffers from lack of communication with other people. The more severe the deafness, the more isolated and withdrawn he becomes. This may lead to depression or, in the elderly, confusion, as yet another channel of information is removed. The person who is hard of hearing frequently mis-hears, giving inappropriate answers and thus causing others to laugh at him, with the result that he hesitates to join in a conversation. People become irritated if they have to repeat themselves frequently and therefore the deaf person may pretend to have heard. There is a lack of sympathy towards the deaf and a tendency to treat them as if they are stupid.

Some patients are assisted by the use of a hearing aid which magnifies all sound in the range of the speech frequency, including background noise. In hospital there is a good deal of noise, and the large area of a ward causes more reverberations, with the result that the patient may not persist with the use of his hearing aid.

The nurse should check that the hearing aid is in good condition. The leads and batteries need to be checked daily and the ear mould should fit snugly to prevent the high-pitched whistle which will otherwise occur. The receiver should be worn outside the clothing to avoid the noise of the clothes moving.

The nurse must recognise that the patient is of normal intelligence and should be treated as such. She should make every effort to ensure that she has made the patient understand any information given. When talking to the patient, she should face him and speak slowly and clearly, but not shout. Some lip-reading will help the patient to understand what is being said, as will visual explanation. Above all, the nurse must make time to communicate with the patient.

EXAMINATION OF THE NOSE

The patient's whole face should be carefully inspected for clues to the underlying condition, e.g. the adenoid facies—mouthbreathing, broad bridge of the nose, arched palate, overlapping incisors. During the examination the nurse should stand behind the patient and steady his head with both her hands. A child may be snugly wrapped in a blanket and sat on the nurse's or his parent's lap, his head steadied by their hands (Fig. 37.7). A nasal speculum is used (Fig. 37.8), and a head mirror worn by the doctor provides reflected light.

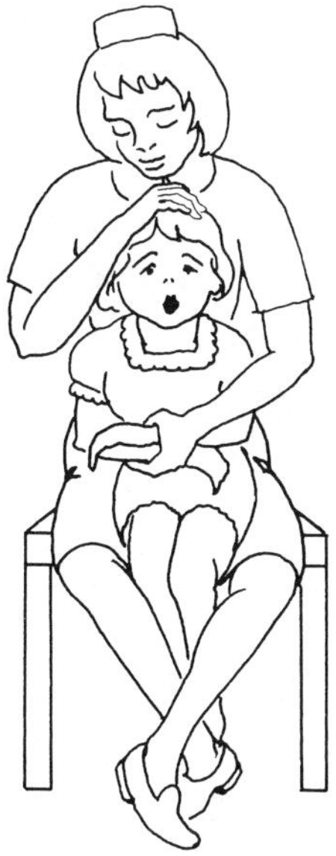

Fig. 37.7 *Position for examination of the nose and throat in a child.*

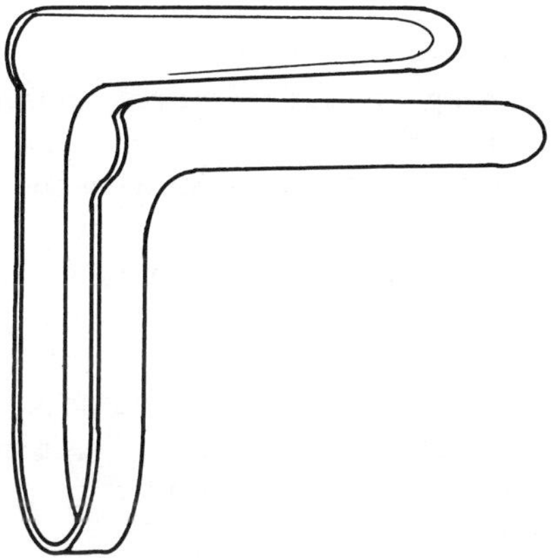

Fig. 37.8 *Nasal speculum.*

PROBLEMS OF THE NOSE AND SINUSES

Foreign body

Objects which children frequently push up their nostrils eventually cause a unilateral discharge if undetected. If they cannot easily be dislodged, a general anaesthetic will be necessary.

Nasal polyps

These are benign growths which develop from the mucous membrane and are usually pedunculated, projecting into the nose. They occur in people suffering from a nasal allergy or chronic infection, and may be removed by means of a snare (Fig. 37.9).

Nasal obstruction—deviated septum

This may be caused by congenital deformity or by trauma. Obstruction of the sinuses and one or both of the nasal passages results and the patient may complain of severe headaches and suffer repeated acute sinus infections. Surgery is not undertaken until the patient is 15 years old, or when the nose has ceased to grow. Correction is effected by submucous resection. The deflected cartilage is removed and the septum is repositioned in the midline. Haemostasis is secured by means of bilateral nasal packs, which are left in place for about 48 hours. A nose bolster may be worn for protection, and the nurse must observe the patient for signs of bleeding. It must be explained to him that he should not blow his nose or mop it with a soiled handkerchief; sterile tissues or gauze should be used instead.

The patient is given analgesia and an ice pack is positioned on the bridge of the nose prior to removal of the nasal packs. The latter both numb the nose and cause vasoconstriction. The patient is sat up with his head well supported. The pack is removed from the unoperated side first, very slowly, the patient lying still afterwards. He should be told to avoid violent exercise for 1 week and to report to the hospital if epistaxis occurs. Occasionally a haematoma may form, if so, this is normally left unless it becomes infected, in which case it is drained.

Epistaxis

This is a common condition, though it may have different causes. In children the most common cause is trauma to the anterior part known as Little's area (Fig. 37.10). Trauma can be caused by

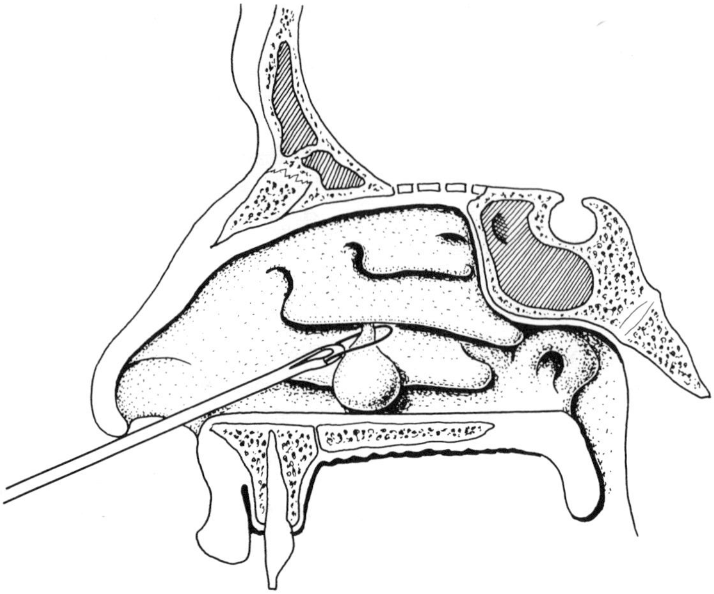

Fig. 37.9 *Removal of a nasal polyp with a snare.*

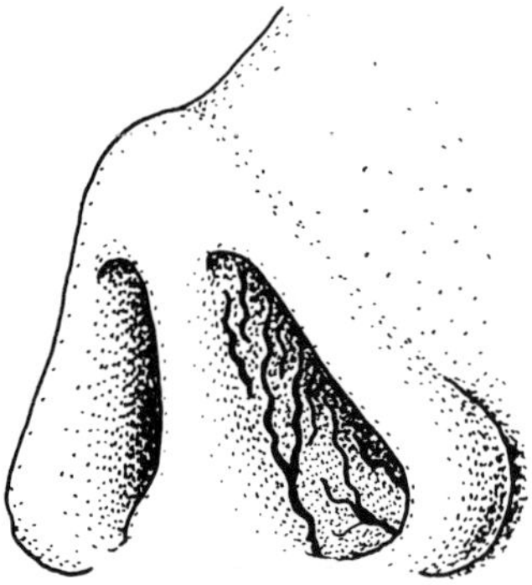

Fig. 37.10 *Little's area.*

nose picking, falls or inflammation. In older people a common cause is hypertension, and the bleeding point is generally in the posterior portion of the nasal cavity. In all age groups it may indicate blood dyscrasias, fevers or may simply be spontaneous.

Treatment commences with first-aid measures to stop the bleeding. The patient is sat with his head inclined forward and downward and the anterior portion of the nose is pinched between finger and thumb for 10 minutes. The patient breathes through his mouth. Clothing is protected against staining. Pressure to the posterior region of the nasal cavity can only be secured by packing with ribbon gauze or by inflating a balloon catheter to exert pressure on the bleeding point (Fig. 37.11). The nurse makes careful and frequent observations of the patient's pulse, blood pressure and mental state. Severe blood loss leads to confusion due to cerebral anoxia. If the pack is left in place for more than 48 hours, antibiotics are usually prescribed to prevent infection.

Acute sinusitis (Fig. 37.12)

Acute sinusitis may be caused by deflection of the nasal septum, infection of the upper respiratory tract, trauma, and dental abscess. The patient reports severe headache, especially on moving his head and stooping. This focus may give rise to secondary infections, or may develop into chronic sinusitis. Treatment may include nasal decongestants, steam inhalations, antibiotic therapy and sniffing salt and sodium bicarbonate solution to clear debris.

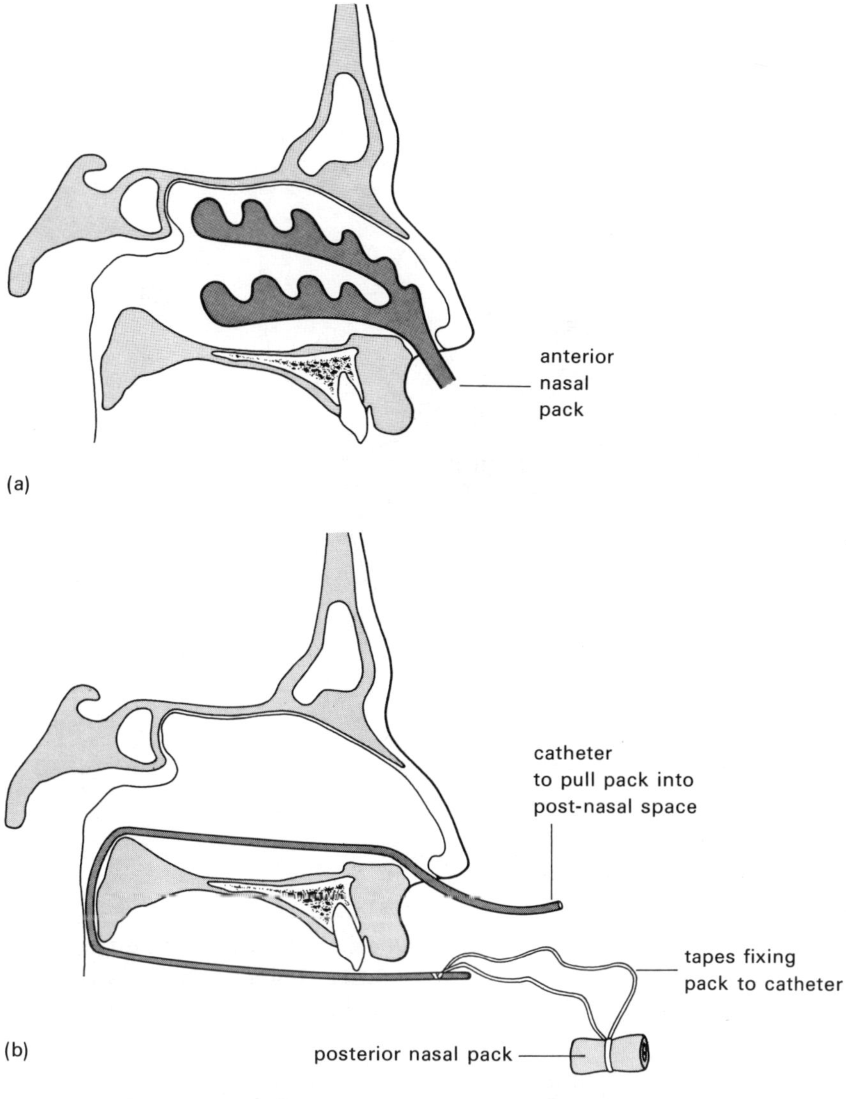

Fig. 37.11 *(a) Anterior nasal pack. (b) Posterior nasal pack.*

Chronic sinusitis

Chronic sinusitis may require drainage as the osteum is no longer patent. A topical anaesthetic is applied, then a Lichtwitz cannula and trocar is used to establish drainage through the antronasal wall (Fig. 37.13). The antrum is then irrigated with sterile physiological saline, using a large plastic syringe or a Higgison's syringe. If other measures prove unhelpful, a Caldwell–Luc operation may be performed. An incision is made above the canine teeth, the antrum is inspected and infected tissue is removed.

Instillation of nose-drops

The patient lies with his head tilted back so that the drops will be retained in contact with the affected

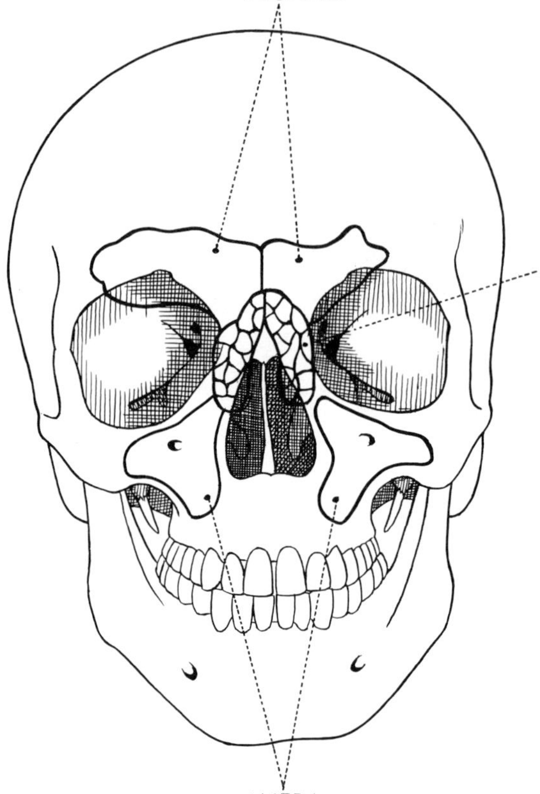

Fig. 37.12 *The sinuses.*

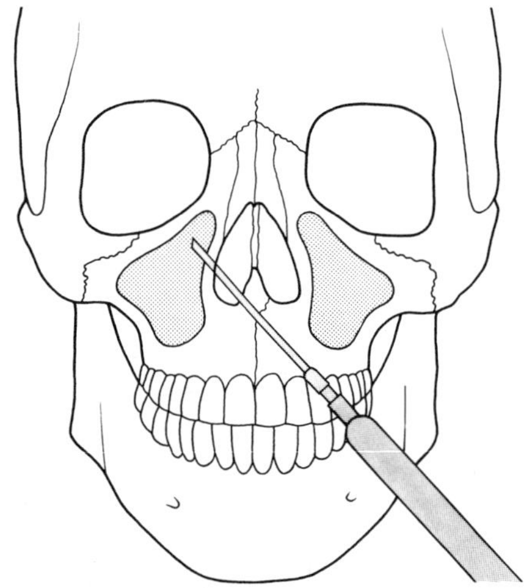

Fig. 37.13 *Insertion of Lichtwitz trocar and cannula into the right antrum.*

part. Following administration of the drops, the patient remains still for a few minutes to allow the medication to take effect.

Steam inhalations

Medicated inhalations are used to reduce mucosal swelling and aid drainage of mucus and pus. Care should be taken to protect the patient. The jug of inhalant is placed on a stable surface in front of the patient, and a towel is drapped around it to form a funnel large enough to admit the patient's nose and mouth. In this way the patient can gain most benefit from the procedure without feeling uncomfortable. The nurse must ensure the patient's safety with regard to the temperature of the water, and prevent spillage.

EXAMINATION OF THE THROAT

Indirect laryngoscopy

The pharynx and larynx are inspected by means of a warmed mirror. The patient is sat up comfortably, with his head supported. The tongue is depressed with a spatula, or the tip wrapped in gauze and hand held. Vocalising 'aah' helps to flatten the posterior part of the tongue. Then the mirror, warmed to prevent misting, is carefully passed over the back of the tongue and the glass is aimed downwards. Vocalisation of 'ee-ee' will approximate the vocal cords.

Direct laryngoscopy

Direct laryngoscopy is carried out by passing a laryngoscope, which combines a spatula and light, which allows the tissues of the pharynx to be moved aside to reveal the larynx. The patient is sedated and a local anaesthetic spray numbs the throat before this procedure. Alternatively, the patient may receive a light general anaesthetic.

SURGERY OF THE THROAT

Tonsillectomy

This operation is performed when the patient's tonsils repeatedly become infected. Hypertrophy of the adenoids causes obstruction of the eustachian tubes and deafness, whereas hypertrophy of the tonsils causes difficulty in swallowing, a condition most common in children.

Preoperatively the patient should be free from infection and apyrexial. It is important to establish whether he has any bleeding disorders, and loose teeth should also be noted. Postoperatively the patient is nursed in the semiprone position with his head positioned so the secretion and blood will drain out of the nose and mouth and not be swallowed, thus masking signs of bleeding. Vital signs are observed and recorded meticulously, as haemorrhage may be brisk. The patient is kept cool and quiet for 24 hours, but allowed to be accompanied to the bathroom. Oral hygiene is very important, gargles and toothbrushing being used, according to the patient's age. Hard foods, such as toast, help deslough the tonsillar bed, but analgesia, such as aspirin mucilage or gum, must be administered beforehand. The patient may be discharged 2 to 5 days postoperatively, but should return, or consult his general practitioner, if haemorrhage or infection occurs.

Once discharged, the patient should remain at home, avoid overheating and infection, and stay away from crowds. He can generally return to normal activity after 3 weeks.

Acute tonsillitis is often followed by quinsy (Fig. 37.14). The infection passes through the tonsil capsule and into the tissue behind it, first causing cellulitis and then an abscess. Thus the affected side of the throat becomes enlarged, red and painful and there is difficulty in swallowing. This will be incised.

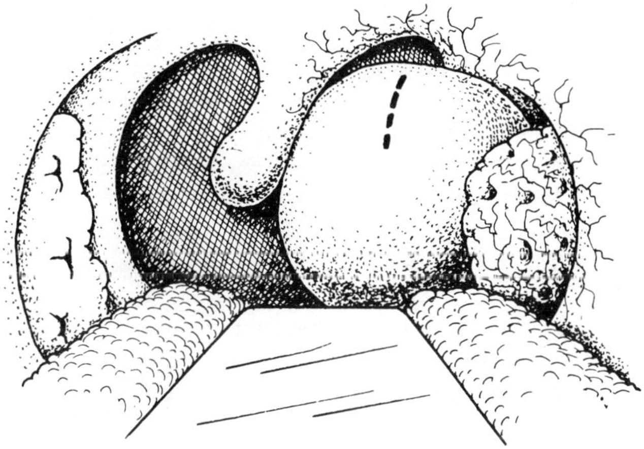

Fig. 37.14 *Quinsy.*

Tracheostomy

This is an emergency procedure to make an artificial opening into the anterior trachea at the level of the second to third cartilaginous rings below the cricoid cartilage. The tracheostomy may be temporary or permanent, and is performed for a number of reasons: to assist breathing for a patient requiring ventilation; to reduce 'dead space' in

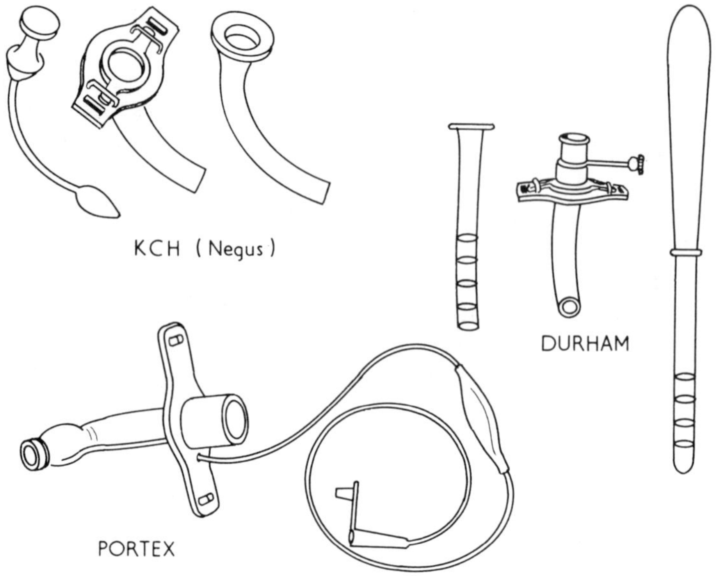

Fig. 37.15 *Tracheostomy tubes.*

respiratory insufficiency; to protect the tracheobronchial tree as, for example, in the case of the comatosed or burned patient; or to preserve life in airway obstruction. The patient will have a tracheostomy tube in place to maintain a patent airway. At first a plastic cuffed tube is used, later being replaced by a non-disposable silver tube (Fig. 37.15). Maintenance of the airway by keeping the tracheostomy patent is the nurse's priority. Initially patients require humidified oxygen or air, as the warming and moistening functions of the nasal cavity have been lost. Suction of the tracheostomy is frequently required in the early stages following surgery, and tracheal dilators should always be at hand in case the tube should come out. Communication by speech is impossible for the patient, so he needs a bell, writing pad and pen to compensate. The nurse should always try to anticipate his needs, and take time to talk to her patient, though he cannot reply.

Laryngectomy

This operation is performed for malignancies of the larynx, which affect men more often than women. Currently radiotherapy is often used as the treatment of first choice. After surgery the tracheostomy is permanent, and normal speech is no longer possible.

The patient is admitted 2 to 4 days preoperatively into a single cubicle. He should be adequately prepared for the loss of his voice, the speech therapist visiting him and explaining how this will be overcome. Rehabilitation is emphasised from the outset. The physiotherapist will teach him breathing exercises and the nurse will seek to improve his state of nutrition. During this period she will make every effort to get to know the patient well and settle him. A nasogastric tube is passed preoperatively and oral hygiene is maintained. Male patients will require a shave. Blood will have been taken for grouping and cross-matching and antibiotics commenced.

Postoperatively the patient requires care of the highest order. He will be 'specialled' initially, being nursed in the intensive care unit or a cubicle on return from theatre. Suction, oxygen and humidification, using a special tracheostomy mask, will be ready for use. Initially, the cuffed tube will be deflated for 5 minutes in every hour to prevent local tissue necrosis caused by pressure. The patient will be sat up as soon as possible, supported by plenty of pillows. Care will include aseptic toilet to the wound in order to keep it clean and dry, the drains being kept vacuumed. Suction apparatus with sterile catheters is kept at the bedside for use as frequently as is required. The nasogastric tube is aspirated as often as is necessary to prevent nausea. As a blood transfusion will be in progress, the patient will be observed for signs of a reaction. A fluid balance chart will be maintained, and frequent mouthwashes given. Analgesia is administered as often as required to keep the patient comfortable and all his daily needs are met by the nurse.

After 2 to 4 days the temporary tube is removed and replaced by a suitable silver tube. Each tracheostomy set consists of a tube, introducer and two inner tubes. An inner tube can be removed if the patient's airway becomes obstructed. The introducer and spare inner tube are kept in a covered sterile container beside the patient. The intravenous infusion is usually discontinued after 24 to 48 hours, and nasogastric feeding is commenced. The first feed is water, in case of inhalation via a fistula. Gradually, full-strength feeds containing all the elements required for correct nutrition are given. Oral diet may commence about 10 days postoperatively. The patient is assisted out of bed on the first or second day, and may sit in a comfortable chair for short periods. The tracheostomy tube is changed daily using an aseptic technique. Two nurses are necessary, one to maintain the patient's airway by the use of tracheal suction and tracheal dilators, if required, the other to change the tube. The drains will be removed when drainage ceases. Sutures are removed when healing has taken place. This varies as preoperative radiotherapy may delay the healing process. Gradually the patient will be taught to care for his own stoma, including tube changes, toilet and care of equipment. A shaving mirror placed on a table in front of him facilitates this procedure.

Physiotherapy is very important to prevent chest infection. The speech therapist will commence teaching the patient to speak again once healing has taken place. He will be shown how to swallow air and then belch it up, forming this into words with his lips and tongue. He may attend group lessons following his discharge home about 3 weeks postoperatively. A silk scarf may be worn loosely around the neck, so hiding the stoma, but on no account should a fluffy one be used. He should be told about the Laryngectomy Society and given the address of the local branch. The one activity which he cannot undertake without special snorkel equipment is swimming. The long-term aim of care is rehabilitation. Curative surgery is not always possible, and surgery may be palliative only. However, the nurse's role is vital, and relief of anxiety and physical symptoms, such as any pain, as well as the support of the patient and his relatives become the primary goal.

SUGGESTED WORK

1. Find out how the current criteria for doing a tonsillectomy are different from those of 20 or more years ago. Why is this?
2. Find out from the speech therapist the different ways in which the loss of a larynx for voice production can be overcome.

SUGGESTED READING

Ashley J. (1973). *Journey into Silence*. London: Bodley Head.

* * *

Mrs JANET CLARK (aged 34 years) is a married woman with two children aged 8 and 4. In the last few years she has become progressively more deaf in both ears, although her left ear is worse than her right. She has been diagnosed as having bilateral otosclerosis.

Medical plan
Left stapedectomy, followed at a later stage by a right stapedectomy if it is successful.

Identification of the patient's needs and problems in the first 48 hours and action arising from these

Management of nausea and vomiting
Administer the antiemetic prescribed regularly and monitor its effectiveness. Arrange that it is given before visiting time to prevent the embar-

rassment of vomiting at this time. It may also be wise for her to have the antiemetic before being mobilised. If she does vomit, ensure that the vomit bowl is removed promptly and that she has a mouthwash afterwards.

Hygiene
As soon as she has fully recovered from the anaesthetic, wash her face and hands and put her own nightdress on her. The first day postoperatively she may have a bowl in bed to wash. A mouthwash will probably be appreciated.

Mobility
Keep Mrs Clark in bed for 24 hours, lying on her unaffected side. She should then be gradually sat up in bed, avoiding sudden movements. Before getting up she should sit on the edge of the bed and dangle her legs. When she takes her first walk, stay with her ready to support her if she loses her balance. Explain that she should not make sudden movements and that if she feels unsteady when walking, she should be escorted by a nurse.

Prevention of infection
Administer the antibiotics as prescribed. Take the temperature 4-hourly and report any rise as this may mean that a different antibiotic will have to be prescribed.

Management of the wound
Advise the patient not to blow her nose until the wound in the eardrum is healed. Remove the packing after 48 hours and insert cotton wool soaked in Cortisporin.

Nutrition
Once the nausea is under control, she will be able to have a light diet, returning to a full diet when she feels she can tolerate it. Loss of taste on one side may interfere with her desire to eat, but taste is still present on the other.

Partial deafness
When talking to Mrs Clark, make sure that she can also see the movements of your mouth. Ensure that she has fully understood what has been said as she may have only heard part of it. Include her in any conversation.

Psychological
If hearing is not restored immediately, Mrs Clark will feel depressed. It should already have been explained to her that it may take up to 2 weeks to be fully restored, but reinforcement at this stage will be necessary. The nausea, vomiting and vertigo may also add to this general feeling of depression and must therefore be adequately controlled. Mrs Clark must be assured that they will go.

Social
She will be concerned about how her two children are managing in her absence. It will be reassuring to her if they can visit once she is feeling like it.

38

Conditions of the Genitourinary Tract

The kidneys are the most important organs in the body for the excretion of waste, which includes the balance of salts and water (Fig. 38.1). They are also involved in maintaining the acid–base balance in the body so that the pH of the blood is kept within narrow limits. Therefore any serious damage to the kidneys will result in a build up of waste substances within the body and a disturbance in the electrolyte balance. They are also very vascular organs.

Infection in the lower part of the urinary tract can ascend to involve the kidneys, and thus it is important to deal promptly with such conditions to prevent this occurring. If the kidneys do become damaged and require surgery, the nurse's role will

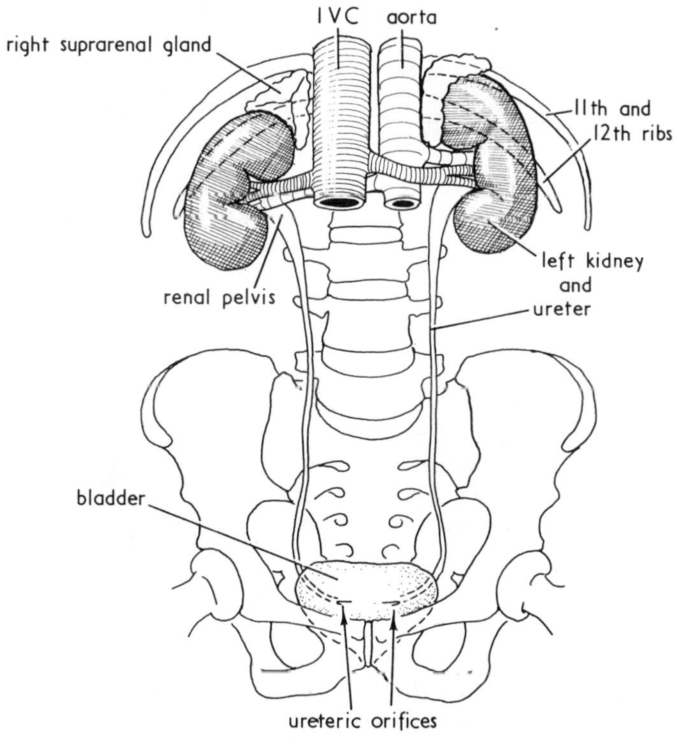

Fig. 38.1 *The urinary tract.*

be to monitor the fluid intake and output of the patient meticulously and to recognise at an early stage any evidence of haemorrhage.

Specific emphasis in the nursing history

Elimination. Test urine for blood and albumin; note output.

Pain. The presence of a dull ache in the loin, renal colic or dysuria.

Vital signs. Note if temperature raised and whether constant or swinging.

General appearance. The presence of lethargy or malaise. Flushed face.

Skin. Pallor or jaundice.

TUMOURS OF THE KIDNEY

Wilm's tumour (nephroblastoma) is a malignant tumour occurring mainly in children. It is usually treated by a combination of surgery, radiotherapy and chemotherapy. Vincristine, actinomycin D and doxorubicin (Adriamycin) are the drugs most commonly employed.

Carcinoma and sarcoma may develop in the kidney in the adult and are also treated with the same therapy combination as above, although the results are not as good as for Wilm's tumour. If the tumour is hormone dependent, progesterone derivations are sometimes given.

Clinical picture

In children a tumour may be felt, but in adults haematuria is usually the first evidence of abnormality. If clots are passed, the patient may suffer from renal colic. There may also be a dull aching pain in the loin, and in the male a varicocele may be present.

Investigations

A specimen of urine is tested in the laboratory for blood and malignant cells. An intravenous pyelogram will demonstrate whether or not the kidney is able to function. Aortography will be done to show any abnormality of the blood supply to the kidney, and lymphangiography will be necessary to demonstrate any spread to the lymph glands. Ultrasound and percutaneous renal cystography (injection of a contrast medium into any cyst present) may also be carried out.

RENAL AND BLADDER CALCULI

Calculi may develop in the kidneys or bladder and are the result of substances being deposited (Fig. 38.2). Metabolic diseases such as gout and endocrine diseases such as hyperparathyroidism may be the underlying cause. The incidence is much higher in those areas of the world where the climate is hot. Those conditions leading to urinary stasis and urinary tract infection will also pre-

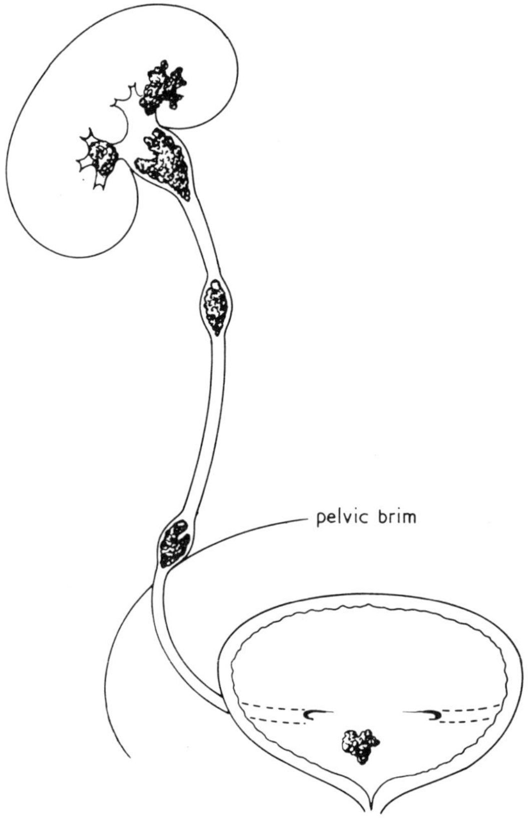

Fig. 38.2 *Calculi.*

dispose to the formation of calculi. Patients who are kept in bed for a long time, such as those receiving lengthy orthopaedic treatment, are also at risk. Having said this, however, in a large proportion of patients with calculi, no cause can be found.

The calculi may be formed from a mixture of ammonium, calcium and magnesium phosphates producing a white or grey stone—the majority are of this type; about 25% consist of calcium-oxalate-producing, dark, irregular stones; and about 10% are smooth brown stones of uric acid. If the last-mentioned are composed entirely of uric acid, they will not be seen on x-ray. Urates and cystine are other substances which can form stones.

There may be just one calculus, of any size, or a large number filling the calyces and pelvis, so forming a staghorn calculus. Tiny calculi may migrate down the ureters to the bladder where they form the basis of a calculus. Those slightly bigger may cause renal colic, thought to be due to the release of prostaglandin.

The presence of a foreign substance such as a calculus in the kidney predisposes to infections such as pyelonephritis, pyelitis or pyonephrosis (pus in the kidney), or cystitis if the calculus is in the bladder.

Clinical features

Calculi in the kidneys or bladder may not cause any symptoms. If the stone is in the kidney, there may be a dull aching pain in the loin which is relieved by lying down. Evidence of infection, such as urgency and frequency, or slight haematuria may be present. A stone passing down the ureter and causing renal colic may give rise to a sudden, acutely distressing pain which comes in waves and moves from the loin to the groin. It may be associated with sweating, vomiting and tenderness in the loin or abdomen on the affected side. Anuria may occur if only one kidney is functioning and a calculus becomes impacted in the other. Impaction of a calculus in a ureter will cause hydronephrosis in which urine accumulates in the pelvis and calyces of the kidney (Fig. 38.3).

Most calculi are radio-opaque and can be seen on x-ray. An intravenous pyelogram, cystoscopy or even retrograde pyelography may be necessary to confirm the diagnosis. A midstream specimen of urine will be taken to detect infection, and urine will be observed for the passage of calculi.

Management

Rest in bed is necessary. Urinary antiseptics such as nitrofurantoin 100 mg 6-hourly will be required if there is any evidence of urinary infection. Renal colic will either be treated by a strong analgesic such as pethidine 100 mg parenterally, which is also a smooth muscle relaxant, or, more recently, by indomethacin 100 mg suppositories which inhibit the production of prostaglandin. Atropine is also given occasionally. Heat applied locally to the loin helps to relieve the pain.

1. *Nephrolithotomy* is the removal of a calculus from the kidney through an incision in the kidney.
2. *Pyelotomy* is the removal of a stone or tumour via an incision in the renal pelvis.
3. *Ureterolithotomy* is the removal of a calculus impacted in the ureter. An x-ray is taken immediately prior to the operation to locate the position of the calculus.
4. *Partial nephrectomy* is the removal of part of a kidney and is used when calculi or disease affect only part of the kidney.
5. *Renal sympathectomy* involves removal of branches of the sympathetic nervous system supplying the renal artery and is used for hypertension or hydronephrosis. In the latter it is done in conjunction with a plastic operation on the pelvis and ureter, a pyeloplasty.
6. *Nephrostomy* involves insertion of a drainage tube into the kidney until further surgery can be done, such as removal of a calculus.
7. *Nephroureterectomy* is excision of the kidney and part or all of the ureter. This may be done in tuberculosis of the kidney or for a tumour of the renal pelvis to prevent spread.
8. *Nephropexy* is an operation to anchor a floating kidney, i.e. one which moves due to insufficient perirenal fat and relaxed abdominal muscles.
9. *Transluminal angioplasty* is carried out if the artery to the kidney is narrowed, leading to a raised

blood pressure. A special catheter is guided under x-ray into the narrowed vessel, the balloon being blown up to widen the artery.

10. *Nephrectomy* is removal of the kidney and may be carried out for any of the following reasons providing the other kidney is healthy.

Injury.
Neoplasm.
Renal calculi, if there is gross damage to the kidney.
Aneurysm.
Ureteric rupture, obstruction or ligation.
Chronic or acute disease of one kidney.

If grafting is to be done, both kidneys may be removed at the same time.

11. *Pyeloplasty* is reconstruction of a narrowed ureter to relieve hydronephrosis (Figs. 38.3, 38.4 and 38.5).

12. *Extracorporeal shock-wave lithotripsy (ESWL)* shock waves are aimed at stones in the kidney or ureter, the anaesthetised patient lying in a water bath. The fragments of stone pass out through the ureter.

Preparation of the patient preoperatively

In a unilateral nephrectomy which is not being done as a surgical emergency, the function of the other kidney must be accurately measured, and for this purpose various renal function tests will be done. These will include an intravenous pyelogram, and possibly a renal biopsy or renal scanning and arteriogram. Blood tests for urea and elec-

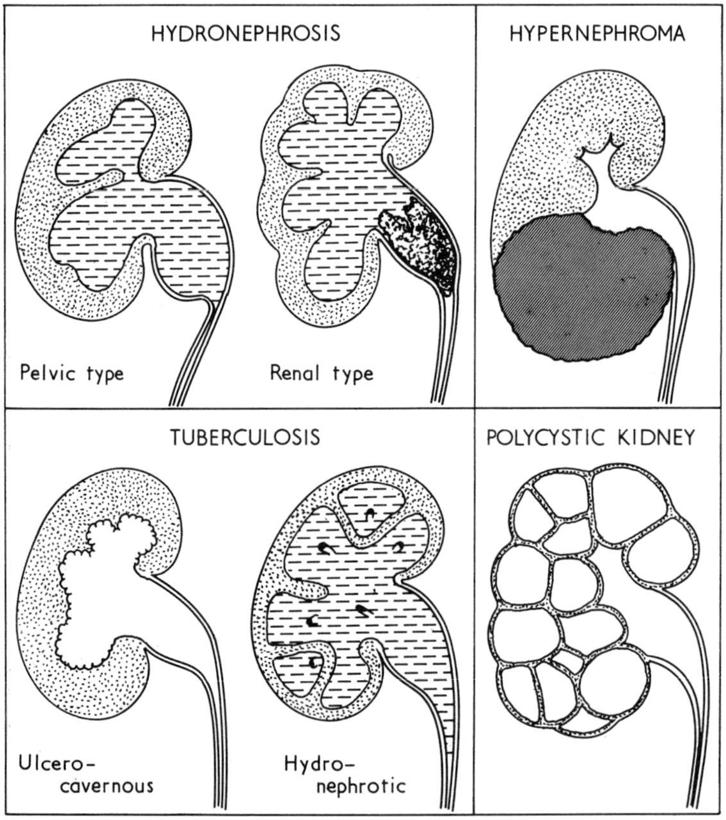

Fig. 38.3 *Hydronephrosis and other kidney disorders.*

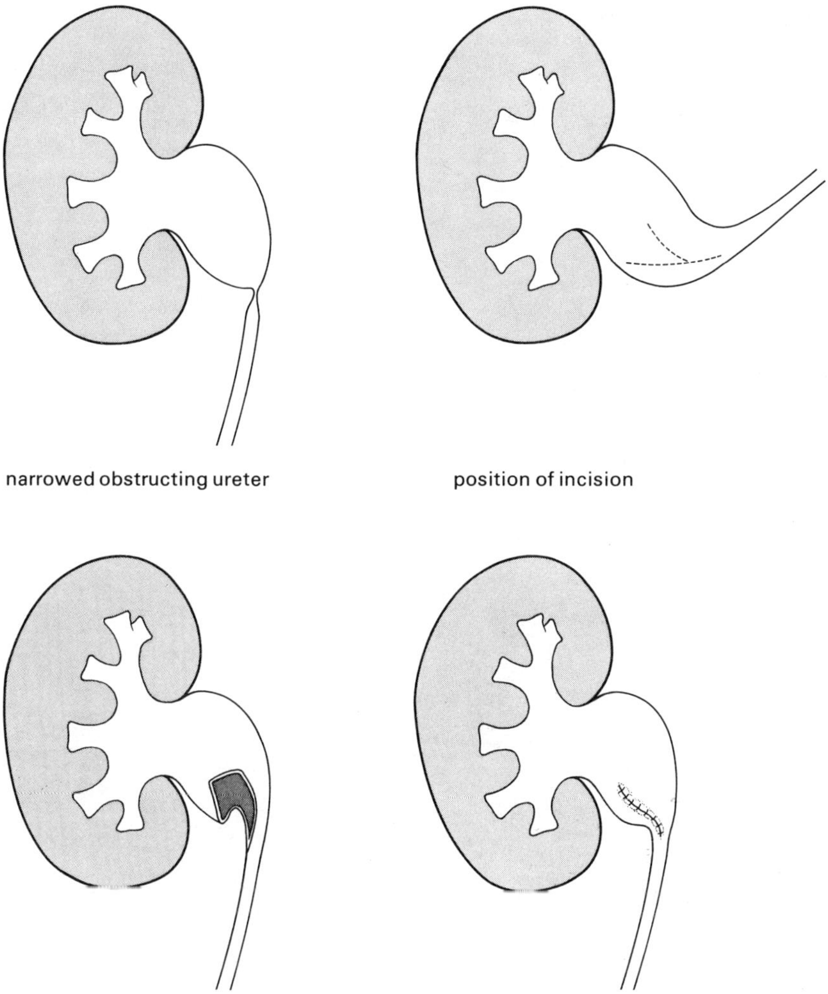

Fig. 38.4 *Foley pyeloplasty: correction of the obstruction without severing the ureter. (This does not diminish the size of the dilated pelvis.)*

trolytes are particularly important. Anaemia may be present and should be corrected, blood also being taken for grouping and cross-matching.

Unless the patient is on restricted fluids, these are encouraged, a strict fluid balance chart being kept. If there is any infection, antibiotics will be commenced. A full shave is required as the approach may be either from behind, as with an adrenalectomy, or abdominally. If only one kidney is being operated on, the appropriate side must be marked by the surgeon.

Postoperative care

Following a nephrectomy there is often a high incidence of shock, therefore it is important that quarter hourly observations of blood pressure and pulse are made. For the same reason the foot of the

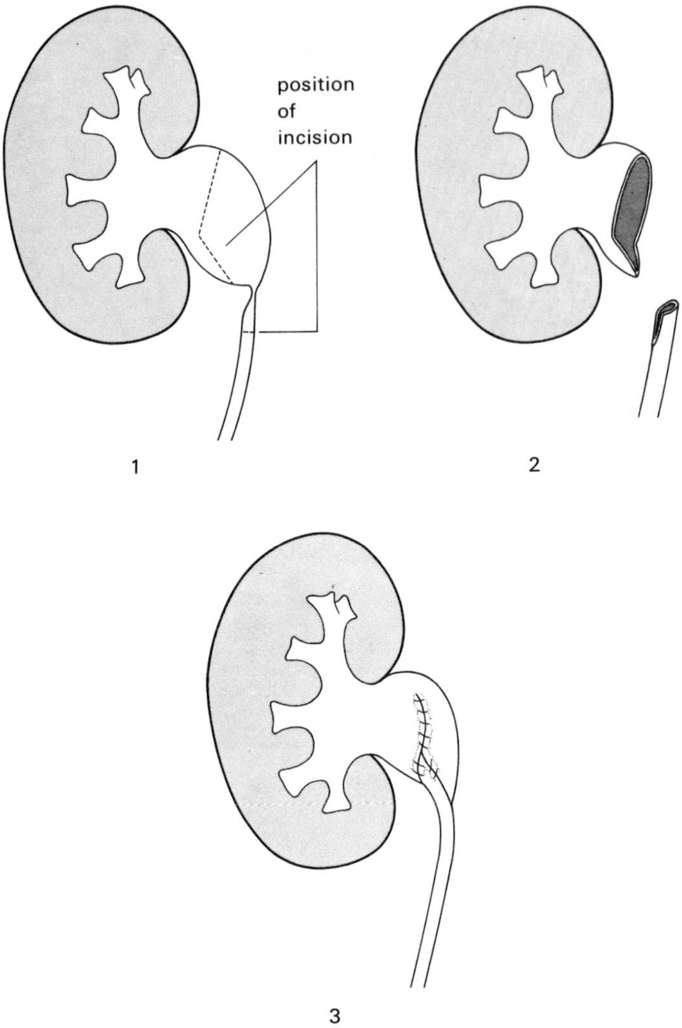

Fig. 38.5 *Hynes–Anderson pyeloplasty. The abnormal ureter and part of the pelvis are excised. The ureter is then anastomosed to the pelvis obliquely.*

bed is elevated. The patient will be receiving either intravenous fluids or blood if there was extensive loss in theatre. On return to the ward the patient is placed in a semirecumbent position, lying toward the affected side in order to assist drainage. A catheter will be in position and all urinary drainage must be measured accurately and recorded. The colour of the urine is carefully noted for bleeding, the previous specimen being kept for comparison.

There will be a drainage tube from the kidney bed to the surface and the drainage from this should be carefully observed. As the patient recovers from the anaesthetic, an analgesic such as morphia is used, particularly if clot colic occurs. However, as morphia causes nausea, an antiemetic may also be required. The dressing is observed for bleeding and repacked as necessary. Mobilisation is gentle, the patient remaining in bed for several days until there is no haematuria. It is essential that the patient realises that he has only one kidney, but that this is sufficient for him to lead a healthy life.

POLYCYSTIC KIDNEYS

This is a hereditary condition often not becoming apparent until middle age. Kidney tissue is replaced by multiple cysts, so that the patient will eventually have insufficient kidney tissue to deal with his waste products and will develop uraemia and die. The only treatment available involves renal dialysis or kidney transplant.

URINARY DIVERSION

In certain conditions it is necessary to bypass the bladder and divert the urine into the bowel or onto the surface of the abdomen. The following are examples of such conditions.

Congenital malformations such as ectopia vesicae.

Meningomyelocele.

Other neurological conditions interfering with bladder control.

Obstruction of the ureters from fibrosis, arising from a chronic infection.

Carcinoma of the bladder or prostate and invasive carcinoma of the uterus or rectum involving the urinary tract.

A large vesicovaginal fistula due to trauma at delivery.

The three main ways of diverting the urine are as follows (Fig. 38.6).

1. The ileal conduit. In this operation, a loop of bowel, such as the ileum or colon, is isolated and

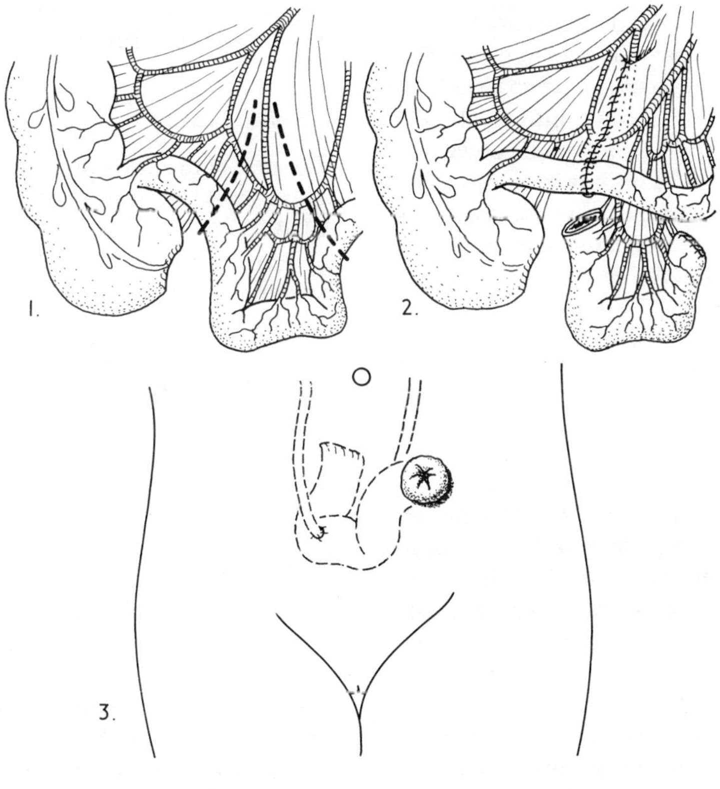

Fig. 38.6 *Urinary diversion.*

brought to the surface of the abdomen to form a stoma. The urine is collected in a bag. Care has to be taken that the urine does not come in contact with the skin and cause excoriation. However, this approach is normally considered superior to other methods, as infection is minimal and there is no reabsorption of waste substances.

2. The original approach was to insert the ureters into the colon, so allowing the urine to mix with the faeces, and preventing the need for a stoma. Unfortunately, not only is the fluid reabsorbed, but also some of the waste products. Ascending infection to the kidneys is also a problem.

3. A modification of the above approach is the rectal bladder in which a colostomy is formed for the excretion of faeces and the ureters are inserted into the rectum.

Preoperative preparation

The patient must be prepared psychologically, particularly if he is to have a colostomy or ileal conduit, and any fears discussed. If married, his wife will also need to be fully informed. The preparation is that for any surgery on the bowel and in particular for a stoma. (This has been discussed in the chapter on the gastrointestinal tract, see Chapter 20). It includes adequate emptying of the bowel, reduction of bacteria with antibiotics, and correct siting of the stoma. The siting of the stoma in an ileal conduit is particularly important to prevent leakage of urine.

Postoperative care

Nursing care is the same as that for any patient undergoing intestinal surgery and a colostomy. Blood is also taken to monitor the electrolyte balance, particularly if the ureters have been inserted into the colon. If an ileal conduit has been performed, the flange of the drainage bag is fixed firmly and smoothly to the abdominal wall so that no leaks can occur. This is usually done in theatre. The bags attached to the flange can be changed daily.

Cystostomy

A catheter is passed and the bladder irrigated with antiseptic lotion after which it is distended with the lotion. An abdominal incision is made, and through this an incision into the bladder. A Winsbury-White suprapubic tube, or a Malecot's or de Pezzer self-retaining catheter, is inserted which enables the bladder to be irrigated. It is usually removed after 3 days with a metal introducer which enables the expanded end to be straightened out.

ENLARGEMENT OF THE PROSTATE

Prostatectomy

The prostate, which encircles the urethra of the male as it leaves the bladder, may become enlarged so causing difficulty on passing urine. If the growth is benign, the gland feels soft and smooth on rectal examination, whereas a carcinoma of the prostate will feel hard and irregular. Enlargement of the prostate occurs primarily in the elderly.

Clinical picture

Because of the position of the prostate, any enlargement will interfere with the emptying of the bladder, so causing difficulty in passing urine, the stream being poor. The patient also has difficulty in starting and finishing. Chronic retention occurs, predisposing to urinary infection, and therefore there may be frequency, urgency and nocturia. This may lead on to uraemia. Patients are frequently admitted with acute retention and may also be suffering from anaemia and dehydration. Diverticula may also develop in the bladder.

Preoperative preparation

The flow of the urine can be measured with a flowmeter, or the doctor may observe the patient passing urine. He will also do a rectal examination. An intravenous pyelogram will be done if the blood urea is not raised. A midstream specimen of urine will be taken to exclude infection which, if present, must be treated before surgery is undertaken.

Blood is taken for haemoglobin, white cell count, urea, electrolytes, ESR, grouping and cross-matching, and serum acid phosphatase. The last-mentioned is raised in carcinoma. If carcinoma is present, x-rays will be taken of the pelvis, lumbar spine, and skull for metastases. A needle aspiration of the prostate may be done to look for malignant cells, and a biopsy of the gland via the perineum or rectum under antibiotic cover.

If the patient is admitted with acute retention of urine, no fluids are given until a catheter has been passed. The patient will then have continuous drainage to the bladder, and fluids are encouraged (unless there is some medical contraindication), and an accurate record kept of fluid balance. The operation will not be done until the blood urea is within normal limits and any anaemia, dehydration or electrolyte imbalance has been corrected. The catheter is removed immediately prior to operation.

Types of operation (Fig. 38.7)

In Britain the most common approach for a benign tumour is a transurethral resection (TUR), in which a rectoscope is passed into the urethra. The rectoscope has a semicircular wire loop through which a cutting electric current is passed and pieces of the prostate are cut away. The blood vessels are coagulated and great care is taken not to damage the external sphincter. If the resection is being done for an early carcinoma, those pieces of tissue resected from the outside of the growth are put into a separate specimen pot to the others. This is to enable the pathologist to estimate the extent of the growth.

In *retropubic prostatectomy* (Millin's operation) an incision is made in the abdominal wall, just above the symphysis pubis. The bladder is moved out of the way and the prostate removed. In a *transvesical prostatectomy* the bladder is opened to remove the prostate.

Postoperative care

An intravenous infusion of sodium citrate, 0.9% sodium chloride or dextrose 5% is run through quickly, up to 3 litres in 24 hours. If much blood is lost at operation, a blood transfusion will be necessary. Occasionally, mannitol is used to induce a diuresis. An accurate record of the fluid balance must be kept. Cyclokapron or epsikapron may be added to the infusion to prevent haemorrhage. The patient is sat up as soon as possible to encourage

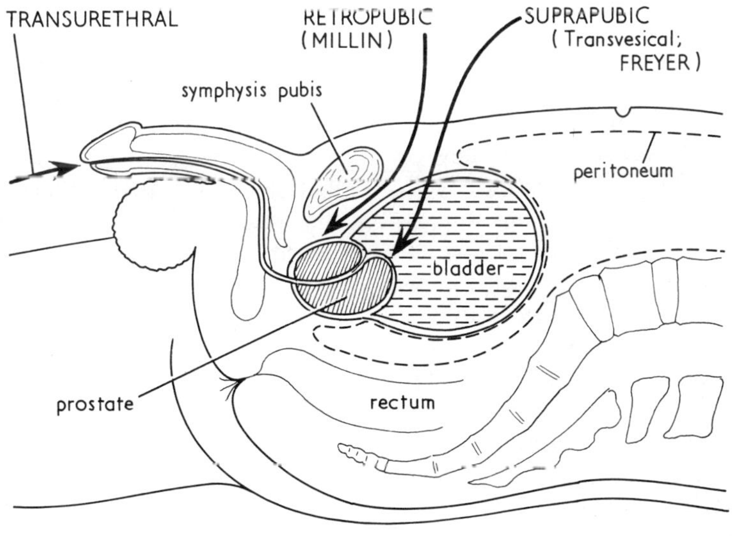

Fig. 38.7 *Types of prostatectomy.*

drainage. A catheter will be in situ and will be on continuous irrigation with sodium citrate or sodium chloride until the urine is clear. The previous drainage bottle is kept for comparison. Catheter toilet will be necessary. If a transvesical operation is done, there will be a suprapubic catheter in position which will need redressing and will require removal in 48 hours.

Other methods of treatment

It is possible that the *laser* will be able to be used through an endoscope to vaporise tissue.

Malignant growths may be treated with chemotherapy, with drugs such as cyclophosphamide, or radiotherapy, particularly if pain is present. Radioactive iodine seeds may be implanted into the prostate in conjunction with the removal of the lymph nodes. Hormone treatment, for example with stilboestrol in small dosages (1 mg three times a day), or orchidectomy, if metastases are present, can also be carried out. Hormone treatment cannot be given to those patients suffering from cardiovascular disease.

RENAL FAILURE (URAEMIA)

This is a condition in which the kidneys are unable to excrete waste substances from the body, and they therefore accumulate in the blood. Acute renal failure may be due to conditions reducing the blood flow to the kidneys, such as dehydration, haemorrhage or shock, or to disease of the kidney or obstruction to the flow of urine from the kidney, as with an enlarged prostate or hydronephrosis. Every system in the body is affected, the patient becoming progressively more drowsy until comatose, from the action on the nervous system. The patient becomes nauseated and vomits, and may have a haematemesis. Hiccoughs and halitosis are other effects due to the action on the gastrointestinal tract. Hypertension and anaemia and changes in the ECG may also be present. The skin becomes pigmented and may itch due to the excretion of urea, which may be seen as a 'frost' on its surface. Acidosis and electrolyte imbalance, polyuria and later oliguria are other signs which develop. The condition may persist and progress to chronic renal failure.

Haemodialysis (Figs. 38.8 and 38.9)

In this procedure blood is taken out of the patient's circulatory system via tubing and diverted into a kidney machine, consisting of semipermeable membranes through which waste products are able to pass. The purified blood is then led back into the patient's circulatory system through tubing. This process is usually carried out for 10 hours at night, and repeated for 3 nights in the week.

Peritoneal dialysis (Fig. 38.10)

In this method, dialysing solution is run into the peritoneal space and allowed to remain there for a certain length of time, during which waste products diffuse out of the adjacent capillaries into the solution. The solution is then syphoned back out of the peritoneal space. This is repeated with fresh solution a number of times. This procedure cannot be carried out if there is infection in the abdominal cavity.

Continuous ambulatory peritoneal dialysis (CAPD)

This is an extension of the previous method and is suitable for those patients who would not be considered for haemodialysis or renal transplants because of age or other medical conditions. The patient has a permanent tube in his abdomen through which he is able to carry out fluid changes. He must be taught to be scrupulous in his management of the tube and fluid or peritonitis will develop.

KIDNEY TRANSPLANTATION

For the patient with chronic renal failure of both kidneys, who is under 55 years old, it may be found more desirable to carry out a kidney transplant than to remain on dialysis.

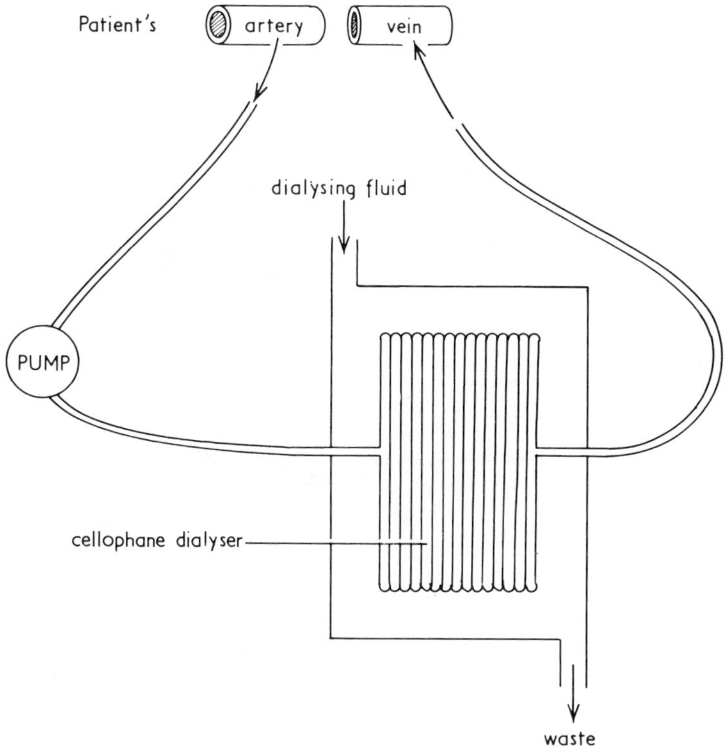

Fig. 38.8 *Haemodialysis.*

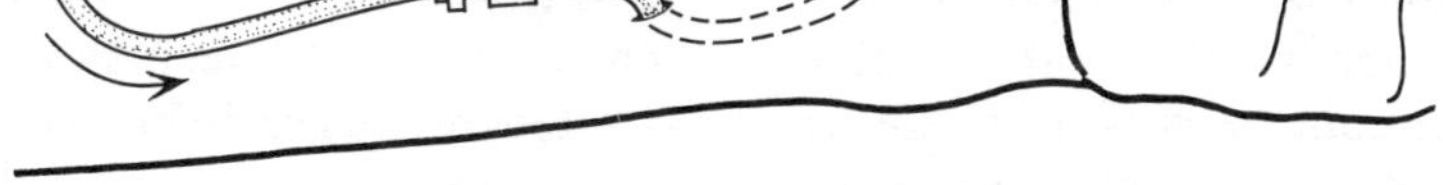

Fig. 38.9 *External arteriovenous shunt for attachment to haemodialysis machine.*

Because of the possibility of rejection, the donor and recipient are tissue typed. They are tested for ABO and Rhesus compatibility as well as leucocyte grouping. An exact match is not possible but the kidneys from a donor are given to that patient with the closest tissue typing. In most instances the kidneys are taken from accident cases after death has been pronounced by a doctor not involved in the transplantation operation (cadaveric donors). Occasionally they are removed from a living donor,

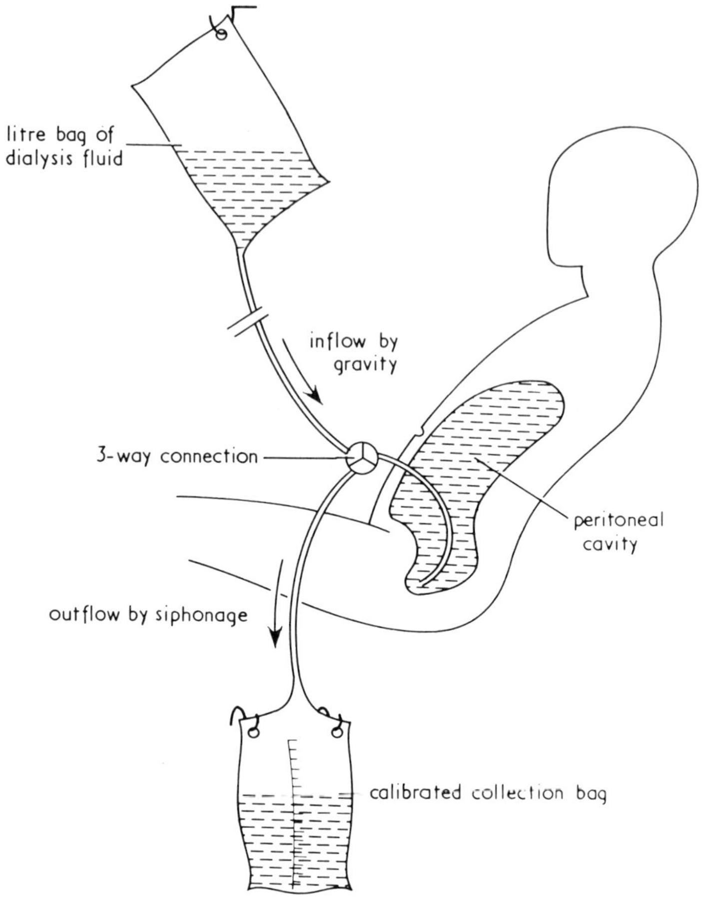

Fig. 38.10 *Peritoneal dialysis.*

usually a close relative. In the latter case it is essential that the donor is completely investigated to ensure the other kidney is fully functioning.

The recipient must be in the best possible condition for the operation; he will therefore be dialysed beforehand. Psychological preparation plays a very important part in this patient's care: there will be the uncertainty of waiting for a donor and possibly several disappointments, and following the operation there is always the possibility of the kidney being rejected. The recipient's kidneys may be removed at an earlier operation, or when the transplant is carried out. However, they may not be removed at all. The donor kidney is placed in the iliac fossa (in the pelvis), to one side of the bladder, the renal artery being anastomosed (end to end) to the internal iliac artery, and the renal vein (end to side) to the external iliac vein. The ureter, which is usually very short, may either be implanted into the recipient's bladder or anastomosed to his ureter.

If the donor is living, the recipient may start immunosuppressive treatment 2 days preoperatively, but this is unlikely to be possible with the cadaveric donor. This treatment is necessary to reduce the possibility of rejection. The drugs most commonly used are azathioprine 75–200 mg in 24 hours, corticosteroids and antilymphocyte serum (ALS). Irradiation may also be used.

The operation is a relatively straightforward one

and the patient will be mobilised on the first postoperative day. He will be able to start eating at an early stage. The urinary output must be measured meticulously, as this may suddenly cease, or large volumes of urine may be excreted causing dehydration. The kidney normally starts functioning within the first 24 hours but in a few patients it takes longer and dialysis will be necessary. The drugs may cause a variety of complications such as susceptibility to infection, agranulocytosis and gastrointestinal disturbances. The patient must therefore be protected by barrier nursing and the limitation of visitors. He should also be observed carefully for any evidence of infection as steroids mask this.

The patient will continue on the drugs following discharge, although the dose will gradually be reduced. He must be told to keep an accurate record of his fluid balance which will be monitored at his twice-weekly visits to the out-patients department. These frequent visits are necessary in the early days to monitor the blood urea and for other tests. If the patient develops an infection, however mild, he must go to his doctor as this could quickly become lethal. He will carry a card or Medic-alert necklet stating that he is on steroid therapy.

URINARY INFECTION

Infection may occur in the bladder from stasis of the urine which may arise from congenital abnormalities, enlarged prostate or damaged nerves supplying the bladder. Pregnancy also predisposes to infection, as does the presence of a catheter. Infection in the bladder (cystitis) may then ascend to the pelvis of the kidneys causing pyelitis, eventually involving the kidneys themselves, pyelonephritis. If pus is present, the condition is called pyonephrosis.

The organisms most commonly involved in urinary infections are *Esch. coli* (95 %), *Proteus* (2–4 %), *Streptococcus faecalis*, *Staphylococcus albus* and *Pseudomonas*.

Cystitis causes frequent micturition with dysuria and pyrexia. If the infection involves the kidneys, there will be pain in the loin with toxaemia.

A midstream specimen of urine is sent to the laboratory for culture and sensitivity tests. This should be an early morning specimen and the patient should not be given large amounts of fluid to drink before passing it as this dilutes the number of organisms. Fluids are encouraged and antibiotics which are concentrated in the urine are given. Examples of these are sulphamethizole (Urolucosil), nalidixic acid, nitrofurantoin and co-trimoxazole (Septrin); other sulphonamides are also used. If the infection involves the kidneys, bedrest will also be essential until the temperature is normal.

PERINEPHRIC ABSCESS

This is an abscess in the fatty tissue around the kidney arising from infection in the kidney or bloodstream. It usually requires incision, although antibiotics may be effective.

TUBERCULOSIS OF THE KIDNEY

This is a chronic infection spreading from the lungs or another focus of infection to affect the cortex of the kidney. Treatment is by antituberculous drugs. If the disease is widespread and there is destruction of the tissue with the formation of pus, drainage of the cavities (cavenotomy) or partial nephrectomy will be indicated. A nephroureterectomy may be required if the kidney is no longer functioning, provided the other kidney is healthy.

PAPILLOMA OF THE BLADDER

This is benign tumour which frequently becomes malignant. The patient presents with episodes of painless haematuria of varying duration. Cystitis generally occurs at a later stage of the condition, but occasionally at an earlier point. Urine is examined microscopically for blood and malignant cells. A cystoscopy and intravenous pyelogram will also be done.

Papillomata may be removed with diathermy on cystoscopy, or with a diathermy knife through a suprapubic cystostomy.

MALIGNANT GROWTHS

These will require either a partial cystectomy or a total cystectomy and transplantation of ureters, treatment by radiotherapy or the implantation of radon seeds around the tumour through a suprapubic cystostomy.

TRAUMA TO THE BLADDER

The bladder may be ruptured by a blow on the abdomen or torn by a fractured pelvis. Gunshot wounds may perforate it.

Intraperitoneal trauma

This is the most common type, the urine escaping into the peritoneal cavity so causing peritonitis. It is treated by surgery to repair the wound, catheter drainage and drainage of the peritoneal cavity.

Extraperitoneal trauma

This type is associated with a fractured pelvis. The urine escapes into the tissues causing cellulitis and a profound toxaemia. The cellulitis requires drainage by incisions accompanied by drainage and surgical repair of the bladder.

DIVERTICULA OF THE BLADDER

A diverticulum is herniation of the bladder mucosa through the muscular coat. It may be congenital or arise as a result of chronic obstruction of the bladder. Calculi frequently develop or become lodged in the diverticulum, and tumours may also form. Until infection becomes evident there may be no signs or symptoms.

Treatment of the obstruction will usually be all that is necessary with small diverticula. However, a large diverticulum will need to be excised, the bladder wall being repaired—diverticulectomy.

FISTULAE OF THE BLADDER

A fistula may develop between the bladder and the skin following the removal of a suprapubic catheter. A *vesicointestinal* fistula may develop between the bladder and the rectum or pelvic colon, and can occur if a carcinoma of the bladder or bowel is present. In this case flatus and faeces are passed in the urine. A *vesicovaginal* fistula is a channel between the bladder and the vagina, usually resulting from trauma during operation or delivery, and occasionally due to carcinoma.

The track has to be removed surgically and the wound repaired. If carcinoma is present, more extensive surgery will be required.

ECTOPIA VESICAE

In this rare congenital condition, there is defective development of the anterior wall of the bladder, the overlying abdominal wall and the pubic bones. The bladder protrudes through the gap in the abdomen. Initially it is treated by transplanting the ureters into the pelvic colon. When the baby is a few months old the bladder is removed and skin grafting is used to close the wound.

VESICOURETERIC REFLUX

This may be a congenital condition or may arise as a result of tuberculosis of the urinary tract or paraplegia. On micturition, when the bladder contracts, some of the urine will return up the ureter due to failure of the valvular action at the junction of the bladder and the ureter. This can be demonstrated with a micturating cystogram. It will lead to recurrent pyelonephritis and therefore the ureters will need resiting.

CONDITIONS OF THE URETHRA

A urethral caruncle

A small mass of granulation tissue which appears as a bright red enlargement at the entrance of the urethra, this is very sensitive to touch and causes dysuria and occasionally haematuria. It is excised with a scalpel or diathermy electrode.

Rupture of the urethra

This may happen in the male if he falls astride a projecting object. It may also be present as a result of a fractured pelvis or gunshot wound. There will be bleeding from the urethra and acute retention of urine.

If this condition is suspected, the patient should not attempt to pass urine as this will leak into the perineal or pelvic tissues (extravasation). The urethra is repaired immediately and a suprapubic catheter inserted. The perineal wound is kept clean by irrigation and then dried.

Stricture of the urethra

Inflammation, trauma or instrumentation may cause fibrosis in and around the urethra in the male. The patient has difficulty in passing urine, overcoming this by straining. Chronic retention of urine occurs, leading to cystitis and calculi. Eventually renal infection and acute epididymo-orchitis may also arise. The condition can be diagnosed by passing a urethroscope, the urethra being distended by air.

Treatment

Dilatation (*bouginage*) A series of plastic or metal bougies of increasing size is introduced into the urethra. Infection frequently follows this procedure, so antibiotics are required.

Urethroplasty This operation is done in two stages, the urethra being laid open in the perineum (Fig. 38.11) and the urine draining through a perineal catheter. The stricture is then excised, and the urethra reconstructed.

Postoperatively a catheter will remain in situ for 14 days and this should not be spigoted at any time. Dilatation with bougies will also be necessary. The wound is kept as clean and dry as possible to prevent breakdown of the wound or abscess formation (periurethral abscess). If the urethra becomes necrosed, urine will escape into the tissues of the perineum and scrotum causing cellulitis, and the patient will become delerious. In this case it will be necessary for the surgeon to make multiple incisions to drain the area.

Phimosis is the inability to retract the foreskin and is either congenital or acquired. It may cause

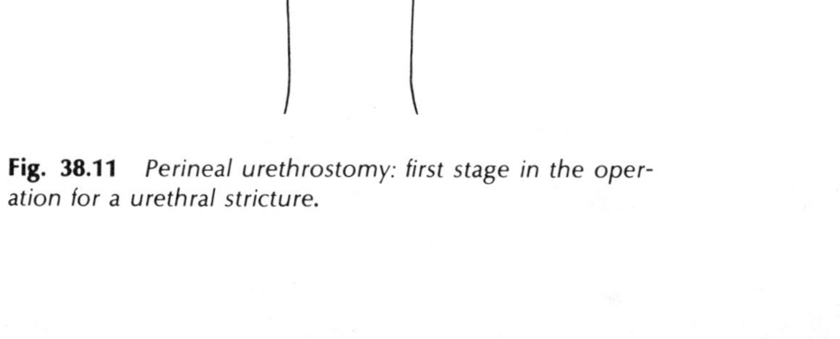

Fig. 38.11 *Perineal urethrostomy: first stage in the operation for a urethral stricture.*

inflammation of the prepuce and glans penis (balanitis). *Paraphimosis* is the inability to replace the foreskin after retracting it, so causing congestion. This condition can be treated by means of a dorsal slit which is made in the foreskin to relieve pressure.

Apart from for religious reasons, circumcision is carried out for phimosis or recurrent paraphimosis. The foreskin is cut away and the skin and mucous membrane sutured with catgut (Fig. 38.12).

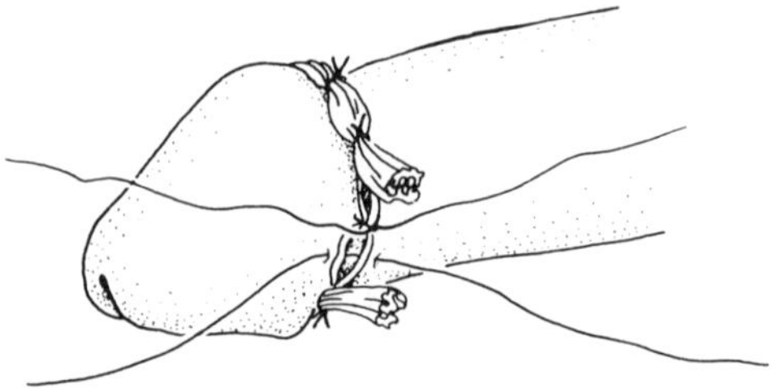

Fig. 38.12 *Circumcision.*

Epispadias is a rare congenital abnormality in which the urethra opens on the upper surface of the penis instead of at the tip. It may be associated with ectopia vesicae. In *hypospadias* there is arrested development of the penis, the urethra opening onto the undersurface of the organ.

Surgical correction of these conditions is necessary, and the operation is usually carried out in two stages, the first to straighten the urethra, the second being a plastic repair (Fig. 38.13). At both stages a catheter is left in position, in the first operation for 2 to 3 days and in the second operation for up to 14 days. The wound must be frequently attended to, to keep it clean and dry.

Carcinoma of the penis is an uncommon condition and requires amputation of the penis and bilateral removal of the inguinal lymph glands, or radiotherapy to them.

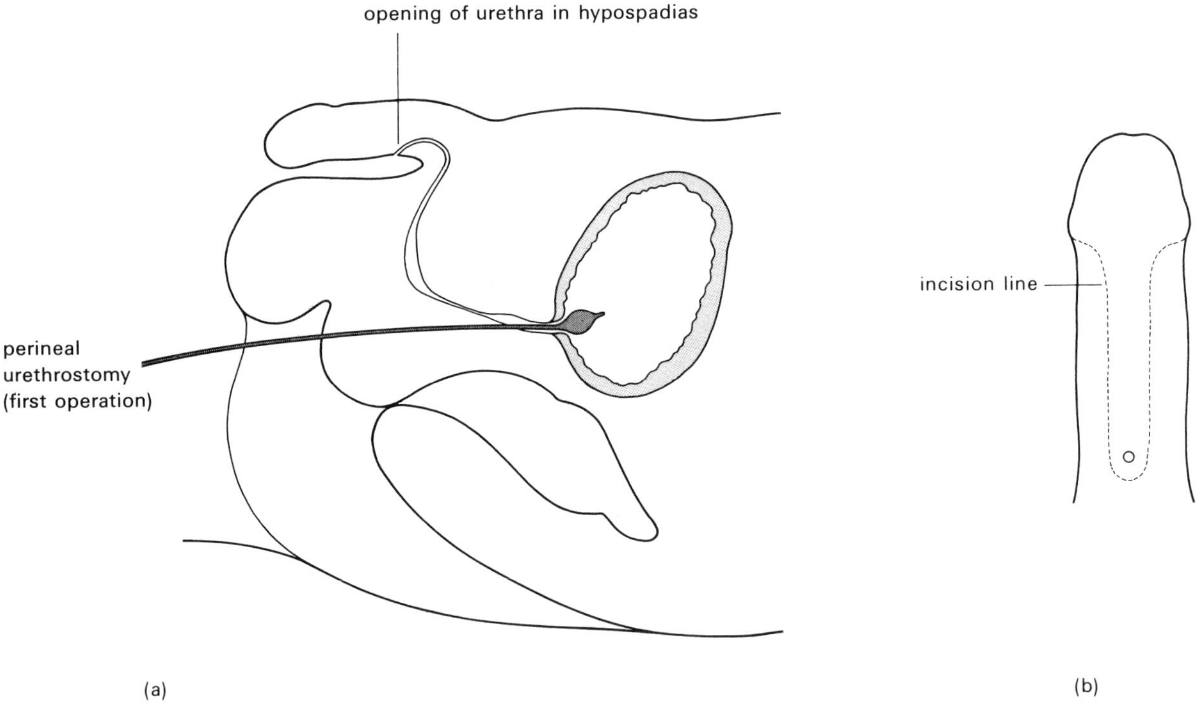

Fig. 38.13 *(a) First stage of treatment for hypospadias. (b) The two flaps are sutured together to form a new urethra.*

Hydrocele

A hydrocele is a collection of serous fluid between the two layers of the tunica vaginalis (the innermost covering of the testis, Figs. 38.14 and 38.15). It may either be unilateral or bilateral and varies considerably in size and shape. Although some are soft and others tightly distended, they are all smooth. Usually a hydrocele is painless, but occasionally it can be tender and painful when touched. The hydrocele is translucent to light on transillumination in a darkened room, which enables it to be differentiated from other conditions.

A small hydrocele will not require treatment. However, as it becomes larger there may be discomfort, embarrassment or even difficulty in passing urine, and fluid will have to be aspirated off (tapping) under a local anaesthetic. The adminis-

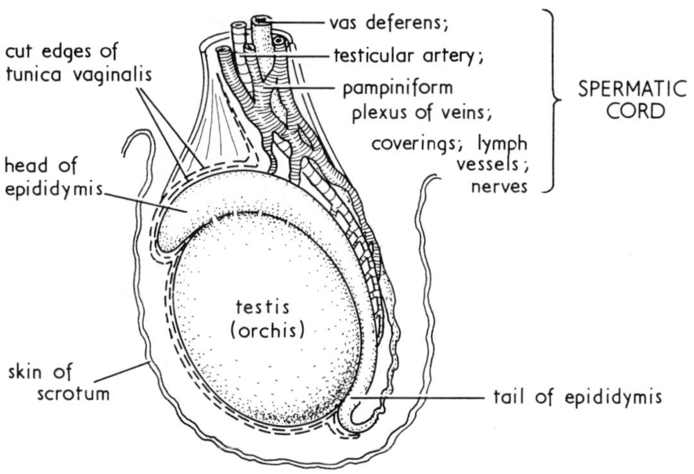

Fig. 38.14 *Testis.*

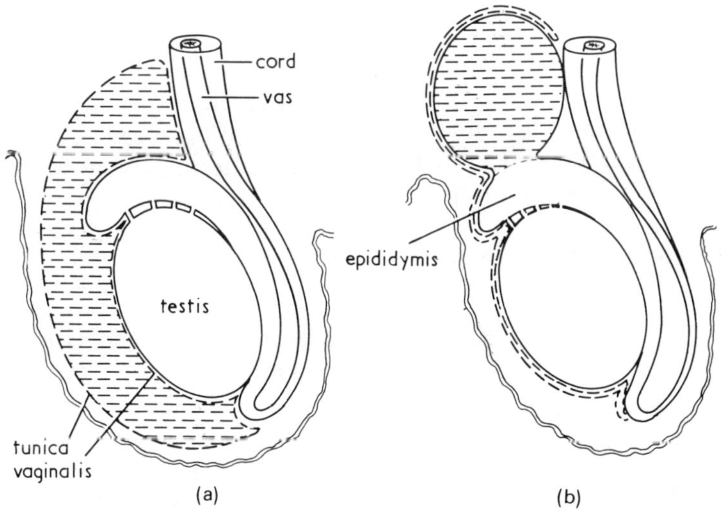

Fig. 38.15 *(a) Hydrocele. (b) Cyst of epididymis.*

tration of sclerosing solution (sodium tetradecyl-sulphate, STD), one to three injections at intervals of 6 weeks, may follow this. While awaiting operation the patient may wear a suspensory bandage. An operation may be done in which the sac of the hydrocele is laid open and a large portion removed. This prevents a recurrence of the condition.

Varicocele

The veins draining the testis become varicosed, usually on the left side. This can happen at any age but may indicate a tumour of the kidney in the older man. Apart from a dragging sensation, there is usually little or no discomfort. Support with a suspensory bandage may be all that is required, although in some cases it may be necessary to remove some of the veins surgically.

Haematocele

Haematocele is escape of blood into the tunica vaginalis due to trauma or malignant disease.

Spermatocele

This is a cyst containing spermatozoa at the upper end of the epididymis. It is translucent on transillumination and is excised if it is causing symptoms.

Teratoma

This tumour of the testis occurs in men around the age of 30 years. These are usually solid tumours which frequently become malignant and spread rapidly. Treatment is by orchidectomy and removal of the spermatic cord followed by radiotherapy.

Seminoma

This carcinoma of the seminiferous epithelium is very sensitive to radiotherapy.

Epididymectomy and orchidectomy

Removal of the epididymis and removal of a testicle may be necessary if tumours are present. Chronic infection, particularly tuberculosis, may require such an operation if it is not responding to chemotherapy. Occasionally it may be done in carcinoma of the prostate as part of the hormonal control.

Postoperatively, any of the operations may have a drain which is removed if no fluid is accumulating. A suspensory bandage may be necessary. Postoperative haematoma and sepsis frequently occur.

Undescended testis

In the fetus the testes are in the abdomen, descending through the inguinal canal into the scrotum during the latter part of development. However, they may not descend, or, more commonly, may only descend part of the way, remaining in the inguinal canal. Occasionally they descend into the scrotal sac but have a tendency to retract up the canal. They may also be found in an abnormal position (ectopic).

Because infertility and malignancy are associated with this condition, operative measures are necessary to free the testes and bring them down to the scrotum, fixing them there (Fig. 38.16). This is usually done when the boy is 6 to 9 years old.

Torsion of the testis

This frequently happens with undescended testes but may also occur when the organ is in its normal position. It is associated with sudden acute pain and vomiting. Because gangrene is usually present, an orchidectomy may be necessary.

Vasectomy

This is usually done following a prostatectomy to prevent ascending infection. It may also be done as a method of birth control once the family is complete, in which case, careful counselling will be required. The man can be reassured that his sexual characteristics and behaviour will not be affected. The operation can be carried out under a local anaesthetic and may therefore take place in the outpatients department. A small incision is made into the scrotum; the vas deferens is then crushed,

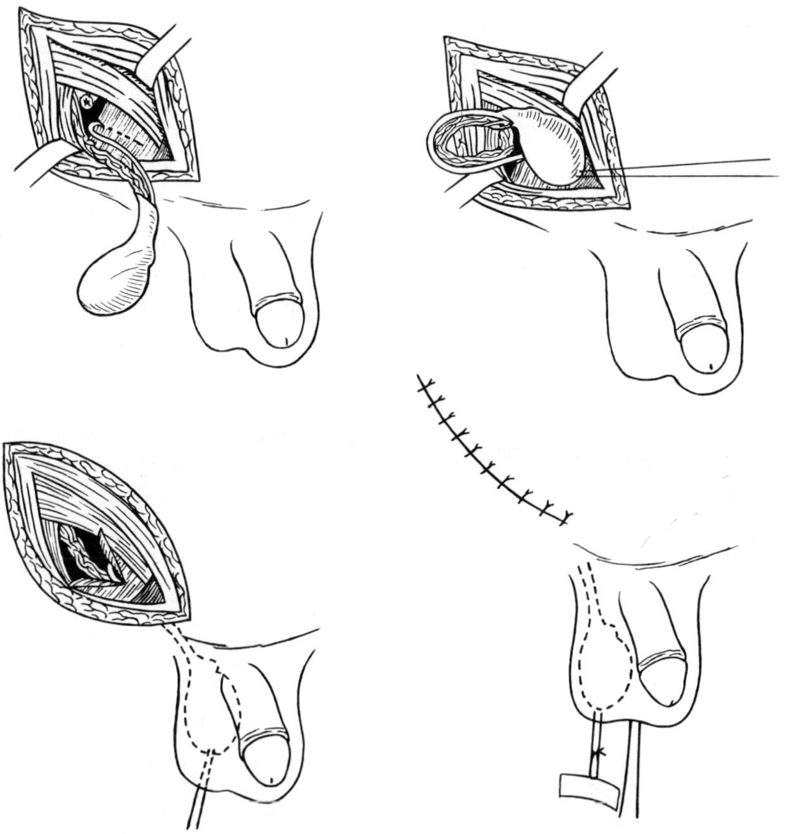

Fig. 38.16 *Operation for undescended testis.*

folded back on itself, and ligated. The operation is repeated on the other side of the scrotum. The patient is advised that contraception must be continued until two specimens of semen have come back from the laboratory negative.

Occasionally a haematoma may develop and this will need evacuating surgically. Wound infection is also likely to occur but this usually resolves without antibiotics.

THE ADRENAL GLANDS

An adrenal gland is situated on the upper pole of each kidney but the two have no physiological relationship.

The cortex (or outer part) of the gland is essential for life and secretes three steroid hormones: the glucocorticoids, such as cortisol which controls the metabolism of carbohydrates, fats and proteins; the mineral corticoids (aldosterone), controlling salt and water balance; and the androgens, involved in sexual functions.

The medulla (or inner part) secretes adrenaline and noradrenaline, the former having a similar effect to the sympathetic nervous system and the latter acting as a vasoconstrictor.

Cushing's syndrome

Hyperplasia of the adrenal cortex leads to Cushing's syndrome, in which the trunk and face become obese but the arms and legs are not affected. Purple striae appear over the abdomen and breasts and there is muscle wasting and a rise in blood pressure. Hirsutism, glycosuria, headache and amenorrhoea are present. Osteoporosis with pathological fractures may also occur.

An adenoma of the cortex may cause an increase in the secretion of aldosterone leading to an electrolyte imbalance.

Adrenogenital syndrome

Tumours or hyperplasia of the cortex frequently cause virilisation of women, hair appearing on the face and the skin becoming coarser. It also causes hypertension.

Phaeochromocytoma

This is a tumour of the medulla of the adrenals or on the sympathetic ganglion chain which causes an increased secretion of adrenaline and noradrenaline, leading to episodes of a raised blood pressure, tachycardia, sweating and pallor.

Adrenalectomy

A unilateral or subtotal adrenalectomy may be done for Cushing's syndrome or primary aldosteronism and this is usually conducted with the patient in the same position as that for a kidney operation, the approach being from the back, and the eleventh or twelfth rib being removed. An abdominal route is preferred if a phaeochromocytoma or carcinoma is to be excised as exploration will also be necessary. If a bilateral adrenalectomy is being done for a hormone-dependent carcinoma of breast, either route may be used, although if a bilateral oopherectomy is to be carried out at the same operation, an abdominal route will be taken.

Before the operation, investigations will have been carried out to diagnose the suspected condition. These will include a 24-hour urine for ketosteroids, a test for plasma cortisol, and x-rays of the adrenals after the introduction of air. There will also be x-rays of the skull to exclude a tumour of the pituitary.

Specific preoperative preparation

The patient is shaved from nipple to knee. It is essential to take the blood pressure for a baseline. Hydrocortisone 100 mg is given either intramuscularly the day prior to the operation or intravenously at operation. An intravenous infusion of sodium chloride or dextrose and sodium chloride is commenced.

Specific postoperative care

Observation of the blood pressure and pulse quarter-hourly is vital and, even if it remains stable, this should be continued for 24 hours because the patient may develop an adrenal crisis up to 12 hours after the operation. If this happens, the blood pressure falls, the pulse becomes rapid and weak, and the patient complains of abdominal pain. He rapidly becomes very shocked, and requires an immediate increase in the amount of intravenous hydrocortisone.

A fluid balance chart must be kept accurately, the doctor also taking blood samples for the electrolytes.

If the posterior route has been used, the patient must be observed for any evidence of a pneumothorax, although there are less likely to be complications with the use of this route.

Where the approach has been via the abdomen, there will inevitably be some degree of paralytic ileus and therefore a nasogastric tube may be required for aspiration as well as the intravenous infusion.

Following removal of a phaeochromocytoma, careful monitoring and control of the blood pressure is even more important.

Intravenous hydrocortisone is continued via the infusion for 48 hours, and then intramuscularly for 12 days. The patient is then discharged on an oral maintenance dose and with a steroid card. He will be advised to attend his doctor with any infection, however mild, as this will alter the dosage required. It must be stressed that the patient must not at any time stop the drug suddenly. If he begins to feel more lethargic or weaker than usual, he should also return to his doctor.

SUGGESTED WORK

1. Discuss with a patient who has had a kidney transplant the period up to and immediately fol-

lowing his operation and the problems he experienced.

2. Find out the preferred method of surgical treatment for an enlarged prostate in your hospital and the reasons for this.

3. Find out what the most common reasons are for the patient with an enlarged prostate to seek medical treatment.

SUGGESTED READING

Beatty R. O. (1979). *Still a Lot of Living. Coping with Cancer*. London: Macmillan.

Grundfest S. (1980). Home parenteral nutrition. *Journal of the American Medical Association*; **244**(15): 1701–03.

* * *

Mr BARRY HARBER (aged 82) lives with his wife of 78. He has had a history of increasing difficulty in passing urine but has done nothing about it. He has now been admitted as an emergency with acute retention of urine. He also has anaemia. This is the first time he has ever been in hospital. He has false teeth.

Medical plan
Relief of the acute retention by catheterisation. Transurethral prostatectomy.

Identification of the patient's needs and problems on admission to hospital and action arising from these

Discomfort due to retention
Careful catheterisation by a skilled male nurse or doctor with an indwelling catheter. If overfilled, the bladder may either be partially emptied initially and emptied further after half an hour or put on slow continuous drainage, a gate clip controlling the flow. Empty the drainage bag as required. Catheter toilet will be necessary. Commence a fluid balance chart.

Anxiety and embarrassment
Ensure that the patient knows exactly what is going to happen and what he is allowed to do. He may prefer a male nurse to attend to his personal needs. Privacy is very important. Lack of embarrassment on the part of the nurse will also help him.

Toxicity from retention of waste products
Encourage copious fluids. Explain to Mr Harber why it is important for him to drink plenty. His wife may bring in some of his favourite drinks. Check his intake frequently.

Control of urinary infection
Send a catheter specimen of urine to the pathological laboratory. Encourage fluids. Administer prescribed antibiotics.

Control of anaemia
Ensure that the latest haemoglobin result is available for the doctor. Administer prescribed iron. Explain to the patient that his stools will be black. Any resulting constipation or diarrhoea will have to be controlled.

Hygiene
Mr Harber will be able to have a general bath with some assistance from a male nurse. He will need a container to put his false teeth in at night, but should be able to clean these himself at the sink.

Mobility
Once Mr Harber's retention has been relieved he will be allowed up, and may move about the ward freely. The urine drainage bag must be securely attached to his pyjamas.

Nutrition
Encourage the choice of a well-balanced diet.

39

Nursing Care of a Patient having Eye Surgery

The general principles which apply to any patient being admitted to hospital and to their preoperative and postoperative care also apply to the patient undergoing eye surgery. Therefore only the specific points which are relevant to ophthalmic nursing care will be discussed here.

On admission, the nurse should greet her patient by name and commence an assessment of his needs. She will note whether the patient focuses upon her face, if the blink reflex is increased, or if there is excess tear production. The last two signs suggest irritation of the eye, although nervousness can increase blinking. Any redness of the eyelids or conjunctiva is also noted and an accurate assessment of visual acuity is made and recorded (Figs. 39.1 and 39.2) in order to be able to monitor progress or lack of it.

The patient is given a brief description of the

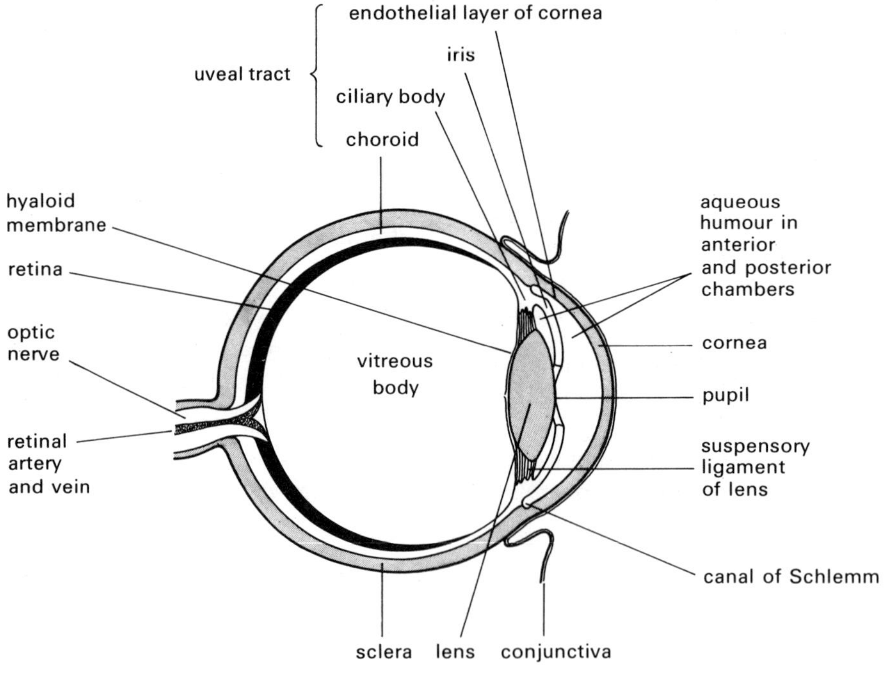

Fig. 39.1 *Diagram of a sagittal (vertical) section through the eye to show its internal structure.*

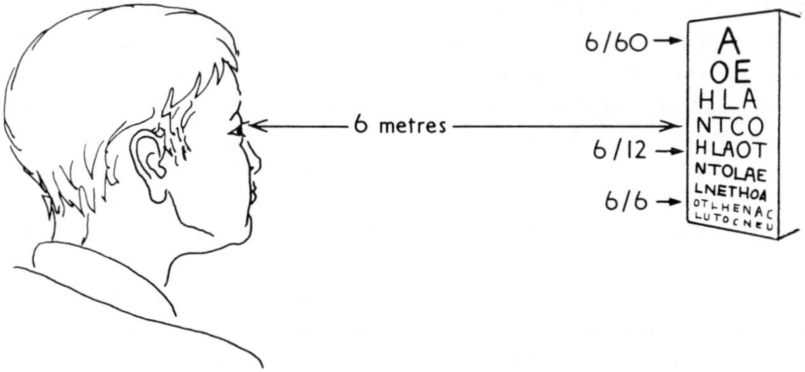

Fig. 39.2 *Eye testing.*

ward geography and a nursing history is taken. A history of the present eye problem is obtained, including when symptoms first began and details of any current treatment. As many of these patients are elderly, an assessment of their social conditions is also made.

It is particularly important prior to eye surgery that there is no focus of infection in the body, because the intact globe of the eye is about to be breached for intraocular surgery, and the entry of bacteria would lead to disastrous results. The nurse should therefore report any sores, ulcers, infected areas, or sinus problems. The presence of a cough is also a contraindication to eye surgery as it may result in postoperative complications.

A patient entering hospital for eye surgery will have many anxieties, which may include fear of an anaesthetic, of death and also of going blind. Therefore careful explanations of what to expect will do much to alleviate these worries. Telling the patient that the eye-drops will blur his vision will prevent him from worrying needlessly.

Specific emphasis in the nursing history

General appearance. Note weight, general nourishment and any sores or infection.

Elimination. Test urine for sugar.

Vital signs. Note blood pressure for signs of hypertension and temperature for infection.

Breathing. Note the presence of a cough or respiratory infection.

Mobility. Find out how much the patient is able to do for himself.

Sight. Is there any diminished vision? Does the patient wear glasses? Note any increase in the production of tears, redness of the eyes, or lack of a blink reflex.

Nose. Notice any sinus problems.

CATARACT EXTRACTION

This is the surgical removal of a lens which has become opaque (Fig. 39.3). A cataract is caused by senile degeneration, trauma, congenital abnormalities and systemic diseases such as diabetes mellitus.

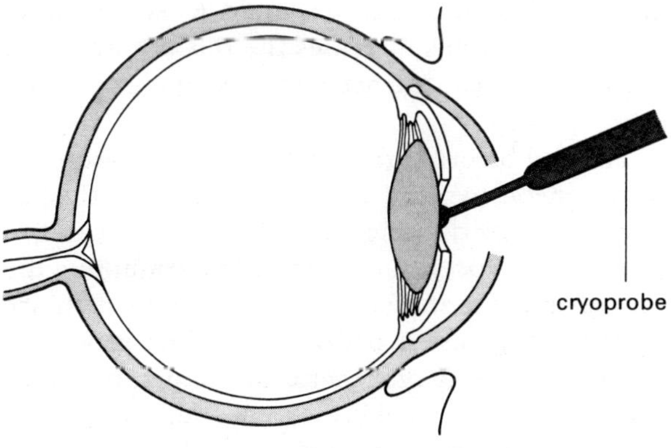

Fig. 39.3 *Removal of a cataract with a cryoprobe.*

The surgical technique used is varied according to the age of the patient, as younger patients have more elastic tissues. At the same time as the extraction, an intraocular lens implant may be performed, but even with this, glasses or contact lenses will still be required. A lens implant involves the insertion of a tiny plastic lens which has a power similar to that of the normal lens of the eye, although it does not have the ability to change its shape and therefore to focus for close work.

The patient is admitted one or two days prior to surgery, thus giving him time to adjust to new surroundings, and to receive information about the surgery proposed. Some surgeons require a conjunctival swab to be taken for culture and sensitivity to enable the appropriate antibiotic to be prescribed. Others prescribe these drops prophylactically, to be instilled in both eyes four times daily for 24 to 48 hours, to reduce the risk of intraocular infection occurring postoperatively. The general fitness of the patient is assessed to ensure the absence of infection or a cough. A local anaesthetic may be given to patients who are unfit for a general anaesthetic.

The education of the patient prior to surgery is very important. He needs to be told that he will wear an eye pad on the operated eye for one or two days as this is often the cause of disorientation. If the sight in the unoperated eye is poor, it makes the situation more difficult, especially as distance judgement is lost. The patient needs to be taught not to rub his eye postoperatively, or to dab it with a handkerchief because of the risk of introducing infection. He must also be warned against bending down because this increases the blood flow to the head and may cause a haemorrhage in the operated eye.

The day before surgery any assistance required with general hygiene is given and, in particular, attention is paid to the cleanliness of the patient's hair. Ocular preparation includes trimming the eyelashes using special curved scissors which are coated with grease to collect them. This is done to prevent any discharged matter accumulating on the eyelashes and so making the eyelids difficult to part. The patient is fasted if he is to have a general anaesthetic, and a night sedation is given.

On the day of surgery the patient is prepared in the usual way. The nurse also ensures that the eye is clean and that the doctor has indicated which eye is to operated on, usually by a mark on the patient's forehead. As well as the normal premedication, an ocular premedication is also prescribed. This is usually a mydriatic eye-drop which will fully dilate the pupil to enable the lens to be delivered through it.

The patient is normally returned to the ward having fully recovered consciousness. Initially he can be nursed in the dorsal position or on his unaffected side, using one pillow. Observations of pulse and blood pressure are recorded half-hourly until the patient's condition is stable. As he recovers and the blood pressure reading returns to a normal level, more pillows may be given gradually until the patient is supported in the sitting position. Vomiting must be avoided as this increases the pressure within the eye and may therefore cause a haemorrhage. For this reason, only sips of water are offered and an antiemetic is given if necessary. The call bell should be within the grasp of the patient to prevent him moving about too much or bending. Analgesia is given as required. The eye pad is checked regularly for leakage and any sudden sharp pain in the eye is reported to the doctor immediately.

As recovery continues, a cup of tea may be offered, but the cup must not be overfilled, and by the evening a light supper may be tolerated. Help may be required as distance judgement is impaired while the eye pad is in position. The elderly may become confused after a general anaesthetic and this is increased by the presence of the eye pad. Added to this they may be deprived of the use of their glasses for the other eye. They must therefore be closely observed and reassured as necessary.

Rest and quiet are important for the first night. Following breakfast on the first day, a trained nurse will carefully assess the condition of the operated eye. The patient is told that his eye pad and shield will be removed and his eye bathed gently. It will then be examined by the nurse using the light from a pencil torch. He is advised to keep his eyes closed gently until the bathing is completed. Before he opens his eyes it is important to point out that his vision will be blurred, as the power to focus is lost, and that colours will be much brighter. Reassurance is needed that the situation will gradually improve and new glasses will be prescribed when the delicate tissues have healed, usually in about 6 weeks.

When the eye has been examined, and if all is well, the prescribed drops may be instilled. These are usually a mydriatic, to rest the eye, and a steroid combined with an antibiotic, to relieve some of the surgically induced inflammation. A new eye pad may then be applied or the patient may wear a pair of dark glasses. He can then be helped up out of bed and taken for a short walk. He is advised to keep his head up and not to bend down. If his slippers are left on his bedside chair, this will enable him to reach them without having to bend down.

Mobilisation is gradually increased over the next few days according to the patient's general condition and the progress of the operated eye. Hygiene needs can be met, although the patient is advised not to clean his teeth vigorously. A few days before discharge from hospital the patient, or a relative, is taught to instil the eye-drops. A plastic shield will be worn to protect the eye at night for about 2 weeks, and this can be washed with soap and water and dried with a tissue. The patient is advised to report any discharge from the eye, pain or redness.

Temporary glasses may be supplied for about 2 months while healing occurs and any oedema settles. These (as nearly as possible) replace the power of the lens in the eye, but it takes a while to become accustomed to them, and this is true also of the later permanent glasses. This is because vision is distorted unless the person looks straight ahead, and distances are difficult to judge at first. Particular care is required when going up or down steps. The glasses magnify by about 25–30%.

The patient is also advised not to lift anything heavy for about 8 weeks. He may gradually increase activities and will return for an out-patient appointment about 2 weeks after his discharge from hospital.

REPAIR OF A RETINAL DETACHMENT

A retinal detachment is the separation of the retina from its attachment with the choroid. This may arise due to a tear in the retina which allows the vitreous to flow through and cause the detachment (Fig. 39.4).

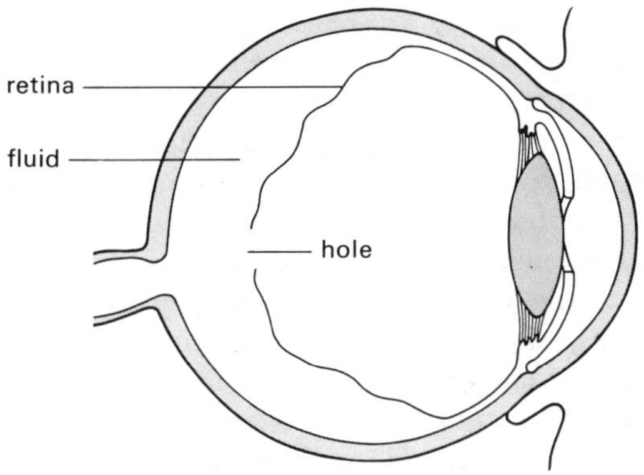

Fig. 39.4 *Detached retina.*

Although the cause may be unknown, trauma (most commonly a temporal head injury) or a tumour may result in a retinal detachment. It may also be secondary to another disease such as diabetes mellitus.

The patient complains of a grey curtain across his vision and of flashes of light. The aim of treatment is to seal the retinal tear and encourage the detached retina to flatten and settle in the normal anatomical position.

Preoperatively the patient is rested in the optimum position to allow the retina to settle, and to prevent further detachment. Boredom and anxiety are particular problems as the patient is discouraged from reading. This bedrest continues for up to a week. Mydriatic drops such as atropine are instilled regularly to enable examination of the retina. Prophylactic antibiotic drops may also be instilled during the 24 hours prior to surgery.

The surgeon may only operate externally, because opening the posterior part of the eye would lead to a loss of vitreous and therefore further damage. He works around the sclera while looking through the well-dilated pupil. However, with the increasing use of high-powered microscopes and fine instruments, surgery can now be performed in the posterior of the eye.

The patient is prepared for surgery in the usual way, the eyelashes being trimmed and the premedication given as prescribed. Surgery is carefully planned to meet the individual need, and there are a variety of techniques available.

Postoperatively the patient's vital signs are monitored half-hourly, and then hourly as his condition stabilises. The position in which the patient is nursed is dictated by the area of detachment. He may be sat up only if this is permitted by the medical staff. Fluids are given as tolerated, and analgesics as required. The patient is allowed out of bed at the surgeon's discretion, but must avoid bending down or any strenuous movements. Mydriatic and antibiotic drops are continued, and the patient is taught how to instil his own drops before discharge. He is usually allowed home within about 10 days and is advised to avoid heavy work, bending or lifting for at least 2 months. Reassurance is given that the drops will cause his vision to be blurred but that this will improve as the retina settles and oedema is resolved. Dark glasses can be used to rest the eye.

The laser beam

Stimulation of a gas, liquid or solid by light or an electrical current produces a light which is then amplified by a series of parallel reflective mirrors. This enables a very high level of energy to be focused on a very small area. Different substances may be used to obtain different effects, and they are particularly useful as a method of treatment to seal a small tear in the retina and so prevent a detachment from occurring. The laser beam may also be used to obliterate the leaking and malformed blood capillaries found in diabetic retinopathy. They can, of course, be used on other parts of the body as well.

GLAUCOMA

This is a rise of pressure within the eye which, if allowed to continue, causes destruction of the optic nerve at the point where it enters the eye (Fig. 39.5). It may arise as a complication of another condition, for example following a haemorrhage into the anterior chamber of the eye which has blocked the normal drainage of aqueous humour.

The condition may be acute or chronic. Acute glaucoma is relieved by surgery once the pressure is under control. Chronic glaucoma is treated medically, however failure to respond will mean that surgical drainage of the aqueous humour will be required.

Acute glaucoma

The onset is sudden, with the patient complaining of a severe pain in the eye and temporal region. Vomiting is commonly present. On examination, the cornea of the eye looks steamy and cloudy, and the conjunctiva red. The patient will complain of cloudy vision and of a rainbow effect around artificial lights.

The patient is admitted to hospital and told that he will receive frequent eye-drops to relieve the pressure and therefore the pain. An analgesic and an antiemetic are often given once the patient is in bed. After the diagnosis has been confirmed, miotic drops are instilled in the eye intensively until the pressure is reduced. They will be continued until surgery is undertaken. A diuretic which reduces the production of aqueous humour by the ciliary body is given orally, if tolerated, or intramuscularly.

Surgery is performed as soon as the pressure has been reduced. The patient is prepared for intraocular surgery as described above. The operation usually involves removing a small portion of the iris to allow escape of aqueous humour.

Postoperative care is the same as that already described. After the first dressing on day one, mydriatic and possibly steroid drops are instilled, to rest the eye. There is no risk of blocking the drainage channel as an iridectomy has been performed. The nurse must take particular care to instil the correct drops into the correct eye as the patient may still be prescribed a prophylactic *miotic*, such as physostigmine or pilocarpine, in the unoperated eye. Many surgeons perform an iridec-

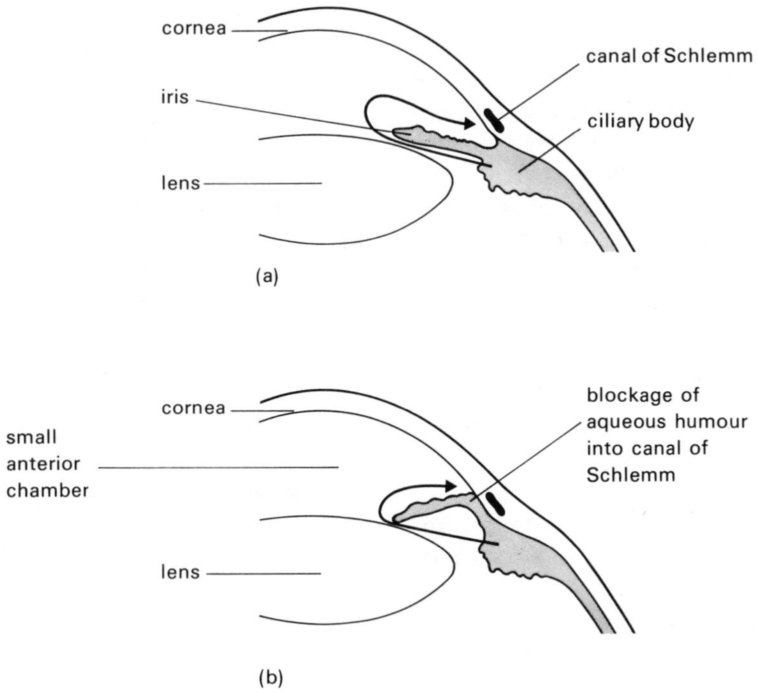

Fig. 39.5 *(a) Normal eye. (The arrows show the normal flow of aqueous humour.) (b) Closed angle glaucoma. The iris is blocking the entrance to the canal of Schlemm.*

tomy on the other eye several days later to prevent glaucoma occurring.

The patient is usually discharged home within a few days, having been taught how to instil drops, and told to avoid heavy work, bending and lifting. An out-patient appointment is given for 2 weeks later.

Chronic glaucoma

If drops fail to control the pressure within the eye, surgery is carried out to open a drainage channel and so allow the escape of aqueous humour. Admission to hospital is planned and the preparation is as described for intraocular surgery. As with acute glaucoma, particular care must be taken when instilling drops. The patient is told that he will not recover vision which has already been lost, but that surgery will prevent further loss.

SQUINT (STRABISMUS)

In this condition the line of vision in one eye deviates from the normal. It may be due to weakness of one or more of the six extrinsic muscles, or to injury of a nerve supplying these muscles, and may occur as a result of a difficult delivery or other trauma, or following inflammatory conditions such as meningitis.

The condition may be treated with glasses and exercises of the muscles. If surgery is necessary, the appropriate muscle is either moved or shortened. The eye is covered postoperatively with a pad for 24 hours. Ten days after discharge, the patient is followed up and may then return to work or school if everything is satisfactory.

CORNEAL GRAFT

This procedure is carried out for patients whose cornea has become opaque following an inflammatory condition. The graft is taken from a donor who has died within the last 4 hours by cutting a circular disc from his cornea. This is kept in a refrigerator for up to 4 days. A similar disc is removed from the patient's cornea with a trephine. The donor disc is then sutured to the patient's cornea. Postoperatively both eyes are kept covered.

NURSING CARE OF A BLIND PATIENT ADMITTED FOR SURGERY

A registered blind person is not necessarily completely without sight, but may be able to distinguish shadows or may have very small areas of good vision. The nurse needs to assess the degree of help that the newly admitted blind patient requires. He will probably have adjusted to his handicap, but this is dependent upon his familiarity with his surroundings.

Admission to hospital promotes anxieties about the illness and also, for the blind patient, a considerable loss of independence. The nurse can help the patient to be familiar with his surroundings. A blind patient should be greeted by name and a handshake, the nurse introducing herself and giving a brief description of the ward layout. She can then escort the patient to his bed area, walking slightly in front and allowing him to take hold of her elbow.

The patient should not be overwhelmed with information initially. He needs to be familiar with the geography around his bed area, be introduced to his neighbours, and understand the nurse call system. His locker should always be placed on the same side of the bed and care must be taken not to leave obstacles such as footstools or cleaning utensils in the way. At meal times the food on a plate can be identified using the face of a clock to locate its position, for example meat at 6 o'clock, peas at 3 o'clock and potatoes at 9 o'clock. Cups should not be overfilled, particularly with hot liquids. Hot and cold taps need to be clearly identified. The nurse can help the patient to build up a picture of where his bed is, in relationship to the rest of the ward, by identifying 'keys' in the ward geography, for example by counting the number of beds to the door and the number of doorways to the toilet.

Communication is of the utmost importance. Unfamiliar sounds will be bewildering to a blind person and therefore he will require frequent explanations to reassure him. A careful explanation is required before any procedures are carried out, including what the patient is expected to do, and what effect the procedure will have on him. He also needs to know what the surgery involves and the expected outcome. All patients need this information of course, but a blind patient will not have any of the non-verbal cues to build on, nor will he see what is going on around him. The apparently trivial things are important, such as the fact that an operating theatre gown ties up at the back. Recovery from an anaesthetic can also be alarming because the patient may forget where he is and be quite disorientated.

Always address a blind patient by name, and use the sense of touch when possible. He should be told when the nurse is moving away or he will feel very foolish when he realises he is talking to himself. Time should be taken to read his correspondence to him if this is desired. He should be involved in the nursing care plan because he may recognise problems or their solutions which the nurse does not. Independence should be encouraged within a safe environment, but at the same time the patient's needs should be anticipated and assistance offered when necessary.

SUGGESTED WORK

1. Discuss with a blind person the problems he experienced either when admitted to hospital or while staying in an unknown hotel.

2. Do a survey on the patients in the eye ward and find out how many suffer from hypertension or diabetes. Are their eye conditions due to their diseases?

SUGGESTED READING

Blackall D. S. (1971). *The Way I See it*. London: J. Baker.
Brace M. (1980). *Where There's a Will*. London: Souvenir Press.
Duguid I. (1971). *Ophthalmology*. London: English Universities Press.
RCN Association of Nursing Practice (1983). *Guidelines for Nurses Working with the Visually Handicapped*. London: Royal College of Nursing.
Ruben M. (1975). *Understanding Contact Lenses*. London: Pitman Press.

* * *

Mrs EMILY WILLS (aged 78) is a widow who lives with her sister aged 86. They are a very independent couple, managing their own cleaning and cooking. They have some difficulty in getting to the shops and, as any relatives they have live some distance away, they do not have any outings. Mrs Wills' vision has become increasingly impaired over the last few years due to cataracts in both eyes.

Medical plan
Cataract extraction.

Identification of the patient's needs and problems prior to discharge and action arising from these

Information
Explain that she should not lift anything heavy for at least 2 months. Advise her to tell the district nurse or her doctor if she develops any discharge, pain or redness of the eye.

Diet
Arrange for the dietitian to look at her normal diet and suggest cheap ways of increasing its nutritive value. The social worker can see if a neighbour would shop for the sisters or if groceries etc. could be delivered.

Social
Check that the social worker has investigated the home and the ability of the sisters to manage.

Supplies
Check that Mrs Wills has the eye shield to wear at night and that she knows about its care. Give her the eye-drops and explain that the district nurse will be coming to put them in.

Mobility
The social worker may be able to arrange for a voluntary worker to take them out occasionally in a car.

Follow-up
Arrange convalescence. Contact the district nurse if she or the district liaison nurse has not already visited, and arrange for Mrs Wills' eye-drops to be instilled. Write down for Mrs Wills and her sister when the district nurse will be visiting. Alert the district nurse to the information that Mrs Wills has received so that she can reinforce it. Arrange an OPD appointment in 2 weeks.

Relatives
Make sure that the sister knows when to expect Mrs Wills and that she has the opportunity to make adequate preparations.

Transport
Arrange for transport to take her home. Check whether she will need transport for her OPD appointment.

40

Care of Patients with Special Problems

MANAGEMENT OF THE SURGICAL PATIENT WITH DIABETES MELLITUS

Before the advent of insulin it was almost impossible to carry out surgical procedures on diabetic patients because the anaesthetic affected the blood sugar levels and the patients invariably suffered from ketosis and electrolyte imbalance.

Diabetics are particularly liable to develop conditions such as gangrene and cataract which require surgery, and they may, of course, develop any of the other surgical conditions. Any infective condition such as peritonitis will cause the diabetes to become unstable, increasing the need for insulin.

Normally the body is able to adjust its production of insulin according to its requirements, but the diabetic has to regulate his insulin by injection, and this is obviously less accurate. It is therefore important to be able to recognise when the amount of insulin required should be adjusted. The patient who is acutely anxious about his operation should have his mind put at rest and, if necessary, should be given sedatives or a night sedation. If he is suffering from an electrolyte imbalance due to vomiting or diarrhoea, not only will this require correction, but his blood sugar will also need to be monitored to ensure an adequate amount of insulin is given.

When in hospital, the patient's diabetes is controlled by the physician already caring for it. Most surgical wards have a set routine for their diabetic patients undergoing surgery.

Elective surgery

Patients who have been controlled by diet or tablets may still require insulin over the operative period if their blood sugar is significantly raised. Those patients already on insulin are admitted for 1 or 2 days prior to the operation to assess the stability of their diabetes and to put them on a quick-acting insulin such as Actrapid or soluble insulin, if they are not already taking this. Any acidosis or electrolyte imbalance is corrected. The most accurate way to monitor the patient's condition is to take regular blood sugar estimates using a Dextrostix and a glucometer. Care must be taken to read the instructions before using the latter.

The patient is starved for 4 to 6 hours prior to the operation, and is the first on the operating list. The morning dose of insulin is given at the usual time to prevent the development of acidosis. It is balanced by the commencement of an intravenous infusion of dextrose, given during the operation and until the patient is able to take food by mouth. The dose of insulin continues to be regulated according to the blood sugar levels, although some doctors still require the urine to be tested 4-hourly. In some units the insulin is given in very small regular amounts intravenously by an automatic injecting device attached to an intravenous infusion. As soon as the patient is able to take food by mouth, this is encouraged, so that he eventually returns to his normal diabetic diet. He will return to his usual regimen of insulin when his blood sugar level has stabilised.

Any alteration in the temperature or blood

pressure in the postoperative phase will alter the amount of insulin required. Wounds should be observed carefully as healing may be impaired.

Emergency surgery

Patients coming in for an emergency operation are frequently already in an unstable state due to the effects of their surgical condition and the fact that they have not felt like eating. Dehydration due to an increased urinary output, ketosis and electrolyte imbalance will probably be present. If it is at all possible, the operation is delayed until the patient is in a more stable state. Intravenous sodium chloride or lactic acid with quick-acting insulin are given initially followed by dextrose–saline. If potassium levels are down, this is added to the intravenous infusion, and antibiotics are given for infection. Blood sugar readings, are taken 2-hourly.

Minor operations

Diabetics are usually admitted for minor operations such as the removal of teeth. A proportion of the normal insulin dose is given in the morning and a light breakfast, the operative procedure being carried out 4 to 6 hours later. In the evening another dose of the quick-acting insulin is given according to the blood sugar levels, followed by a light meal. The next day a normal routine will be followed.

Hypoglycaemia

This arises as a result of too much insulin or too little carbohydrate. It may develop unnoticed in the anaesthetised patient, who becomes restless, pale and sweaty. When conscious, he may complain of abdominal discomfort. He will appear mentally confused, weak and have a tachycardia. Oral glucose is given if the patient is able to swallow it; if not, intravenous glucose is given.

Ketosis

If infection or persistent vomiting is present, there is an electrolyte imbalance and the diabetic state will become unstable. The breakdown products of fat metabolism—ketone bodies—will circulate in the blood causing acidosis, and will be excreted in the urine and on the breath. These act as a poison to the brain, causing the patient to become drowsy and eventually go into a coma. The treatment is to give intravenous sodium chloride or sodium lactate and a quick-acting insulin. Regular estimation of the blood sugar is maintained. Potassium is given as required.

MANAGEMENT OF THE SURGICAL PATIENT UNDER STEROID TREATMENT

Any patient undergoing an operation should be checked to see whether he is taking steroids or has been taking them during the past 2 years. If so, it should be clearly marked on his case notes. This is particularly important in emergency cases. If the patient has been on steroids in the past and there is any doubt as to the ability of the adrenals to respond in a stress situation, a corticotrophin test will be done.

Preoperatively the patient should be checked for any side-effects from the steroids, such as electrolyte imbalance or diabetes mellitus by the doctor. The blood pressure is taken to act as a baseline for further readings, and an intramuscular injection of 100–200 mg hydrocortisone is given. Postoperatively intramuscular injections of hydrocortisone are continued 12-hourly, according to the patient's blood pressure. Once the patient has fully recovered the dose is gradually tailed off until he either returns to his former steroid regimen or is taken off medication altogether.

Emergency surgery

Preoperatively the patient is given the larger intramuscular dose of 200 mg hydrocortisone. During the operation a further 100 mg is given via the intravenous infusion of sodium chloride. Postoperatively the hydrocortisone is continued 12-hourly, according to the blood pressure.

Smaller doses of hydrocortisone are required for

minor surgery. Observation of the wounds of these patients is important as they do not heal very well, and may therefore break down. Infection may be masked by the use of steroid, the temperature not rising, so the patient must be watched carefully for other signs of infection.

THE CARE OF CHILDREN UNDERGOING SURGERY

Children are admitted to hospital for the shortest time possible and may therefore have most investigations carried out on an out-patient basis and be admitted on the day of operation. In some hospitals they may be sent home on the day of surgery after straightforward operations, providing the initial recovery is uneventful and the home conditions are suitable.

On admission it is important to obtain all the information from the parents as the child may be unable to provide this. The nurse should find out what method of feeding is being used and any particular likes or dislikes. She also needs to know whether the child is clean and if he uses a pot or the toilet. Any special names for the latter are also noted. The consent form will be signed after the doctor has explained what is to be done to the child. If one of the parents can stay in the hospital, this will help the younger child to settle. A special toy will also provide comfort in a strange environment. Before the parents leave, the child must have an identity bracelet securely attached to an ankle or wrist.

Only those x-rays and diagnostic tests which are really necessary will be done and they should be carried out by experienced staff to avoid distressing the child. Blood specimens are normally taken from a prick rather than an intravenous injection. The haemoglobin is checked and if it is reduced below 70% of normal, either the operation will be postponed or a blood transfusion will be given. A raised temperature contraindicates surgery.

The child is weighed in order to estimate the dosage of drugs to be given. If there is any electrolyte imbalance or acidosis as a result of vomiting or dehydration, this is corrected. The child is starved for up to 6 hours, but not longer because this may cause an acidosis or hypoglycaemia. A mild aperient may be given to empty the bowel but purgatives and enemas are avoided. A record must be made of when the child last passed urine and had a bowel motion. Nasal hygiene is important as children find difficulty in blowing their noses.

Atropine to dry the secretions is all that is required in the child aged under a year. Older children usually need some form of sedation which is best given either orally or rectally, such as Nepenthe, Vallergan or Omnopon. Trimeprazine and diazepam are alternative drugs used. A simple explanation is always given to the child old enough to understand before any procedure. It may help the child to overcome his fears if he can play a game to act out the procedures involved in the operation.

Postoperative care

For the infant, great care must be taken to maintain the body heat and this is why babies may be wrapped in cotton wool, a space blanket or nursed in an incubator. The baby is encouraged to cry in order to expand the lungs and clear the airway. Noisy breathing will indicate a partially obstructed airway. The normal respiratory rate in an infant is 30–40 breaths per minute, and a marked increase in this rate and cyanosis suggest respiratory embarrassment. However, there may be no other indication than an increasing exhaustion. The infant breathes with the diaphragm and therefore distension of the abdomen may interfere with respirations.

An intravenous infusion may be necessary to counteract shock or fluid loss. If this is so, it is essential that a paediatric infusion set is used with a smaller drop and a 100-ml chamber so that the rate is carefully controlled. It is very easy to overload the circulation of a small baby and cause a strain on the heart, leading to pulmonary oedema, therefore an accurate fluid balance chart must be kept.

Postoperative analgesia is first administered before the child leaves the theatre. Later, if it is required, Nepenthe or Omnopon may be given. The baby can be given sips of boiled water or 5%

glucose solution during the first 3 to 4 hours postoperatively. He will then go on to half-strength feeds and eventually back to his normal regimen, if there is no vomiting. Breast-fed babies can usually return to the breast within 12 hours. Any dressings must be completely sealed or the child will explore under them.

The mother is often the best person to be with the child while he is still feeling the main effects of the operation. Once he feels fit enough, the child himself will want to move around and start to play. There should therefore be suitable play materials provided for his age and activity. Most children enjoy play more if there is someone to share it with, and if the mother or other relative is not available, there should be a nursery nurse or 'play lady' to help guide and encourage play. If the older child is to be in hospital any length of time, he may also require the attention of a teacher.

SUGGESTED WORK

1. Find out the regimen in your hospital for patients with diabetes mellitus who are undergoing major surgery. Compare it with that described in the chapter. Does it vary significantly? If so, can you find out why?

2. Find out the regimen in your ward for patients who are receiving steroid therapy and compare it with that described in this chapter.

3. Discuss with a mother the fears and problems she has experienced when her child has had to undergo surgery.

SUGGESTED READING

Abdurrahman M. B. (1978). Parents' understanding of their children's illnesses. *Journal of Tropical Paediatrics*; **24**(5): 233–5.

Bibace R., Walsh M. E. (1980). Development of children's concepts of illness. *Pediatrics*; **66**(6): 912–17.

Lewer H., Robertson L. (1983). *The Essentials of Nursing*. London: Macmillan.

Peterson M. C. (1979). Preparation of the cardiac child and the family for surgery. *Issues in Comprehensive Paediatric Nursing*; **3**(7): 61–71.

Rupert and his Friends—A Guide for the Young Diabetic (1977). Slough: Ames Co., Miles Laboratories.

Schrader E. S. (1979). Preparation play helps children in hospital. *Association of Operating Room Nurses Journal*. **30**(2): 336, 340–41.

Schrader E. S. (1980). Preparing children for surgery. *National Association of Theatre Nurses News*; **17**(6): 11–14.

Appendix

Care Charts

Care Chart

Patients with Appendicitis, Peritonitis or Obstruction

SPECIFIC NURSING ASSESSMENT

Pain — where
what type
changes

Vital signs — temperature
pulse
blood pressure

Nutrition — appetite
vomiting

Elimination — bowel function
constipation
diarrhoea
urine output

SPECIFIC POINTS FOR NURSING CARE PLANS

Preoperative — emergency
nasogastric tube
possible intravenous infusion
nil by mouth

Postoperative — observations, particularly of temperature and vomiting
nil by mouth usually until bowel sounds return
movement to be encouraged
pain relief

Care Chart

Patients Requiring Gastric Surgery

SPECIFIC NURSING ASSESSMENT

Social — divorce
bereavement
family stress

Occupation — type
attitude to it

Nutrition — type of food eaten
nutritive value
regularity of meals
nausea
vomiting

General appearance— weight change
Attitude — tenseness, why?
anxiety

Breathing — smoking
cough
sputum

Pain — relation to meals

Previous medication — antirheumatic
steroids
aspirin

SPECIFIC POINTS FOR NURSING CARE PLANS

Preoperative — nasogastric tube
? stomach washout
stop smoking

Postoperative — nil by mouth
graduated fluids
nasogastric tube–aspiration
intravenous infusion
fluid balance chart
deep breathing
leg exercises

Care Chart

Patients with a Hernia or Intestinal Obstruction

SPECIFIC NURSING ASSESSMENT

General appearance — abdomen
colour

Pain — character
position
strength

Elimination — bowel action
blood
mucus

Vomiting — character
amount

Vital signs — blood pressure
pulse
temperature

SPECIFIC POINTS FOR NURSING CARE PLANS

Hernia

Preoperative — no smoking
deep breathing exercises

Postoperative — hold wound when coughing
note urine for haematuria

Obstruction

Preoperative — emergency
nasogastric tube
intravenous infusion

Postoperative — nasogastric tube
intravenous infusion
graduated fluids
drainage tube
deep breathing

Care Chart

Patients with Carcinoma of Colon and Rectum

SPECIFIC NURSING ASSESSMENT

Elimination — alteration of bowel habit
blood
mucus

Nutrition — roughage
food avoided

General appearance — weight

Attitude — anxiety

Skin — soreness

Vital signs — temperature
pulse

Previous medication — steroids

SPECIFIC POINTS FOR NURSING CARE PLANS

Preoperative — psychological–ileostomy, colostomy
reduction of bowel bacteria,
non-absorbed antibiotics,
clear bowel, mannitol, Hartmann's,
rectal washout, aperients, enema
booster dose of steroids
position of stoma

Postoperative — colostomy } skin, action, colour,
ileostomy } protusion

wounds — abdominal
perineal–vacuum
drain, keep dry

catheter
nil by mouth–nasogastric tube,
intravenous infusion

Care Chart

Patients with Haemorrhoids, Fistulae, Fissures and Abscesses

SPECIFIC NURSING ASSESSMENT

Elimination — bowel habits
blood
mucus

Nutrition — roughage
fluid intake

General appearance — energy

Skin — colour
irritation

Mobility — amount of exercise taken

Previous medication — aperients
constipating drugs

SPECIFIC POINTS FOR NURSING CARE PLANS

Preoperative — clear bowel–bulk laxative, suppositories, low residue diet
perineal shave

Postoperative — lateral position
observations–haemorrhage
urinary output
analgesia–entonox
saline baths
dilatation
high-fibre diet
check haemoglobin

Care Chart

Patients with Diseases of the Biliary Tract

SPECIFIC NURSING ASSESSMENT

Elimination — colour of urine
colour of stools

Nutrition — avoidance of fat

Vomiting — relationship to pain
relationship to fatty food

General appearance — weight

Pain — when
where
type

Vital signs — temperature

SPECIFIC POINTS FOR NURSING CARE PLANS

Preoperative — nasogastric tube

Postoperative — sit up
analgesia
observe breathing,
temperature
remove drain around 48 hours,
T tube 8–10 days
deep breathing

Care Chart

Patients having Vascular Surgery

SPECIFIC NURSING ASSESSMENT

Mobility — pain

Vital signs — limb pulses
temperature extremities

Pain — factors increasing it
factors relieving it

Excretion — glycosuria

Skin — colour of extremities

SPECIFIC POINTS FOR NURSING CARE PLANS

Preoperative — test urine for sugar
stop smoking
nasogastric tube

Postoperative — observe for haemorrhage–pulse, blood pressure

urinary output
nasogastric tube
observe limbs–colour
temperature
pulses

breathing
limb strengthening exercises

Care Chart

Patients undergoing Thoracic Surgery

SPECIFIC NURSING ASSESSMENT

Breathing — history of smoking–dyspnoea
cough–sputum, type
amount
halitosis

Vital signs — temperature
pulse
respiration

General appearance — weight
malaise
prominent veins

Pain — relation to breathing

Social — background

Nutrition — anorexia
vomiting

Mobility — effect on breathing

Skin — colour of extremities and lips

SPECIFIC POINTS FOR NURSING CARE PLANS

Preoperative — general health
oral hygiene

Postoperative — vital signs
sat up
breathing–hold wound
analgesia before physiotherapy
steam inhalations
oxygen
blood transfusion
drainage tubes — apical
basal
breathing exercises
coughing
arm movements

Care Chart

Patients having Surgery of the Breast

SPECIFIC NURSING ASSESSMENT

Skin — nodules, ulceration, peau d' orange
nipple–fissures, eczema, discharge

Sexuality — relationships

Breathing — smoking
infection

Pain–elsewhere in body–back

SPECIFIC POINTS FOR NURSING CARE PLANS

Preoperative — psychological–husband
introduction to another patient with condition
prosthesis

Postoperative — pressure bandage
sit up
arm supported
note–shock
chest pain
dyspnoea
analgesia
intravenous infusion
psychological support
posture
arm exercises
breathing
prosthesis
mastectomy nurse specialist
mastectomy association
posture
arm exercises
breathing exercises

Care Chart

Patients undergoing Neurosurgery

SPECIFIC NURSING ASSESSMENT

Mental — vertigo
fits
headaches
alertness
behaviour

Nutrition — nausea
vomiting

Communication — expression
understanding

Mobility — ataxia
movement–loss
abnormal

Skin — sensation

Vital signs — pulse
respiration
blood pressure

Special senses — sight
hearing
smell
taste

SPECIFIC POINTS FOR NURSING CARE PLANS

Preoperative — baseline neurological observations
shave head and cover

Postoperative — recumbent position
simple analgesics
neurological
observations–pupils
blood pressure
pulse
respiration
level of consciousness
observe fits
hemiplegia
intravenous infusion

Care Chart

Patients with Fractures and Dislocations

SPECIFIC NURSING ASSESSMENT

General appearance — limbs–position, shortening
shock

Pain — position
related to movement

Skin — swelling, bruising
altered sensation

Mobility — loss
abnormal

Social — help
accommodation

SPECIFIC POINTS FOR NURSING CARE PLANS

Plaster of Paris — keep cool
elevate limb 24 hours
check list–pain
temperature of limb
pulse
colour
loss of movement
sensation
exercise of extremities

Skeletal traction — check site of pin
weights hanging free
check feet–sensation
colour
movement
Thomas splint–skin
exercise of good limb

Skin traction — allergy
sores
foot drop
slipping extension

Care Chart

Patients with Injuries to Upper Limbs and Chest

SPECIFIC NURSING ASSESSMENT

General appearance — limbs–position
shortening
shock

Pain — position
movement

Skin — swelling, bruising
sensation

Mobility — loss
abnormal

Social — help required

Plaster of Paris — keep cool
support arm
check list–pain
temperature of limb
pulse
colour of limb
loss of movement
sensation

Internal fixation — support arm
check–pain
temperature of fingers
pulse
colour of fingers
loss of movement
sensation
finger movements
joint movements

Care Chart

Patients with Injuries to the Lower Limb and Pelvis

SPECIFIC NURSING ASSESSMENT

General appearance—limbs–position
shortening
shock

Pain — position
relation to movement

Skin — swelling
bruising
sensation

Mobility — loss
abnormal

Social — help required

SPECIFIC POINTS FOR NURSING CARE PLANS

Meniscectomy

Preoperative — quadriceps exercises
povidine compress

Postoperative — rest joint
observe – pain
pyrexia
swelling of foot
exercises
weight on foot

Arthroplasty

Preoperative — check correct limb marked
trochanteric area shaved

Postoperative — recumbent
abduction pillow
vacuum drainage
check foot – sensation
movement
no straight leg raising
early mobilisation
crutches
sticks
quadriceps exercises

Care Chart

Patients with a Condition of the Vertebral Column

SPECIFIC NURSING ASSESSMENT

General appearance — posture
spine

Mobility — bending
joints
paralysis
gait

Breathing — abnormal respiration
infection

Pain — back
sciatica

Skin — sensation–feet

Elimination — micturition
bowel action

Sexual — activity affected

Social — young children
assistance required

Employment — lifting
redeployment

SPECIFIC POINTS FOR NURSING CARE PLANS

Preoperative — mark side
slipper pan
stabilising spine

Postoperative
Prolapsed Intravertebral Disc
spine straight
strong analgesia
feet—temperature
sensation
movement
no sitting in chair

Osteotomy or Spinal Fusion
nasogastric tube
intravenous infusion
underwater seal
plaster bed—turning–prone
pressure areas–knees
limbs–movement
sensation
pulses
strong analgesia
Stryker bed
flexion/extension exercises

Care Chart

Patients with Congenital and Acquired Deformities

SPECIFIC NURSING ASSESSMENT

General appearance — posture
physical progress

Mobility — joints
muscle strength
movement

Pain — joints
extremities

Social — finance
other children
patient's work
distance from hospital

Skin extremities — sensation
colour

Nutrition — type

Elimination — habits
language

SPECIFIC POINTS FOR NURSING CARE PLANS

Protection of plaster
Hygiene
Prevention of sores
Mobility
Occupation
Observation of feet

Care Chart

Patients with Rheumatoid or Osteoarthritis

SPECIFIC NURSING ASSESSMENT

Pain — at rest
movement

General appearance — weight
shape of limbs
joints
colour
energy
growth in children

Mobility — gait
extent
chairs
toilet

Skin — intact
nodules

Vital signs — temperature

Social — housing
relatives

SPECIFIC POINTS FOR NURSING CARE PLANS

Preoperative — check correct limb marked
trochanteric area shaved

Postoperative — recumbent position
abduction pillow
vacuum drainage
check foot–sensation
movement
no straight leg raising
early mobilisation–walking
crutches
sticks

Care Chart

Patients with Burns

SPECIFIC NURSING ASSESSMENT

General appearance — other injuries

Skin — extent of burns
depth

Vital signs — temperature, pulse, respiration
blood pressure

Breathing — difficulty

Excretion — urinary output

Mobility — joints affected
bedfast

Social — relatives
visiting

Leisure pursuits — recovery

SPECIFIC POINTS FOR NURSING CARE PLANS

Burns — oral fluids in small amounts
fluid chart
catheter
analgesics

monitor–temperature, pulse, respiration
blood pressure

wound–open
non-stick dressings
saline baths
sterile room

splints
elevation limbs
nasogastric tube

Skin grafting — wound–non-stick dressings
firm bandage
elevate limb
snip blisters
lanoline
leisure pursuits
breathing exercises
movement of limb

Care Chart

Patients with a Condition of the Thyroid

SPECIFIC NURSING ASSESSMENT

General appearance — flushed
weight
eyes

Vital signs — pulse

Breathing — rate

Mobility — activity

Nutrition — appetite

Attitude — irritable
easily upset

Social — attitude to family

SPECIFIC POINTS FOR NURSING CARE PLANS

Preoperative — careful handling
sedatives
cool position
eyes–lubricant
dark glasses

Postoperative — sat up
vacuum drainage
sutures 2–3 days
check–dyspnoea
haematoma
oedema
pulse
temperature
voice
deep breathing
coughing

Care Chart

Patients undergoing Surgery of the Face and Mouth

SPECIFIC NURSING ASSESSMENT

General appearance — symmetry of face
weight
salivation
weakness

Pain — degree
progression
other sites

Nutrition — swallowing
problems in mouth

Breathing — smoker
dyspnoea

Vital signs — temperature, respiration

Social — relatives
finance
travel

SPECIFIC POINTS FOR NURSING CARE PLANS

Preoperative — antibiotics
removal of dental caries
oral toilet

Postoperative — observe airway
oral hygiene
suction
oxygen
nasogastric tube
? parenteral feeding
sutures 4th or 5th day
psychological support–relatives

Care Chart

Patients with Conditions of the Ear, Nose and Throat

SPECIFIC NURSING ASSESSMENT

General appearance — run down
mouth breathing
vertigo

Excretion — glycosuria

Vital signs — temperature

Pain — rubbing ears
headaches

Ears — tinnitus
loss of hearing–one or both ears
nausea
vomiting

SPECIFIC POINTS FOR NURSING CARE PLANS

Tonsillectomy
Preoperative — no infection
no loose teeth
no bleeding disorders

Postoperative — semi-prone
swallowing blood
vital signs
oral hygiene
hard food

Submucous Resection
Postoperatively — pack 48 hours
ice pack
analgesia
nose bolster
sit up

Ear Surgery
Postoperative — bed 24 hours
flat (stapedectomy)
antiemetic
wound drain pack

Care Chart

Patients with a Condition of the Renal Tract

SPECIFIC NURSING ASSESSMENT

Elimination — blood
albumin
output

Pain — renal colic
ache in loin
dysuria

Vital signs — temperature
blood pressure

General appearance — lethargy
malaise

Skin — flushed
pallor
jaundice

SPECIFIC POINTS FOR NURSING CARE PLANS

Preoperative — blood balance chart
fluids as prescribed

Postoperative — blood pressure
pulse
foot of bed elevated
blood transfusion
semi-recumbent–towards affected side
catheter
fluid balance chart
note colour urine
drainage tube
analgesia
antiemetic
repack dressing

Care Chart

Patients having Eye Surgery

SPECIFIC NURSING ASSESSMENT

General appearance — weight
nourishment
sores
infection

Elimination — urine–glycosuria

Vital signs — blood pressure
temperature

Breathing — cough
respiratory infection

Mobility — independence

Nose — sinus

Eyes — glasses
diminished vision
tears
red eyes
blink reflex

SPECIFIC POINTS FOR NURSING CARE PLANS

Preoperative — conjunctival swab
eye drops
education–rubbing eye
bending down
clean hair
trim eyelashes
check correct eye marked

Postoperative — position–unaffected side
dorsal, sitting
blood pressure
pulse
avoid vomiting–sips of water
antiemetic
report pain in eye
avoid bending
check eye pad
eye drops–mydriatic
antibiotic
steroid

Index